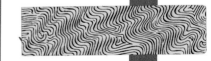

BRADDOM'S
REHABILITATION
CARE
A Clinical Handbook

BRADDOM'S
REHABILITATION
CARE
A Clinical Handbook

David X. Cifu, MD
Chairman
Department of Physical Medicine and Rehabilitation
Herman J. Flax, MD Professor
Virginia Commonwealth University School of Medicine
Principal Investigator
Veterans Affairs/Department of Defense Chronic Effects of Neurotrauma Consortium
Richmond, Virginia

Henry L. Lew, MD, PhD
Tenured Professor, University of Hawaii School of Medicine
Chair, Department of Communication Sciences and Disorders
Honolulu, Hawaii
Adjunct Professor, Department of Physical Medicine and Rehabilitation
Virginia Commonwealth University School of Medicine
Richmond, Virginia

ELSEVIER

ELSEVIER

1600 John F. Kennedy Blvd.
Ste 1800
Philadelphia, PA 19103-2899

BRADDOM'S REHABILITATION CARE:
A CLINICAL HANDBOOK   ISBN: 978-0-323-47904-2

Notices

Knowledge and best practice in this field are constantly changing. As new research and experience broaden our understanding, changes in research methods, professional practices, or medical treatment may become necessary.

Practitioners and researchers must always rely on their own experience and knowledge in evaluating and using any information, methods, compounds, or experiments described herein. In using such information or methods they should be mindful of their own safety and the safety of others, including parties for whom they have a professional responsibility.

With respect to any drug or pharmaceutical products identified, readers are advised to check the most current information provided (i) on procedures featured or (ii) by the manufacturer of each product to be administered, to verify the recommended dose or formula, the method and duration of administration, and contraindications. It is the responsibility of practitioners, relying on their own experience and knowledge of their patients, to make diagnoses, to determine dosages and the best treatment for each individual patient, and to take all appropriate safety precautions.

To the fullest extent of the law, neither the Publisher nor the authors, contributors, or editors, assume any liability for any injury and/or damage to persons or property as a matter of products liability, negligence or otherwise, or from any use or operation of any methods, products, instructions, or ideas contained in the material herein.

Library of Congress Cataloging-in-Publication Data
Names: Cifu, David X., editor. | Lew, Henry L., editor.
Title: Braddom's rehabilitation care : a clinical handbook / [edited by]
    David X. Cifu, Henry L. Lew.
Other titles: Rehabilitation care | Supplement to (expression): Braddom's
    physical medicine & rehabilitation. Fifth edition.
Description: Philadelphia, PA : Elsevier, [2018] | Includes bibliographical
    references and index.
Identifiers: LCCN 2017021675 | ISBN 9780323479042 (pbk. : alk. paper)
Subjects: | MESH: Rehabilitation—methods | Handbooks
Classification: LCC RM700 | NLM WB 39 | DDC 617.03—dc23 LC record available at
https://lccn.loc.gov/2017021675

Senior Acquisition Editor: Kristine Jones
Content Development Specialist: Meghan Andress
Publishing Services Manager: Patricia Tannian
Senior Project Manager: Claire Kramer
Design Direction: Amy Buxton

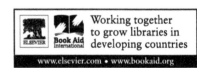

Working together
to grow libraries in
developing countries

www.elsevier.com • www.bookaid.org

Last digit is the print number: 9   8   7   6   5   4   3   2   1

Contributors

Mohd Izmi Bin Ahmad, MBBS, MRehabMed, CIME (USA)
Rehabilitation Physician
Head, Department of Rehabilitation Medicine
Hospital Pulau Pinang
George Town, Penang, Malaysia

Eleftheria Antoniadou, MD, FEBPMR, PhDc
Consultant
Rehabilitation Clinic for Spinal Cord Injury
Patras University Hospital
University of Patras
Patras, Greece

Jason Bitterman, MD
Department of Physical Medicine and Rehabilitation
Rutgers New Jersey Medical School
Newark, New Jersey

Joseph Burris, MD
Associate Professor of Clinical Physical Medicine and Rehabilitation
University of Missouri
Columbia, Missouri

Maria Gabriella Ceravolo, MD, PhD
Professor of Physical and Rehabilitation Medicine
Department of Experimental and Clinical Medicine
Politecnica delle Marche University
Director of Neurorehabilitation Clinic
University Hospital of Ancona
Ancona, Italy

Chein-Wei Chang, MD
Professor
Department of Physical Medicine and Rehabilitation
National Taiwan University
Taipei, Taiwan

Shih-Chung Chang, MD, MS
Department of Physical Medicine and Rehabilitation
Chung Shan Medical University
Department of Physical Medicine and Rehabilitation
Chung Shan Medical University Hospital
Taichung, Taiwan

Carl Chen, MD, PhD
Director
Department of Physical Medicine and Rehabilitation
Chang Gung Memorial Hospital
Taipei, Taiwan

Chih-Kuang Chen, MD
Assistant Professor
Department of Physical Medicine and Rehabilitation
Chang Gung Memorial Hospital
Taoyuan, Taiwan

Shih-Ching Chen, MD, PhD
Deputy Dean and Professor
School of Medicine
College of Medicine
Taipei Medical University
Professor and Attending Physician
Department of Physical Medicine and Rehabilitation
Taipei Medical University Hospital
Taipei, Taiwan

Chen-Liang Chou, MD
Director and Clinical Professor
Department of Physical Medicine and Rehabilitation
National Yang-Ming University
Taipei Veterans General Hospital
Taipei, Taiwan

Willy Chou, MD, HRMS
General Secretary, Superintendent Office
Chief Director, Physical Medicine and Rehabilitation
Chi Mei Medical Center
Associate Professor
Recreation and Health Care Management
Chia Nan University of Pharmacy
Tainan, Taiwan

Tze Yang Chung, MBBS, MRehabMed
Senior Lecturer, Department of Rehabilitation Medicine
University of Malaya
Rehabilitation Physician
Department of Rehabilitation Medicine
University of Malaya Medical Centre
Kuala Lumpur, Malaysia

David X. Cifu, MD
Chairman
Department of Physical Medicine and Rehabilitation
Herman J. Flax, MD Professor
Virginia Commonwealth University School of Medicine
Principal Investigator
Veterans Affairs/Department of Defense Chronic Effects of Neurotrauma
    Consortium
Richmond, Virginia

Andrew Malcolm Dermot Cole, MBBS (Hons), FACRM, FAFRM
Chief Medical Officer
HammondCare
Sydney, Australia
Associate Professor (Conjoint)
Faculty of Medicine
University of New South Wales
Kensington, Australia
Senior Consultant Rehabilitation Medicine
Greenwich Hospital
Greenwich, Australia

Rochelle Coleen Tan Dy, MD
Assistant Professor
Department of Physical Medicine and Rehabilitation
Baylor College of Medicine
Houston, Texas

Blessen C. Eapen, MD
Section Chief, Polytrauma Rehabilitation Center
TBI/Polytrauma Fellowship Program Director
South Texas Veterans Health Care System
Associate Professor
Department of Rehabilitation Medicine
UT Health San Antonio
San Antonio, Texas

Julia Patrick Engkasan, MBBS (Mal), MRehabMed (Mal)
Associate Professor
Department of Rehabilitation Medicine
University of Malaya
Kuala Lumpur, Malaysia

Gerard E. Francisco, MD
Department of Physical Medicine and Rehabilitation
University of Texas Health Science Center (UTHealth)
McGovern Medical School
NeuroRecovery Research Center
TIRR Memorial Hermann
Houston, Texas

Francesca Gimigliano, MD, PhD
Associate Professor of Physical and Rehabilitation Medicine
Department of Mental and Physical Health and Preventive Medicine
University of Campania "Luigi Vanvitelli"
Naples, Italy

Elizabeth J. Halmai, DO
Medical Director, Section Chief
Division of Polytrauma
South Texas Veterans Health Care System
Assistant Professor
Department of Physical Medicine and Rehabilitation
University of Texas Health Science Center San Antonio
San Antonio, Texas

Nazirah Hasnan, MBBS, MRehabMed, PhD
Deputy Director (Clinical)
University of Malaya Medical Centre
Associate Professor and Rehabilitation Consultant
Department of Rehabilitation Medicine
University of Malaya
Kuala Lumpur, Malaysia

Ziad M. Hawamdeh, MD
Senior Fellowship of the European Board of Physical Medicine and
    Rehabilitation
Jordanian Board of Physical Medicine and Rehabilitation
Professor of Physical Medicine and Rehabilitation
Faculty of Medicine
University of Jordan
Amman, Jordan

Joseph E. Herrera, DO, FAAPMR
Chairman and Lucy G Moses Professor
Department of Rehabilitation Medicine
Mount Sinai Health System
Icahn School of Medicine at Mount Sinai
New York, New York

Ming-Yen Hsiao, MD
Lecturer
Department of Physical Medicine and Rehabilitation
National Taiwan University Hospital
College of Medicine
National Taiwan University
Taipei, Taiwan

Lin-Fen Hsieh, MD
Professor
School of Medicine
Fu Jen Catholic University
New Taipei City, Taiwan
Director
Department of Physical Medicine and Rehabilitation
Shin Kong Wo Ho-Su Memorial Hospital
Taipei, Taiwan

Rashidah Ismail Ohnmar Htwe, MBBS, M MED Sc (Rehab Med), CMIA
Associate Professor
Rehabilitation Unit
Department of Orthopedics and Traumatology
Associate Research Fellow
Tissue Engineering Centre
Faculty of Medicine
Universiti Kebangsaan Malaysia
Consultant Rehabilitation Physician
Rehabilitation Unit
Department of Orthopedics and Traumatology
Hospital Canselor Tuanku Muhriz
Kuala Lumpur, Malaysia

Yu-Hui Huang, MD, PhD
Associate Professor
School of Medicine
Chung Shan Medical University
Director
Physical Medicine and Rehabilitation
Chung Shan Medical University Hospital
Taichung, Taiwan

Chen-Yu Hung, MD
Attending Physician
Physical Medicine and Rehabilitation
National Taiwan University Hospital, Beihu Branch
Taipei, Taiwan

Norhayati Hussein, MBBS, MRehabMed, Fellowship in Neurorehabilitation
Rehabilitation Physician
Department of Rehabilitation Medicine
Cheras Rehabilitation Hospital
Kuala Lumpur, Malaysia

Elena Milkova Ilieva, MD, PhD, Prof.
Head of Department
Physical and Rehabilitation Medicine
Medical Faculty
Medical University of Plovdiv
Head of Department
Physical and Rehabilitation Medicine
"Sv Georgi" University Hospital
Plovdiv, Bulgaria

Lydia Abdul Latif, MBBS, MRM
Professor and Consultant Rehabilitation Physician
Department of Rehabilitation Medicine
Faculty of Medicine
University of Malaya
Kuala Lumpur, Malaysia

Wai-Keung Lee, MD
Chief, Department of Physical Medicine and Rehabilitation
Tao Yuan General Hospital
Tao Yuan, Taiwan

Henry L. Lew, MD, PhD
Tenured Professor, University of Hawaii School of Medicine
Chair, Department of Communication Sciences and Disorders
Honolulu, Hawaii
Adjunct Professor, Department of Physical Medicine and Rehabilitation
Virginia Commonwealth University School of Medicine
Richmond, Virginia

Chia-Wei Lin, MD
Attending Physician
Department of Physical Medicine and Rehabilitation
National Taiwan University Hospital, Hsin Chu Branch
Hsin Chu, Taiwan

Ding-Hao Liu, MD
Department of Physical Medicine and Rehabilitation
Taipei Veterans General Hospital, Yuanshan Branch
Yilan, Taiwan

Mazlina Mazlan, MBBS, MRM
Associate Professor
Department of Rehabilitation Medicine
Faculty of Medicine
University of Malaya
Kuala Lumpur, Malaysia

Matthew J. McLaughlin, MD, MSB
Assistant Professor
Division of Pediatric Rehabilitation Medicine
Children's Mercy Hospital
Kansas City, Missouri

Amaramalar Selvi Naicker, MBBS (Ind), MRehabMed (Mal)
Professor of Rehabilitation Medicine and Head of Rehabilitation Medicine Unit
Department of Orthopedics and Traumatology
Associate Research Fellow
Tissue Engineering Centre
Faculty of Medicine
Universiti Kebangsaan Malaysia
Kuala Lumpur, Malaysia

Mooyeon Oh-Park, MD, MS
Director of Geriatric Rehabilitation
Kessler Institute for Rehabilitation
Vice Chair of Education
Research Professor
Department of Physical Medicine and Rehabilitation
Rutgers New Jersey Medical School
Newark, New Jersey

Vishwa S. Raj, MD
Director of Oncology Rehabilitation
Department of Physical Medicine and Rehabilitation
Carolinas Rehabilitation
Chief of Cancer Rehabilitation
Department of Supportive Care
Levine Cancer Institute
Carolinas Healthcare System
Charlotte, North Carolina

Renald Peter Ty Ramiro, MD
Dean, College of Rehabilitative Sciences
Cebu Doctors' University
Mandaue City, Cebu, Philippines,
Head, Physical and Rehabilitation Medicine
Cebu Doctors' University Hospital
Cebu City, Cebu, Philippines
Head, Rehabilitation Medicine
Mactan Doctors' Hospital
Lapu-lapu City, Cebu, Philippines

Reynaldo R. Rey-Matias, PT, MD, MSHMS
Chair, Department of Physical Medicine and Rehabilitation
St. Luke's Medical Center and College of Medicine
Quezon City, Metro Manila, Philippines
Clinical Associate Professor
Department of Rehabilitation Medicine
University of the Philippines–College of Medicine
Manila, Philippines

Desiree L. Roge, MD
Assistant Professor
Department of Physical Medicine and Rehabilitation
Baylor College of Medicine
Assistant Professor
Department of Physical Medicine and Rehabilitation
Texas Children's Hospital
Houston, Texas

Shaw-Gang Shyu, MD
Department of Physical Medicine and Rehabilitation
National Taiwan University Hospital
Taipei, Taiwan

Clarice N. Sinn, DO, MHA
Assistant Professor
UT Southwestern Medical Center/Children's Health
Dallas, Texas

Anwar Suhaimi, MBBS, MRehabMed (Malaya)
Rehabilitation Medicine Specialist
Department of Rehabilitation Medicine
University of Malaya Medical Centre
Senior Lecturer
Department of Rehabilitation Medicine
University of Malaya
Kuala Lumpur, Malaysia

Yi-Chian Wang, MD, MSc
Department of Physical Medicine and Rehabilitation
National Taiwan University Hospital
Taipei, Taiwan

Chueh-Hung Wu, MD
Department of Physical Medicine and Rehabilitation
National Taiwan University Hospital
Taipei City, Taiwan

Yung-Tsan Wu, MD
Attending Physician and Assistant Professor
Department of Physical Medicine and Rehabilitation
Tri-Service General Hospital and School of Medicine
National Defense Medical Center
Taipei, Taiwan

Tian-Shin Yeh, MD, MMS
Attending Physician
Department of Physical Medicine and Rehabilitation
National Taiwan University Hospital, Yun-Lin Branch
Yun-Lin, Taiwan
Graduate Institute of Clinical Medicine
National Taiwan University College of Medicine
Taipei, Taiwan

Mauro Zampolini, MD
Chief
Department of Rehabilitation
Italian National Health Service, USL UMBRIA 2
Foligno, Perugia, Italy

Tunku Nor Taayah Tunku Zubir, MBBS
Consultant Rehabilitation Physician
Department of Rehabilitation
Gleneagles Hospital
Kuala Lumpur, Malaysia

Preface

Over the past 4 years, we have worked diligently with more than 200 authors from across the international community to create (1) the fifth edition of the textbook *Braddom's Physical Medicine & Rehabilitation* and (2) *Braddom's Rehabilitation Care: A Clinical Handbook*. These complementary resources compile key elements of the field of disability medicine, ranging from the basic sciences to clinical care. While the *Braddom's* textbook is the premier reference for all academicians and practitioners in physical medicine and rehabilitation, this new clinical handbook represents the first comprehensive practical guide for trainees and practitioners across all elements of health care. Any student or clinician who sees, evaluates, manages, or refers individuals with disability should use this handbook as his or her key source for information. Whether the patient is a young adult with an acute combat-related musculoskeletal injury, a teen with a sports medicine injury, an elderly person with joint or neurologic dysfunction, a child with specialized equipment needs, or a middle-aged individual after a life-altering trauma, this text can serve as a guide for each patient's clinical care. In addition to practical information and clinical pearls, this handbook also features accompanying online slides and training materials to enhance understanding, to serve as part of core educational modules, and to expand on the key points of the text. We are indebted to the authors of *Braddom's Physical Medicine & Rehabilitation* for providing the comprehensive materials from which this clinical handbook was abstracted, the more than 50 authors who worked meticulously to develop this special edition, and the editorial support staff at Elsevier. We are hopeful that this handbook will be used throughout the world to support the training of health care professionals working with individuals with disabilities and to enhance the clinical care of those individuals with disabilities. It is a resource that we would see in any health care and training setting and used by the full range of trainees and practitioners. We also welcome feedback from readers and users of it to improve the quality and usability of future iterations and editions.

David X. Cifu, MD, and Henry L. Lew, MD, PhD

Foreword

There are more than 1 billion individuals with some degree of disability, physical or mental, in the world, and there are a growing number of practicing clinicians and trainees to assist them in achieving and maintaining their independence. However, there has not been a single, easy-to-use clinical guide to specifically assist these practitioners to optimize their care. This handbook brings together all the key elements of practical clinical care in physical and rehabilitation medicine found in the fifth edition of *Braddom's Physical Medicine & Rehabilitation* into a single, convenient source. The compact size, clinical focus, and state-of-the-art online resources make it the must-have guide. It has been designed to be invaluable at the bedside, in the clinic, in the office, and even in the patient's home. Written in a straightforward style, supported by online slides, and packed with clinical pearls, this handbook is perfect for the full range of professionals, from the beginning student to the advanced practitioner. Created by two of the leading international educators in the field of physical medicine and rehabilitation, Drs. David Cifu and Henry Lew, this book was carefully compiled by more than 50 professionals in physical medicine and rehabilitation from more than 25 countries across the globe to reflect the latest in the field, while remaining consistent with the *Braddom's* reference textbook. It is truly the must-have resource for all trainees and clinicians who see individuals with acute and chronic disabilities.

Jianan Li, MD, Immediate Past President, International Society of Physical and Rehabilitation Medicine (ISPRM)
Jorge Lains, MD, President, ISPRM

Contents

SECTION III COMMON CLINICAL PROBLEMS

Video Contents

BRADDOM'S
REHABILITATION
CARE
A Clinical Handbook

EVALUATION

The Physiatric History and Physical Examination

Shaw-Gang Shyu

The physiatric history and physical examination are the basis for precise diagnosis and recognition of the patient's impairment, and they help in the development of a comprehensive treatment plan. They also serve as a medicolegal record and a basis for physician billing. They are documents used for communication between rehabilitation and nonrehabilitation health care professionals. The essential elements of the physiatric history and physical examination are summarized in this chapter and the accompanying eSlides.

• THE PHYSIATRIC HISTORY

The World Health Organization classification defines *impairment* as any loss or abnormality of body structure or a physiologic or psychological function. *Activity* is the nature and extent of functioning at the level of the person. *Participation* refers to the nature and extent of a person's involvement in life situations in relation to impairments, activities, health conditions, and contextual factors. One of the unique aspects of physiatry is the recognition of functional deficits caused by illness or injury. Identifying and treating the primary impairments to maximize performance becomes the primary thrust of physiatric evaluation and treatment. Physicians in training tend to overassess, but with time the experienced physiatrist develops an intuition regarding the detail needed for each patient, given a particular presentation and setting. The time spent in taking a history also allows the patient to become familiar with the physician, establishing rapport and trust. This initial rapport is critical for a constructive and productive doctor–patient–family relationship. Patients are the primary source of information, but if patients are not able to fully express themselves, the history takers might also rely on the patient's family members and friends; other physicians, nurses, and professionals; or previous medical records.

Chief Complaint

The chief complaint is the symptom or concern that caused the patient to seek medical treatment. Unlike the relatively objective physical examination, the chief complaint is purely subjective, and the physician should use the patient's own words.

History of the Present Illness

The history of the present illness details the chief complaint(s), and it should include some or all of these eight components related to the chief complaint: location, time

3

of onset, quality, context, severity, duration, modifying factors, and associated signs and symptoms.

Functional Status and Activities of Daily Living

The patient's functional status provides a better understanding of mobility, activities of daily living (ADL), instrumental activities of daily living (I-ADL) (eSlide 1.1), communication, cognition, work, and recreation. Assessing the potential for functional gain or deterioration requires an understanding of the natural history, cause, and time of onset of the functional problems.

It is sometimes helpful to assess functional status with a standardized scale. No single scale is appropriate for all patients, but the Functional Independence Measure (FIM) is the scoring system most commonly used in the inpatient rehabilitation setting. Each of 18 different activities is scored on a scale of 1 to 7 (total score: 18 to 126) (eSlide 1.2), and FIM serves as a kind of rehabilitation shorthand among team members to quickly and accurately describe functional deficits.

MOBILITY

Mobility is the ability to move about in one's environment. Bed mobility includes turning from side to side, changing from the prone to supine positions, sitting up, and lying down. Transfer mobility includes getting in and out of bed, standing from the sitting position, and moving between a wheelchair and another seat.

Wheelchair mobility can be assessed by asking if patients can propel the wheelchair independently, how far or how long they can go without resting, whether they need assistance with managing the wheelchair parts, and the extent to which they can move about at home, in the community, and up and down ramps. Whether the home is potentially wheelchair accessible is particularly important in cases of new onset of severe disability.

Ambulation and stair mobility can be assessed by the patient's walking distance and endurance, the patient's requirement for assistive devices and need for breaks, the number of stairs the patient must routinely climb and descend at home or in the community, and the presence or absence of handrails in their daily lives. Identifying associated symptoms during ambulation and a history of falling or instability are also important.

Driving (a type of community mobility) is a crucial activity for many people, and older adults who stop driving face increased depressive symptoms. The risks of driving are weighed against the consequences of not being able to drive.

COGNITION

Cognition is the mental process of knowing. Because persons with cognitive deficits often cannot recognize their own impairments (agnosia), it is important to also gather information from other individuals who are familiar with the patient. Cognitive deficits interfere with the patient's rehabilitation and safety.

COMMUNICATION

Communication skills are used to convey information, including thoughts, needs, and emotions. Verbal-expression deficits can be subtle. Patients who have deficits in verbal expression might or might not be able to communicate through other means, known as augmentative communication strategies. These strategies include writing and physicality (e.g., sign language, gestures, and body language) and the use of communication aids (e.g., picture, letter, word board, and electronic devices).

Past Medical and Surgical History

The past medical and surgical history allows the physiatrist to understand how pre-existing illnesses affect the patient's current status, the precautions and limitations that will be necessary during a rehabilitation program, and the impact on rehabilitation outcomes. Particularly, cardiopulmonary deficits can severely compromise mobility, ADL, I-ADL, work, and leisure.

All medications should be documented, including prescription medications, over-the-counter drugs, nutraceuticals, supplements, herbs, and vitamins. Drug and food allergies should be noted. Particular attention should be paid to commonly prescribed medications, such as nonsteroidal antiinflammatory agents.

Social History

Understanding the patient's home environment and living situation includes asking whether the patient lives in a house or an apartment and whether elevators, stairs, or handrails are present. These factors, in conjunction with the level of support from the patient's family and friends, will help determine the discharge plans.

Patients should be asked in a nonjudgmental manner about their history of smoking, alcohol use or abuse, and drug abuse. Sexuality is particularly important to patients in their reproductive years. Sexual orientation and safer sex practices should be addressed when appropriate.

VOCATIONAL ACTIVITIES
Vocation is a source of financial security and provides self-confidence and even identity. The history should include the patient's education level, recent work history, and ability to fulfill job requirements subsequent to injury or illness.

FINANCES AND INCOME MAINTENANCE
A social worker may help patients with financial concerns. Whether a patient has the financial resources or insurance to pay for adaptive devices can significantly affect discharge planning.

RECREATION
Loss or limitation of the ability to engage in hobbies and recreational activities can be stressful to most people. Recreation is also a primary outcome in sports medicine. A recreational therapist can be helpful.

PSYCHOSOCIAL HISTORY, SPIRITUALITY, AND BELIEFS
Patients with impairment may feel a loss of overall health, body image, mobility, independence, or income. Providing assistance in developing coping strategies, especially for depression and anxiety, can help accelerate the process whereby the patient learns to adjust to a new disability.

Health care providers should be sensitive to the patient's spiritual needs and provide appropriate referral or counseling.

LITIGATION
Litigation (active or pending) can be a source of anxiety, depression, or guilt. Patients should be asked in a nonjudgmental manner whether they are involved in litigation. The answer should not change the treatment plan.

Family History

Patients should be asked about the health, or cause and age of death, of parents and siblings. The family history will help identify genetic disorders within the family and potential assistance that may be obtained from family members.

Review of Systems

The review of systems identifies problems or diseases that have not yet been reviewed during the history taking.

• THE PHYSIATRIC PHYSICAL EXAMINATION

Neurologic Examination

Neurologic problems are common in rehabilitation medicine. The precise location of the lesion should be identified from an organized neurologic examination. An accurate and efficient neurologic examination requires that the examiner have a thorough knowledge of both central and peripheral neuroanatomy *before* the examination. Weakness may be seen in both upper motor neuron (UMN) and lower motor neuron (LMN) disorders. UMN lesions involving the central nervous system are typically characterized by hypertonia and hyperreflexia. LMN defects are characterized by hypotonia, hyporeflexia, significant muscle atrophy, fasciculations, and electromyographic changes. UMN and LMN lesions often coexist, as seen in amyotrophic lateral sclerosis or traumatic brain injury with a brachial plexus injury.

MENTAL STATUS EXAMINATION

The mental status examination (MSE) should be performed in a comfortable setting where the patient is not likely to be distracted by external stimuli. Bedside MSE might need to be supplemented by observations in therapy and evaluation by a neuropsychologist.

The Folstein Mini-Mental Status Examination is a brief and convenient tool to test general cognitive function. It is useful for screening patients for dementia and brain injuries. Of a maximum of 30 points, a score of 24 or above is considered within the normal range. The clock-drawing test is a quick and sensitive test of cognitive impairment. This task uses memory, visual spatial skills, and executive functioning. The use of the three-word recall test in addition to the clock-drawing test, which is known collectively as the Mini-Cog Test, has recently gained popularity in screening for dementia.

Level of consciousness. Consciousness is the state of awareness of one's surroundings. A functioning pontine reticular activating system is necessary for normal conscious functioning.

Lethargy is the general slowing of motor processes, such as speech and movement, in which the patient can easily fall asleep if not stimulated but is easily aroused. *Obtundation* is a dulled or blunted sensitivity in which the patient is difficult to arouse and is still confused after arousal. *Stupor* is a state of semi consciousness characterized by arousal only by intense stimuli, such as sharp pressure over a bony prominence (e.g., sternal rub); the patient also has few or even no voluntary motor responses.

In *coma*, the eyes are closed, sleep-wake cycles are absent, and there is no evidence of a contingent relationship between the patient's behavior and the environment. *Vegetative state* is characterized by the presence of sleep-wake cycles but still no contingent relationship. *Minimally conscious state* indicates a patient who remains severely disabled but demonstrates sleep-wake cycles and inconsistent, nonreflexive, contingent behaviors in response to a specific environmental stimulus. In acute settings, the Glasgow Coma Scale is the most commonly used objective measure to document level of consciousness (eSlide 1.3).

Attention. Attention is the ability to address a specific stimulus for a short period of time without being distracted by internal or external stimuli. Vigilance is the ability to hold one's attention over longer periods. Attention is tested by digit recall; repeating seven numbers in the forward direction is considered normal, with fewer than five indicating significant attention deficits.

Orientation. Orientation is composed of four parts: person, place, time, and situation. Sense of time is usually the first to be lost, and sense of person is typically the last. Temporary stress can account for a minor loss of orientation, but major disorientation usually suggests an organic brain syndrome.

Memory. The components of memory include learning, retention, and recall. The patient is typically asked to remember three or four objects or words and then asked to repeat the items immediately to assess immediate acquisition (encoding) of the information. Retention is assessed by recall after a delayed interval, usually 5 to 10 minutes. Normal individuals younger than 60 years should be able to recall three of four items. Recent memory can be tested by asking questions about the past 24 hours. Remote memory is tested by asking where the patient was born or which school or college the patient attended.

General fundamentals of knowledge and abstract thinking. Intelligence is a global function encompassing both basic intellect and remote memory. The examiner should note the patient's highest level of education. Abstraction is a higher cortical function and should always be considered in the context of intelligence and cultural differences. It can be tested by asking the patient to interpret a common proverb or explain a humorous phrase or situation.

Insight and judgment. Insight has been conceptualized into three components: awareness of impairment, need for treatment, and attribution of symptoms. Recognizing that one has an impairment is the initial step necessary for recovery. A lack of insight can severely hamper a patient's progress in rehabilitation.

Judgment is an estimate of a person's ability to solve real-life problems, and it is related to the patient's capacity for independent functioning. Judgment can be evaluated by simply observing the patient's behavior or by noting the patient's responses to hypothetical situations.

Mood and affect. The examiner should document reactivity and stability of mood. Mood can be described in terms such as being happy, sad, euphoric, blue, depressed, angry, or anxious. Affect describes how a patient feels at a given moment, which can be described by terms such as blunted, flat, inappropriate, labile, optimistic, or pessimistic.

COMMUNICATION
Aphasia. Aphasia involves the loss of production or comprehension of language. Naming, repetition, comprehension, and fluency are the key components. Testing

comprehension of spoken language should begin with single words, progress to sentences that require only yes/no responses, and then progress to complex commands. Visual naming, repetition of single words and sentences, word-finding abilities, reading and writing from dictation, and then spontaneous reading and writing should also be assessed. Some standardized aphasia measures include the Boston Diagnostic Aphasia Examination and the Western Aphasia Battery (see Chapter 3).

Dysarthria. Dysarthria refers to defective articulation but unaffected content of speech. Key sounds include "ta ta ta," which is made by the tongue (lingual consonants); "mm mm mm," which is made by the lips (labial consonants); and "ga ga ga," which is made by the larynx, pharynx, and palate.

Dysphonia. Dysphonia is a deficit in sound production, which can be secondary to respiratory disease, fatigue, or vocal cord paralysis. Indirect laryngoscopy is the best method to examine the vocal cords. Patients are asked to say "ah" to assess vocal cord abduction and "e" to assess adduction. Patients with weakness of both vocal cords will speak in a whisper and exhibit inspiratory stridor.

Verbal apraxia. Apraxia of speech involves a deficit in motor planning without impaired strength or coordination. It is characterized by inconsistent errors when speaking. Oromotor apraxia is seen in patients with difficulty organizing nonspeech oral motor activity. It can adversely affect swallowing. Tests for verbal and oral motor function are listed in Chapter 3.

Cognitive linguistic deficits. Cognitive linguistic deficits involve the pragmatics and context of communication, such as confabulation. Cognitive linguistic deficits are distinguished from fluent aphasias (e.g., Wernicke aphasia) by the presence of relatively normal syntax and grammar.

CRANIAL NERVE EXAMINATION

Cranial nerve I: olfactory nerve. Both perception and identification of smell should be tested with aromatic, nonirritating materials that avoid stimulation of the trigeminal nerve. The olfactory nerve is the most commonly injured cranial nerve (CN) in head trauma.

Cranial nerve II: optic nerve. The optic nerve is assessed by testing visual acuity and visual fields. Visual acuity refers to central vision. Visual field testing assesses the integrity of the optic pathway. Testing visual fields is most commonly performed by confrontation. For patients with deficits, further assessment by a neuro-optometrist or visually trained occupational therapist can be helpful.

Cranial nerves III, IV, and VI: oculomotor, trochlear, and abducens nerves. The oculomotor nerve innervates the medial rectus muscle (adductor of the eye), superior rectus and inferior oblique muscles (elevators of the eye), and inferior rectus muscle (depressor of the eye). The trochlear nerve innervates the superior oblique muscle, which is responsible for the downward gaze, especially during adduction. The abducens nerve controls the lateral rectus muscle, which abducts the eye. The examiner should assess the alignment of the patient's eyes while the eyes are at rest and when the eyes are following an object, observing the full range of horizontal and vertical eye movements in the six cardinal directions. The optic (afferent) and oculomotor (efferent) nerves are involved with the pupillary light reflex, which normally results in constriction of *both* pupils when a light stimulus is presented to either eye separately. A characteristic head tilt when looking downward is sometimes seen in CN IV lesions.

Cranial nerve V: trigeminal nerve. The three sensory branches of CN V can be tested along the forehead (ophthalmic branch), cheeks (maxillary branch), and jaw (mandibular branch) bilaterally. The motor branch of the trigeminal nerve innervates the muscles of mastication, which include the masseters, pterygoids, and temporalis muscles. The corneal reflex tests the ophthalmic division of the trigeminal nerve (afferent) and the facial nerve (efferent).

Cranial nerve VII: facial nerve. The facial nerve is first examined by observing the patient while he or she is talking, smiling, closing the eyes, flattening the nasolabial fold, and elevating one corner of the mouth. The patient is then asked to wrinkle the forehead (frontalis muscle function), close the eyes while the examiner attempts to open them (orbicularis oculi function), puff out both cheeks while the examiner presses on the cheeks (buccinator function), and show the teeth (orbicularis oris function). A peripheral injury to the facial nerve, such as Bell palsy, affects both the upper and lower face, whereas a central lesion typically affects mainly the lower face.

Cranial nerve VIII: vestibulocochlear nerve. The vestibulocochlear nerve comprises two divisions: the cochlear nerve, which is responsible for hearing, and the vestibular nerve, which is related to balance. The cochlear division can be tested by checking gross hearing by rubbing the thumb and index fingers near each ear of the patient. Patients with dizziness or vertigo associated with changes in head position or suspected of having benign paroxysmal positional vertigo should be assessed with the Dix-Hallpike maneuver (eSlide 1.4).

Cranial nerves IX and X: glossopharyngeal nerve and vagus nerve. Hoarseness is usually associated with a lesion of the recurrent laryngeal nerve, a branch of the vagus nerve. Normally, the soft palate should elevate symmetrically, and the uvula should remain in the midline when the patient says "ah." In UMN vagus nerve lesions, the uvula will deviate toward the side of the lesion, but in LMN lesions, the uvula will deviate to the contralateral side. Gag reflex can be tested by touching the pharyngeal wall with a cotton tip applicator until the patient gags. The examiner should compare the sensitivity of each side (afferent: glossopharyngeal nerve) and observe the symmetry of the palatal movement (efferent: vagus nerve). The presence of a gag reflex does *not* imply the ability to swallow without risk of aspiration.

Cranial nerve XI: accessory nerve. Atrophy or asymmetry of the patient's trapezius and sternocleidomastoid muscles should be checked. Trapezius atrophy results in a laterally migrated scapula ("open door" winging). To test the strength of the sternocleidomastoid muscle, the patient should be asked to rotate the head against resistance.

Cranial nerve XII: hypoglossal nerve. The hypoglossal nerve is tested by asking the patient to protrude the tongue and noting evidence of atrophy, fasciculation, or deviation. Fibrillations in the tongue are common in patients with amyotrophic lateral sclerosis. The tongue typically points to the side of the lesion in peripheral hypoglossal nerve lesions but away from the lesion in UMN lesions.

SENSORY EXAMINATION (eSlides 1.5 and 1.6)
Evaluation of the sensory system requires testing both superficial sensation (light touch, pain, and temperature) and deep sensation (position and vibration).

Light touch can be assessed with a fine wisp of cotton or a cotton tip applicator. Pain is assessed with a safety pin. Thermal sensation can be checked with two different cups, one filled with hot water and one filled with cold water and ice chips.

Proprioception is tested by passive vertical movement of the toes or fingers when the patient's eyes are closed. The patient is asked whether the digit is being moved in an upward or downward direction. It is important to grasp the sides of the digit rather than the nailbed to avoid the patient perceiving pressure in this area.

Vibration is tested with a 128-Hz tuning fork, which is placed on a bony prominence, such as the dorsal aspect of the malleoli, olecranon, or terminal phalange of the great toe or finger. The patient is asked to indicate when the vibration ceases.

Two-point discrimination is tested by calipers with blunt ends. The patient (with closed eyes) is asked to indicate whether one or two stimulation points are felt. Commonly tested two-point discrimination areas and their normal values are as follows: lips (2–3 mm), fingertips (3–5 mm), dorsum of the hand (20–30 mm), and palms (8–15 mm).

Testing for graphesthesia, the ability to recognize numbers, letters, or symbols traced onto the palm, is performed by writing recognizable numbers on the patient's palm while the patient's eyes remain closed. Stereognosis is the ability to recognize common objects, such as keys or coins, when placed in the hand.

MOTOR CONTROL
Strength. Manual muscle testing (eSlides 1.7 and 1.8) provides an important method of quantifying strength. Pain can result in give-way weakness. It is important to recognize the presence of substitution when muscles are weak or movement is uncoordinated. Patients who cannot actively control muscle tension (e.g., those with spasticity) are not appropriate for standard manual muscle testing methods. A muscle grade of 3 is functionally important because antigravity strength implies that a limb can be used for activity. Females' strength typically increases up to 20 years, plateaus through the twenties, and then gradually declines after age 30 years. Males increase strength up to age 20 years and then plateau until older than 30 years before declining.

Tables 1.13 and 1.14 in *Braddom's Physical Medicine and Rehabilitation*, Fifth Edition (ISBN: 978-0-323-28046-4), summarize joint movements, innervation, and manual strength testing techniques for all major muscle groups of the extremities. Examples of tests for shoulder abduction are shown in eSlide 1.9.

Coordination. Ataxia or coordination deficits can be secondary to deficits of sensory, motor, or cerebellar connections. Dysdiadochokinesia describes an inability to perform rapidly alternating movements.

Lesions affecting the midline cerebellum usually produce truncal ataxia, whereas lesions that affect the anterior lobe of the cerebellum usually result in gait ataxia. Lateral cerebellar hemisphere lesions produce limb ataxia, which can be tested by the finger-to-nose test and heel-to-shin test.

The Romberg test can be used to differentiate a cerebellar deficit from a proprioceptive deficit. If loss of balance is present when the eyes are open or closed, it is indicative of cerebellar ataxia. If loss of balance occurs only when the eyes are closed, it is a positive Romberg sign, which indicates a proprioceptive (sensory) deficit.

Apraxia. Apraxia is the loss of the ability to carry out programmed or planned movements despite adequate understanding of the task and no weakness or sensory loss. Ideomotor apraxia occurs when a patient cannot carry out motor commands but can perform the required movements under different circumstances. Ideational apraxia refers to the inability to carry out sequences of acts, although each component can be performed separately. Dressing apraxia and constructional apraxia are the result of neglect rather than actual deficits in motor planning.

Involuntary movements. Tremor, the most common type of involuntary movement, is a rhythmic movement of a body part. Myoclonus is a quick jerking movement of a muscle or body part. Chorea constitutes movements that consist of brief, random, nonrepetitive movements in a fidgety patient who is unable to sit still. Athetosis consists of twisting and writhing movements and is commonly seen in cerebral palsy. Dystonia is a sustained posturing that can affect small or large muscle groups. Hemiballismus occurs when there are repetitive violent flailing movements.

Tone. Tone is the resistance of a muscle to stretch or passively elongate (see Chapter 23). Spasticity is a velocity-dependent increase in the stretch reflex, whereas rigidity is the resistance of the limb to passive movement in the relaxed state (non–velocity-dependent).

Tone can be quantified by the Modified Ashworth Scale (MAS). A pendulum test can also be used to quantify spasticity. The Tardieu Scale has been suggested as a more appropriate clinical measure of spasticity than the MAS. Measurements are usually taken at three velocities (V1, V2, and V3). V1 is measured as slow as possible, V2 is measured at the speed of the limb falling under gravity, and V3 is measured when the limb is moving as fast as possible. Responses are recorded at each velocity and at the angles (in degrees) at which the muscle response occurs.

REFLEXES

Superficial reflexes (eSlide 1.10). The normal plantar reflex consists of flexion of the great toe or no response. With dysfunction of the corticospinal tract, there is a positive Babinski sign, which consists of dorsiflexion of the great toe with an associated fanning of the other toes. A positive Chaddock sign refers to dorsiflexion of the great toe after stroking from the lateral ankle to the lateral dorsal foot. A positive Stransky sign refers to an upgoing great toe after flipping the little toe outward.

Muscle stretch reflexes (eSlide 1.11). Muscle stretch reflexes, which were called deep tendon reflexes in the past, are assessed by tapping the skin overlying the muscle tendon with a reflex hammer. The response is assessed as 0, no response; 1+, diminished but present and might require facilitation; 2+, usual response; 3+, brisker than usual; and 4+, hyperactive with clonus. Reinforcement maneuvers, such as the Jendrassik maneuver, assist examination.

Primitive reflexes. Primitive reflexes are abnormal reflexes that represent developmental regression, indicating significant neurologic abnormalities in adults. Examples of primitive reflexes include the sucking reflex, rooting reflex, grasp reflex, snout reflex, and palmomental response.

GAIT

Gait is a series of rhythmic, alternating movements of the limbs and trunk that result in the forward progression of the center of gravity. Gait is dependent on input from several systems, including the visual, vestibular, cerebellar, motor, and sensory systems. Gait disorders have stereotypical patterns that reflect injury to various aspects of the neurologic system (eSlide 1.12).

Musculoskeletal Examination

The musculoskeletal (MSK) examination incorporates inspection, palpation, passive and active range of movement (ROM), assessment of joint stability, manual muscle testing, joint-specific provocative maneuvers, and special tests. Readers may view Table 1.9 in *Braddom's Physical Medicine and Rehabilitation*, Fifth Edition, for details and reliability of joint-specific provocative maneuvers.

INSPECTION

Inspection includes observing mood, signs of pain or discomfort, functional impairments, or evidence of malingering (e.g., Waddell signs). The spine should be inspected for scoliosis, kyphosis, and lordosis, whereas limbs should be examined for symmetry, circumference, and contour. Muscle atrophy, masses, edema, scars, skin breakdown, and fasciculations should also be checked. Joints should be inspected for deformity, visible swelling, and erythema.

Kinetic chain refers to the summation of individual joint movements linked in a series, leading to the production of a larger functional goal. A change in movement of a single joint may affect the motion of adjacent, as well as distant, joints in the chain. This may result in asymmetric patterns causing disease at seemingly unrelated sites.

PALPATION

Palpation is used to identify tender areas and localize trigger points, muscle guarding, or spasticity. Joints and soft tissues should be assessed for effusion, warmth, masses, tight muscle bands, tone, and crepitus.

Assessment of joint stability. Bilateral examination is critical because assessment of the "normal" side establishes a patient's unique biomechanics. Joint play or capsular patterns assess the integrity of the capsule in positions of minimal bony contact, sometimes referred to as an open-packed position.

Assessment of range of movement general principles. ROM testing is used to assess the integrity of a joint, monitor the efficacy of treatment regimens, and determine the mechanical cause of impairment. Normal ROM varies according to age, gender, conditioning, body habitus, and genetics. Passive ROM should be performed through all planes of motion. Active ROM is performed by the patient through all planes of motion, without assistance from the examiner. Range is measured with a universal goniometer (eSlide 1.13). Correct patient positioning and planes of motion for testing shoulder and hip joint ROM are shown in eSlides 1.14 and 1.15.

For more comprehensive and detailed information regarding measurements of each joint, the reader may refer to Chapter 1 in *Braddom's Physical Medicine and Rehabilitation, Fifth Edition.*

• ASSESSMENT, SUMMARY, AND PLAN

Only after completing a thorough physiatric history and physical examination is the physiatrist able to develop a comprehensive treatment plan. The organization of the initial treatment plan and goals should clearly state the impairments, performance deficits (activity limitations), community or role dysfunction (participation level), medical conditions that can affect achieving both short-term and long-term functional goals, and goals for the interdisciplinary rehabilitation team. Follow-up treatment plans and notes are likely to be shorter and less detailed, but they *must* address important interval changes since the last documentation and any significant changes in treatment or goals.

Clinical Pearls

A comprehensive rehabilitation physiatric history and physical examination help develop a treatment plan with proper goals.

The physiatric history and physical examination begin with the standard medical format but go beyond that to assess impairment, activity limitation (disability), and participation (handicap).

Identifying and treating the primary impairments to maximize performance is the primary thrust of physiatric evaluation and treatment.

Physiatrists' understanding of the MSK principles and MSK examination distinguishes them from neurologists and neurosurgeons. Bilateral examination is critical.

Physiatrists' understanding of neurology and the neurologic examination distinguishes them from orthopedists and rheumatologists.

BIBLIOGRAPHY
The complete bibliography is available on ExpertConsult.com.

2 History and Examination of the Pediatric Patient

Chia-Wei Lin

• HISTORY

Birth History (eSlide 2.1)

Birth history should include any issues during pregnancy or during labor and delivery. Maternal complications during pregnancy, such as seizures, febrile illnesses, hypertension, or hyperglycemia, should be evaluated. Any medications or drugs that the mother took during pregnancy and any substances the infants were exposed to should be reviewed. The duration of gestation, presence of multiple fetuses, fetal movements, and presentation at birth are also important factors.

The child's birth weight and length, as well as the Apgar score, should be noted. The Apgar score consists of five components: activity, pulse, grimace, appearance, and respiration. Postnatal complications, such as hyperbilirubinemia, retinopathy of prematurity, respiratory difficulties, feeding difficulties, and duration of respiratory support, may provide clues to underlying disease and functional impact. Complications during the mother's previous pregnancies, such as stillbirths, miscarriages, or fetal anomalies, should be recorded.

History of Presenting Problem (eSlide 2.2)

The physician should determine the onset, progression, and associated factors of the current problem. It is important to determine which diagnostic tests have been performed, as well as any treatments that have been initiated. The child's medical history, including any significant illnesses, hospitalizations, surgeries, procedures, previous trauma, medications taken, allergies, and immunization status, should be reviewed.

Developmental History

Developmental history is one of the most important aspects of pediatric history. Illnesses, injuries, and different disease processes can have a profound impact on the attainment of developmental milestones. Delays may be noted in gross motor, fine motor, speech and language, and/or psychosocial areas. A thorough understanding of developmental milestones (eSlides 2.3, 2.4, 2.5, and 2.6) and the age at which the child attained them can assist with diagnosis and treatment protocols. If delays are noted in motor skills, a neuromuscular disorder is more likely, and if delays are primarily noted in speech and language skills, assessment of the child's hearing is warranted. A discussion of the developmental milestones is helpful in educating the family regarding what the child should be doing and what skills he or she should be working on. It should be emphasized that there is a wide range of normal for attaining certain skills, and the family may notice that the child progresses at different rates in different areas.

Family History

The family history should include any history of early stroke, early myocardial infarction, peripheral neuropathy, joint or tissue abnormalities, myopathies, bony abnormalities, gait abnormalities, or developmental delays; a history of these conditions should be ascertained through multiple generations. If a genetic disorder is suspected, the child and family should be referred for genetic testing, which can help with planning future pregnancies and provide counseling to the extended family.

Social and Educational History

The examiner should inquire about the child's environment, including who lives with the child, who the caregivers are, and the layout and accessibility of the home. The child's peer interactions, extracurricular activities, current educational history, and history of receiving early intervention services can give insight into the child's social skills, personality, and learning abilities.

• PHYSICAL EXAMINATION (eSlide 2.7)

There is no standardized approach to the physical examination of the pediatric patient. It should be tailored to the age and developmental level of the child. Developing a rapport by playing or talking with the child can be helpful. Very young children are typically most comfortable on their parent's lap during the examination.

Growth

Height and weight should be monitored as the child grows. The average full-term newborn measures 50 cm in length and weighs 3400 g. Height increases 50% by the first year and doubles by the fourth year. Children's adult height can be estimated by doubling their height at age 2 years. Body weight doubles by 5 months and triples by 1 year. Growth may be arrested early as a result of precocious puberty, with premature closure of the growth plate. Precocious puberty is defined as the onset of puberty in girls younger than 8 years and boys younger than 9 years. Decreases in the velocity of height or weight growth, as well as actual weight loss, may be associated with poor nutrition or malabsorption. Significant increases may indicate a pituitary tumor, metabolic disorder, or poor diet. The average head circumference at birth is 35 cm and increases to 47 cm by 1 year. Macrocephaly and microcephaly are defined as a head circumference greater than 2 standard deviations above and below the mean, respectively. With institution of the "Back to Sleep" program, there has been an increase in the presence of flattening of the occiput, brachycephaly, and plagiocephaly; these conditions resolve spontaneously.

Inspection

The child's general appearance, movements, degree of engagement, skin, cranial deformities, facial dysmorphisms, joint abnormalities, and asymmetry of stature should be examined. The presence of certain physical abnormalities is linked with some common syndromes (eSlide 2.8).

Musculoskeletal Assessment

Inspect and palpate the bones, joints, and muscles, and perform passive and active range of movement (ROM) of all joints. Loss of ROM may be attributable to joint contracture, and hypermobility may be due to connective tissue disorders. The back and spine examination should focus on any bony abnormalities, as well as any muscular asymmetries. The most common form of scoliosis is a right thoracic curve in adolescent girls.

It is not unusual for the child's foot to be flat until 3 to 5 years of age. However, if the foot is rigid or painful, it may be the result of a tarsal coalition (eSlide 2.9). If the child has pes cavus (eSlide 2.9), the presence of a neuromuscular disease, such as Charcot-Marie-Tooth disease, should be investigated. The most common causes of intoeing are metatarsus adductus in infancy, tibial torsion in the toddler, and femoral anteversion in the older child. Children have normal, physiologic bow legs up to age 2 years, but rickets or Blount disease could account for pathologic genu varus position. If there is significantly reduced ROM at the hip or a leg length discrepancy, the hip may be subluxed or dislocated. An anteroposterior pelvis film will delineate the degree of subluxation.

Neurologic Assessment

Neurologic assessment evaluates cranial nerve function, sensory function, strength, movement, reflexes, coordination, balance, gait (eSlide 2.10), and cognitive function. Infants will track an object to the midline at 1 month of age and from side to side at 3 months. Auditory evaluation should be reassessed in any child who demonstrates speech and language delays, articulation errors, inattentiveness to sound, a history of recurrent ear infections, or a history of brain injury.

Evaluations of primitive reflexes (eSlide 2.11) and postural responses (eSlide 2.12) are helpful tools in assessing an infant's motor responses. Any asymmetry in responses may reflect an underlying stroke or peripheral nerve disorder, such as a brachial plexus injury. A true manual muscle examination is not very accurate before the age of 5 years. A child's muscle tone will change during development. Hypotonia with associated areflexia in a newborn is consistent with spinal muscular atrophy. Hypertonia may be subdivided into spasticity, dystonia, and rigidity. Hypertonia indicates a central nervous system disorder. A child's gait pattern changes and progresses from the age of 1 year to approximately 7 years: the base of support narrows, the stride length increases, and the cadence decreases.

Functional Assessment

Developmental skills can be formally assessed with a variety of tools, such as the Denver Developmental Screening Test II (DDST-II), Bayley Scales of Infant Development, and Gesell Developmental Schedule (eSlide 2.13). A children's version of the Functional Independence Measure (WeeFIM) was developed to evaluate a child's functional progression. Cognition and potential for academic achievement can be assessed in the preschooler and school-age child with several tests (eSlide 2.14). It is also important to evaluate a child's social and adaptive skills and his or her perceived quality of life (eSlide 2.15). Disability-specific assessment tools include the Gross Motor Function Measure (GMFM) and the Manual Abilities Classification Scale (MACS), which measure motor function in patients with cerebral palsy.

Clinical Pearls

It is important to obtain a thorough history and detailed physical examination of pediatric patients. Future research may focus on how to improve the clinical skills during daily practice, as well as on establishing the reliability and validity of various examination techniques.

BIBLIOGRAPHY
The complete bibliography is available on ExpertConsult.com.

3 Adult Neurogenic Communication and Swallowing Disorders

Ming-Yen Hsiao

Communication and swallowing disorders are among the most common impairments resulting from various neurologic diseases or injuries. They impose great impact on a patient's medical condition, psychological health, social integration, and overall quality of life. The pathophysiology, clinical presentation, evaluation, and management of aphasia, cognitive communicative disorders, motor speech disorders, and swallowing disorders are summarized in this chapter and the accompanying eSlides.

• REHABILITATION OF PATIENTS WITH COMMUNICATION DISORDERS (eSlides 3.1 and 3.2)

Rehabilitation of patients with communication disorders focuses on *restorative* as well as *compensatory* strategies and techniques [augmentative and alternative communication (AAC)]. When the attempt is made to restore deficit areas, early implementation of AAC and incorporation of family and caregivers in the treatment plan to ensure participation of the affected individual are essential.

Aphasia (eSlides 3.3 and 3.4)

Common causes of aphasia include stroke (most common, 20% to 40% of people with stroke have aphasia), traumatic brain injury, dementia, and other progressive neurologic disorders. Aphasia types include Broca, Wernicke, conduction, global, transcortical motor, transcortical sensory, anomic, and crossed and primary progressive aphasia. Assessment involves identification of the specific areas of deficit.

SPECIAL CONSIDERATIONS: HANDEDNESS AND LANGUAGE DOMINANCE

Language control is in the left hemisphere in 99% of right-handed individuals. Of left-handed individuals, 70% have language control in the left hemisphere, 15% have it in the right hemisphere, and 15% have it in both hemispheres. Overall, 97% of the population has language control in the left hemisphere.

Cognitive Communication Disorders

Cognitive communication disorders impair memory, new learning, awareness, problem solving, organizing, planning, and all other areas of executive function.

The following sections describe the management of these disorders, which result mostly from right hemisphere strokes, brain injuries, and dementia.

RIGHT HEMISPHERE STROKE

Common disorders of right hemisphere strokes include impairments in memory, attention, and problem solving; decreased awareness or insight into the severity of the deficits; reduced ability to process and express higher level or abstract language concepts; decreased or flat affect; and impairments in organizing, planning, and other executive functions. The most common deficits are seen in attention, neglect, perception, and learning or memory.

TRAUMATIC AND NONTRAUMATIC BRAIN INJURY (eSlide 3.5)

Penetrating injuries often cause focal damage, and closed head injuries often result in diffuse axonal damage. Interventions focus on supporting and optimizing the progressions through different stages; these stages are often described with the Rancho Los Amigos Levels of Cognitive Functioning Scale.

Early Stage of Recovery (Rancho Levels I–III): The treatment focuses on stimulating or shaping responses for basic communication and identifying the transition to localized responses.

Middle Stage of Recovery (Rancho Levels IV–V): The treatment initially focuses on structuring the environment to facilitate participation. This stage of recovery is particularly important with regard to speech recovery, and the focus is to increase orientation, insight, memory, and new learning; manage language confusion and confabulations; and increase functional participation. AAC will be implemented for those who remain nonspeaking.

Late Stage of Recovery (Rancho Levels VI–VIII): The intervention focuses on increasing orientation, memory, carryover of new learning, and eventually higher-level executive functions.

Mild brain injury. High level cognitive communication disorders can affect social reintegration. Impairments of executive function are common. Intervention focuses on increasing awareness and education.

ALZHEIMER DISEASE AND OTHER DEMENTIAS

Definitive diagnosis hinges on evidence of short-term and long-term memory impairment in addition to the presence of at least aphasia, apraxia, agnosia, or impaired executive functioning. Treatment often occurs in bouts, occurring at crucial times during the patient's disease progression.

Motor Speech Disorders

DYSARTHRIA (eSlide 3.6)

Dysarthria is a major source of disability and involves impairments of respiration, phonation (larynx), resonance (velopharynx), and articulation (tongue and lips). It can be categorized into several types: flaccid, spastic, ataxic, hypokinetic, hyperkinetic, and mixed. Management of dysarthria depends on subsystem involvement and severity, and extensive practice is necessary for optimal recovery.

APRAXIA

Apraxia of speech is characterized by a slow speaking rate, lengthened sounds and durations between sounds, sound distortions, consistent errors, abnormal prosody, difficulty in initiating speech, and a preference for automatic speech. The assessment includes an oral mechanism and a motor speech examination. Therapy typically involves behavioral therapy that focuses on the position or movement of the articulators and is based on principles of motor learning.

• REHABILITATION OF PATIENTS WITH SWALLOWING DISORDERS

Swallowing disorders, or dysphagia, can lead to malnutrition, dehydration, respiratory compromise, and a decrease in quality of life. This section provides an overview of the neurophysiology, common assessment tools, disorders, and treatments related to dysphagia.

Physiology and Pathophysiology (eSlides 3.7, 3.8 and 3.9)

A normal swallow is divided into oral preparatory, oral transit, pharyngeal transit, and esophageal stages. It depends on a coordinated sucking, swallowing, and breathing pattern regulated by a swallow central pattern generator. Both food transport and airway protection should be considered when assessing dysphagia.

1. Oral preparatory and transit stages: the food is prepared for transport to the pharyngeal cavity. Natural mastication includes the following stages: (1) the preparatory series, when the food is transported between the molar teeth; (2) the reduction series, when the food is broken down; and (3) the preswallowing series, when the food is transported into a "swallow-ready" position. Disorders of this stage include retention of the bolus, anterior spillage (due to an inadequate labial seal), pocketing in the lateral sulcus (weak cheeks or buccal walls), and premature leakage (impaired tongue–palate contact).

2. Pharyngeal stage: the soft palate and pharyngeal wall achieve a velopharyngeal seal. The base of the tongue retracts, the pharyngeal walls contract, and the upper esophageal sphincter (UES) opens to allow the bolus to pass through. Disorders at this stage may include impaired swallow initiation, ineffective bolus propulsion, bolus retention in the pharyngeal recesses or vallecula, nasal regurgitation (due to an inadequate velopharyngeal seal), and aspiration. To protect the airway, the true vocal folds adduct, the arytenoids tilt to the base of the epiglottis, and the hyolaryngeal mechanism moves upward and forward. *Laryngeal penetration* is defined as passage of material into the larynx but not through the vocal folds. *Aspiration* is defined as passage of material through the vocal folds. Impaired opening of the UES can be caused by increased stiffness of the UES, failure of relaxation of the cricopharyngeus muscle, weakness of the muscles of sphincter opening (related to hyolaryngeal elevation), discoordination, and inadequate pressure of the bolus.

3. Esophageal stage: the esophagus is composed of striated muscle proximally and smooth muscle distally, both of which propel the bolus by peristalsis. The lower esophageal sphincter (LES) relaxes during a swallow. Esophageal dysfunction can lead to retention of material, regurgitation, and aspiration. Structural disorders should be ruled out.

Dysphagia is found in half of individuals with a recent stroke (most recover in less than 2 weeks). It is characterized by discoordination, reduced laryngeal elevation, insufficient UES opening, and weakness of the vocal fold and oropharyngeal muscles. Dysphagia is typically more severe in bilateral cerebral and brainstem lesions.

Evaluation (eSlide 3.10)

The purpose of a swallowing evaluation is to assess dysphagia and make recommendations for diet, swallowing strategies, and interventions. Silent aspiration occurs in 25% to 30% of patients with dysphagia, and pharyngeal disorders should be evaluated with instrumentation; however, note that the instrumentation results will represent only a snapshot of the patient's swallowing function. It is imperative to interpret the results in conjunction with the overall clinical picture of the patient.

BEDSIDE/CLINICAL SWALLOW ASSESSMENTS

Swallow screening. The purpose of swallow screening is to identify individuals at risk of dysphagia and to refer them for further evaluation. The screening protocol should be quick and minimally invasive. In the Yale Swallow Protocol, the individual must consume 3 ounces of water uninterrupted without overt signs of aspiration.

Clinical swallow examination. The clinical swallow examination (CSE) has five basic components: (1) medical history and medical status; (2) cognitive/mental status; (3) oral motor function: strength, tone, symmetry, movement of the lips, tongue, and palate, and dentition and oral mucosa; (4) laryngeal and pulmonary function: strength of the cough and vocal quality and respiratory rate; and (5) trial swallows: saliva, followed by ice chip, and then other bolus sizes and consistencies. Submandibular, hyoid bone, and laryngeal movements are assessed. Any clinical signs of aspiration usually trigger a referral for instrumental assessment.

Blue dye clinical swallow examination. The blue dye clinical swallow examination (BDCSE) is performed by adding food coloring to the ingested substance to allow detection of aspiration through the tracheostomy. It has a low sensitivity in detecting aspiration.

Cervical auscultation. Cervical auscultation enables evaluation of swallowing and airway sounds. It has limited interrater reliability and correlation with physiologic events (e.g., aspiration).

INSTRUMENTAL SWALLOW ASSESSMENT

Videofluoroscopic swallow study. The videofluoroscopic swallow study (VFSS), which uses various consistencies of barium sulfate to evaluate swallowing function, is considered the gold standard for diagnosing dysphagia. It allows evaluation of the integrity of airway protection in all swallowing phases, as well as assessment of the effectiveness of bolus modifications, postural changes, and swallowing maneuvers.

Fiberoptic endoscopic examination of the swallow procedure. The fiberoptic endoscopic examination of the swallow (FEES) is the second most common instrumental assessment and allows for an evaluation of the related anatomic structures, secretion levels, swallowing ability, sensory input and airway protection, and effect of compensatory strategies. Endolaryngeal secretions and reduced vocal fold mobility are predictive of aspiration.

Comparison of VFSS and FEES. Both VFSS and FEES procedures are valuable methods to evaluate swallowing function. The selection is usually driven by specific patient characteristics or instrument availability.

High resolution manometry. High resolution manometry measures pressure events along the entire length of the pharynx and esophagus, providing a more comprehensive picture of how bolus volumes affect swallowing function.

Ultrasonography. The advantages of ultrasonography include no exposure to radiation, noninvasiveness, and portability. Submental placement assesses bolus transport during the oral phase and hyoid bone displacement in the pharyngeal phase. It has inadequate reliability in detecting aspiration.

Electromyography. Electromyography (EMG) of the muscles of the pharynx and larynx is a reliable method for detecting lower motor neuron dysfunction and aberrant central motor patterning. It can be used with biofeedback. EMG should be used only as an adjunct to other instrumental assessments.

Treatment of Dysphagia

Early treatment of dysphagia reduces the risk of aspiration pneumonia, the likelihood of medical complications related to malnutrition and dehydration, and the length of hospital stay. Equally important is to increase an individual's ability to participate in and enjoy the pleasures of eating orally.

RESTORATIVE: EXERCISE TRAINING AND PLASTICITY CONSIDERATIONS (eSlide 3.11)

The oropharyngeal system exhibits considerable plasticity. Strength training follows the principles of specificity and overloading. Examples include the Mendelsohn and Masako exercises, isometric lingual exercises, expiratory muscle strength training (EMST), effortful swallowing, and Shaker exercises.

COMPENSATORY STRATEGIES IN SWALLOWING REHABILITATION (eSlides 3.12 and 3.13)

Compensatory strategies can be divided into postural strategies, maneuvers, and diet modification. Postural strategies successfully address 80% of all swallowing disorders. Modification of food should be viewed as a treatment of last resort. Thermal tactile stimulation is recommended in cases of delayed pharyngeal swallow, but it should be viewed as a short-term compensatory strategy.

SURGERY FOR DYSPHAGIA

Surgery is rarely indicated, but it may be needed for large Zenker diverticulum. Cricopharyngeal myotomy can reduce UES pressure. Botulinum injections can help patients with dystonia, trismus, or cricopharyngeal dysfunction. In severe and chronic aspiration, a permanent tracheostomy with a laryngectomy can be necessary.

PHARYNGEAL BYPASS (eSlide 3.14)

Pharyngeal bypass procedures provide alternative means for achieving nutrition and hydration.

PREVENTION OF ASPIRATION PNEUMONIA (eSlide 3.15)

Measures to minimize aspiration include upright positioning, head elevation, oral hygiene, proper meal duration, and use of slow and continuous tube feedings. Education of family and caregivers is important. Neither tube feedings nor tracheostomies prevent aspiration pneumonia. Tracheostomy alters normal aerodynamics, eliminating positive subglottic pressure and hampering laryngeal protective reflexes. An inflated cuff, likewise, does not fully eliminate the risk of aspiration.

PSYCHOLOGICAL CONSIDERATIONS

Treatment focuses on providing education regarding the risk and management (e.g., Heimlich maneuver) of airway obstruction in the short term and on social and community reintegration in the chronic stages. Psychological consultation should be requested when appropriate.

Given the variety of disorders that can cause communication and swallowing disorders, as well as the serious impacts and complications that can result, a comprehensive understanding of normal and abnormal physiology and prognosis is essential. A team approach to addressing the medical, cognitive, physical, and psychosocial aspects of these disorders facilitates as near a return to independence as possible.

Clinical Pearls

Communication disorders (including aphasia, cognitive communication disorders, dysarthria, and apraxia) and dysphagia are major sources of disability. Rehabilitation focuses on *restorative* and *compensatory* strategies and techniques.

Early implementation of AAC strategies and incorporation of family and caregivers in the treatment plan to ensure participation of individuals with communication disorders are essential.

Interventions for patients with brain injury focus on optimizing the progressions through different stages; these stages are often described using the Rancho Los Amigos Levels of Cognitive Functioning Scale.

Normal swallowing is divided into oral preparatory, oral transit, pharyngeal transit, and esophageal stages. Swallowing disorders result in retention of the bolus, anterior spillage, lateral pocketing, premature leakage, impaired initiation, nasal regurgitation, and aspiration.

The purpose of CSE is to identify individuals at risk so that they can be referred for instrumental assessment (e.g., VFSS and FEES). Silent aspiration occurs in 25% to 30% of patients with dysphagia.

The results of instrumental assessments represent only a snapshot of swallowing function. It is imperative to interpret the results in conjunction with the overall clinical picture.

Neither tube feedings nor tracheostomy tubes prevent aspiration pneumonia. Measures to minimize aspiration include upright positioning, head elevation, oral hygiene, proper meal duration, and use of slow and continuous tube feedings.

BIBLIOGRAPHY

The complete bibliography is available on ExpertConsult.com.

4 Psychological Assessment and Intervention in Rehabilitation

Willy Chou

Health is a complex interaction between three components: body structures and functions, activities and participation, and environmental and personal factors. Psychologists with specialty training in rehabilitation are equipped to provide assessment and intervention within all three health-related components, including cognitive remediation, social participation through behavioral management, and psychotherapeutic services for family members.

• HEALTH COMPONENTS (eSlide 4.1)

The health components are listed on the eSlide.

• PSYCHOLOGICAL ASSESSMENT IN REHABILITATION

A core competency of a psychologist working in rehabilitation is the capability to select and interpret psychometric tests and measures.

Assessment in the Acute Care Setting

Premorbid demographic information and injury characteristics, such as duration of loss of consciousness, Glasgow Coma Scale score, and duration of posttraumatic amnesia, are often some of the only empirically supported data points available for use in predicting long-term outcomes of short-term inpatients.

Acute Phase (eSlide 4.2)
ASSESSMENT IN THE INPATIENT REHABILITATION SETTING
Careful assessment of preinjury and current psychological functioning is necessary to identify facilitators or barriers to recovery, track clinical changes, predict reemployment, and determine the patient's capacity to make medical or financial decisions. These assessments include preinjury and postinjury psychological function evaluation, orientation and cognition determination (e.g., O-Log and Cog-Log), neuropsychological assessment, the Independent Living Scale, and the Financial Capacity Instrument.

Inpatient Phase (eSlide 4.3)
ASSESSMENT IN THE POSTACUTE REHABILITATION SETTING
Psychological assessment in the postacute rehabilitation setting involves an evaluation of the individual's participation and quality of life. Careful assessment of

potential environmental facilitators and inhibitors is essential to optimize success-ful reintegration into the community. Psychologists can contribute to the reha-bilitation process by assessing and monitoring negative and positive psychological factors that can affect outcome and life satisfaction. Assessment or reassessment of cognitive functioning is also important in the postacute rehabilitation setting. Neuropsychological testing will facilitate the prediction of various long-term outcome-related variables, such as return to work in individuals with an acquired neurological insult. One of the most important roles of the psychologist may be the translation of information obtained by these tests into plans to help the patients reintegrate back into society and improve their quality of life.

Postacute Phase (eSlide 4.4)

Please see the eSlide for the purpose and assessment during the postacute phase.

• PSYCHOLOGICAL MANAGEMENT OF COGNITIVE, EMOTIONAL, AND BEHAVIORAL PROBLEMS

The goal of this section is to allow the reader to become an educated consumer of psychological and neuropsychological intervention services so that appropriate referral of patients can be made.

Interventions for Cognitive Problems
COGNITIVE PROBLEM (eSlide 4.5)

Impaired awareness. Impaired awareness refers to the lack of ability to recog-nize deficits. Crosson et al. described a hierarchy of awareness levels that have implications for the level of intervention needed. Intellectual awareness refers to having a basic understanding. Emergent awareness refers to the ability to recog-nize a problem in real time. Anticipatory awareness refers to the ability to predict that a particular problem may occur in specific situations and settings.

Because impaired awareness can represent a safety risk, the minimum require-ment is to modify the environment to reduce these risks. In the outpatient set-ting, impairments in emergent or anticipatory awareness are the most common awareness deficits. Milieu-oriented therapy is a way to address impaired awareness. Metacognitive strategies are those that improve one's ability to self-monitor and alter cognitive functions. Cicerone et al. recommended the use of metacognitive strategies to improve executive functioning for patients after a traumatic brain injury (TBI) or stroke.

Hierarchy of Awareness (eSlide 4.6)
IMPAIRED AWARENESS (eSlide 4.7)

Attention. The most basic level of attention is focused attention, which is the ability to respond discretely to specific sensory stimuli. Sustained attention is the ability to maintain a consistent behavioral response during a continuous repetitive activity. A higher level of attention is selective attention, which is the ability to maintain cognitive or behavioral set in the face of competing or distracting stimuli. Alternating attention refers to the ability to shift focus between tasks that have dif-ferent cognitive or behavioral requirements. This ability is also known as cognitive flexibility. The highest level on the attention hierarchy is divided attention. This refers to the ability to respond spontaneously to multiple task demands. A person who has impairments at one of the lower levels of attention will necessarily have impairment at all of the higher levels as well.

Cicerone et al. concluded that there is insufficient evidence to recommend direct attention training during acute and inpatient rehabilitation. However, they recommend direct attention training in the postacute period as a practice standard. Attention process training is a form of attention training in which patients complete a series of hierarchical computer tasks to improve attention. They also recommend supplementing direct attention training with training in compensatory (such as use of checklists or memory notebooks) and metacognitive strategies (such as self-monitoring, self-verbalization, and problem-solving) to improve generalization to real-world activities.

Attention Hierarchy (eSlide 4.8)
ATTENTION IMPAIRMENT (eSlide 4.9)

Memory. Typical manifestations of memory problems include difficulty keeping track of belongings and forgetting what, how, and when. Interventions targeting memory can be classified into two broad areas: restorative and compensatory. Restorative treatments are based on the concept that memory abilities can be restored through practice. They are not recommended in the TBI or stroke inpatient or outpatient settings because of their lack of effectiveness. Compensatory strategies can be classified as internal or external. Internal strategies rely on internal processes to learn and remember information. External memory strategies rely on cues outside of people to remind them of important information. Cicerone et al. recommended memory strategy training using either internal or external strategies for people with mild to moderate memory impairment. External memory strategies are the practice guidelines for people with severe memory impairment.

Interventions for Memory Impairment (eSlide 4.10)
PROBLEM-SOLVING

Impairments can manifest at any level of problem-solving, including analyzing problematic situations, generating potential solutions, evaluating alternatives, choosing a solution, and evaluating the real-world consequences of solutions. The best evidence is for interventions that combine the use of self-monitoring and emotional regulation for effective problem-solving orientation with training in systematic analysis and solution of problems.

Problem-Solving Level (eSlide 4.11)
INTERVENTIONS FOR EMOTIONAL AND BEHAVIORAL PROBLEMS

Emotional problems. Depression and anxiety disorders are the most common emotional problems experienced by rehabilitation populations. CBTs are based on the theory that thoughts, emotions, and behaviors are founded on an underlying belief system, and that emotional symptoms arise from negative, maladaptive, and underlying beliefs. Behavioral therapies focus on helping patients identify current patterns of coping, particularly how they may exacerbate emotional symptoms, and develop improved coping patterns and greater access to reinforcing and pleasant life events. The focus of supportive psychotherapy is on improving psychological functioning and reducing dysfunction in a positive therapeutic relationship. CBTs will likely be more effective for people with intact cognition, whereas supportive psychotherapy may be more appropriate for people with severe cognitive deficits.

Intervention Strategy for Emotional Problems (eSlide 4.12)

BEHAVIORAL PROBLEMS

Behavioral problems, such as agitation, disinhibition, aggression, and impulsivity, may need a combination of pharmacologic and nonpharmacologic interventions. The first step in effective behavioral intervention is to complete an individualized functional behavioral analysis. Problem behavior should be described in terms of its nature, frequency, severity, and duration. The observations of antecedents and consequences are essential in the subsequent treatment of problem behavior. Behavioral interventions often include management of both antecedents and consequences. Manipulation of the antecedents can prevent problem behavior from occurring, and contingency management, which is the systematic and planned manipulation of consequences, can increase or decrease specific behaviors.

Interventions for Behavioral Problems (eSlide 4.13)

CONTINGENCY MANAGEMENT OF PROBLEM BEHAVIOR (eSlide 4.14)

Antecedent Management of Problem Behavior (eSlide 4.15). Psychologists not only focus on treatments to reduce distress and dysfunction but also capitalize on opportunities to promote well-being and positive emotional adjustment following an injury.

Clinical Pearls

Psychological assessment is one of the core competencies of a psychologist working in rehabilitation.

Psychologists collect information to predict outcomes, identify facilitators and barriers, and measure community participation and quality of life in the acute, inpatient, and postacute phases of an injury.

Cognitive assessment and modification of the environment for awareness impairment can reduce the risk of inpatient injury.

Compensatory and metacognitive strategies to improve generalization to real-world activities for attention impairment are recommended.

Patients with mild to moderate memory impairment can be trained in the use of internal and external compensatory strategies, whereas patients with more severe memory impairment should use external memory strategies.

CBTs for emotional impairment are effective for people with intact cognition, whereas supportive psychotherapy may be more appropriate for people with severe cognitive deficits.

Manipulation of the antecedents can prevent problem behavior from occurring, and contingency management can increase or decrease specific behaviors.

BIBLIOGRAPHY
The complete bibliography is available on ExpertConsult.com.

5 Practical Aspects of Impairment Rating and Disability Determination

Maria Gabriella Ceravolo

Specialists in physical medicine and rehabilitation (PM&R) can expect to be called on to make formal assessment of the disabilities of their patients. This chapter summarizes the information needed to address the patients' health care needs through acquisition of the conceptual foundation and terminology of disablement and application of the same to the practices of impairment rating and disability determination.

TERMINOLOGY AND CONCEPTUALIZATION OF DISABLEMENT (eSlides 5.1, 5.2, and 5.3)

The medical model still serves as the fundamental basis for Social Security disability determinations and physician-rating schedules that remain largely anatomically and diagnostically based. A "biopsychosocial model" of disability is now the preferred model and has gained wide acceptance when disability is conceptualized. The *biological* component refers to the physical or mental aspects, or both, of an individual with a given health condition; the *psychological* component recognizes personal beliefs, coping strategies, and emotional and other psychological factors that may affect functioning; and the *social* component recognizes contextual, infrastructural, and other environmental factors that may also affect functioning in any given case. The World Health Organization introduced the International Classification of Functioning, Disability, and Health (ICF), which underlines the interactive (i.e., nonlinear) relationships between the impairment and the potential functional consequences of impairment with respect to the individual's personal and social sphere, and contextual factors that may mitigate or amplify these consequences.

AMERICANS WITH DISABILITIES ACT AND IMPLICATIONS (eSlides 5.4, 5.5, and 5.6)

According to the Americans with Disabilities Act (ADA), disability is "a physical or mental impairment that substantially limits one or more of the major life activities of such individual, a record of such impairment or being regarded as such impairment." "Title 1" of the ADA (Employment) recognizes employment as a major life activity and views disability within the context of performance of the *essential functions* of an employment position with or without *reasonable accommodation*. *Reasonable accommodation* can include structural modifications of the work site to improve accessibility, availability of modified duty options, and acquisition of adaptive equipment or devices to enable an otherwise qualified worker with a disability to perform the essential functions of the job. Accommodation under the ADA is a fundamental social environmental modifier mandated by statutes to mitigate the disabling consequences of impairment in the workplace, in terms of accessibility related to activity limitations and participation restrictions. However, the employer is ultimately responsible for determining *reasonable accommodation*. It is not the responsibility of the disability-evaluating physician to determine the essential functions of a job, devise accommodation, or determine reasonableness of any accommodation proposed by the employer.

RELATING IMPAIRMENT TO DISABILITY AND COMPENSATION FORMULAS

All the major current disability systems are designed with the intent to compensate individuals financially for losses due to their qualifying disablement. The impairment rating represents the keystone to any disability determination for the following several reasons:
- It serves as a standard reference point in terms of linking a specific diagnosis to an associated percentage of physical and functional loss in compensable injury claims.
- It enables the impaired individual to exit the system of temporary disablement at maximum medical improvement (MMI).
- It provides a diagnosis-based classification of severity to segue to alternative systems for the management of long-term disablement.

Social Security Disability Insurance and Supplemental Security Income

Social Security Disability Insurance (SSDI) provides benefits to individuals who have worked in a qualified job for at least 5 of the 10 years before onset of disability, paid into the Social Security system, and subsequently become disabled before age 65 years. Eligibility for SSDI requires that the disability prevents the affected individual from engaging "in any substantial gainful activity (SGA) ... for a continuous period of not less than 12 months." Supplemental Security Income (SSI) provides income for medically indigent people who are blind, disabled, or older (>65 years). Eligibility is determined according to a means test and does not require a work history. SSI also requires that a "medically determinable impairment" be established.

Federal and State Workers' Compensation Systems (eSlide 5.7)

In the United States, four major federal workers' compensation programs provide wage replacement benefits, medical treatments, vocational rehabilitations, and other benefits to injured workers (or their dependents) who experience a work-related injury or an occupational disease. At the individual state level, each state has enacted a workers' compensation law. The PM&R physician can be involved in four situations: (1) initial evaluation and treatment of the injury, either as an approved and designated attending physician or as an authorized consultant; (2) overseeing rehabilitation, including return-to-work or stay-at-work issues; (3) determination of any residual impairment (permanent) or disability (work restrictions); and (4) estimation of long-term care needs in catastrophic injuries (e.g., limb amputations, spinal cord injuries, and major multiple trauma), including participation in life care planning.

• IMPAIRMENT RATING GUIDES FOR PHYSICIANS WITH ATTENTION TO GUIDES, SIXTH EDITION (eSlides 5.8, 5.9, and 5.10)

The American Medical Association's *Guides to the Evaluation of Permanent Impairment* is a standardized and objective reference and reporting guide for physicians and other professional stakeholders. It is the preferred reference for the US Department of Labor and for many domestic personal injury claims. The sixth edition has adopted the *ICF* terminology, definitions, and conceptual framework of disablement, defining impairment rating as a "consensus-derived percentage estimate of loss of activity reflecting severity of a given health condition and the degree of associated limitations in terms of activities of daily living." As such, the AMA *Guides* has adopted metrics sensitive and specific to medical (i.e., anatomic and physiologic) aspects of organ system disease, as well as functional aspects (mobility and self-care) of losses that can occur; both an ADL-based functional history and ordinal measures of ADL assessment serve as important modifiers of the final impairment rating, when applicable.

Four key issues guide the physician in evaluation of patients' reports:
• What is the clinical diagnosis?
• What difficulty does the patient report (symptoms, functional loss)?
• What are the examination findings?
• What are the results of clinical studies?

• INDEPENDENT MEDICAL EXAMINATION: ELEMENTS AND REPORTING REQUIREMENTS

An independent medical examination (IME) is a one-time evaluation performed by a physician for the purpose of, answering a series of interrogatory questions posed by the referring party to achieve claim settlement. The opinions set forth by the independent medical examiner must be expressed in terms of medical possibility versus probability. The physician examiner is expected to provide the specific diagnosis for each and all allowed conditions relevant to a specific claim, and to help determine both *medical* and *legal causation*. *Medical causation* is biological in nature and is established through scientific analysis of sufficient rigor to demonstrate a cause-and-effect relationship with a high degree of certainty. *Legal causation* is determined on two bases: first, if an injury would have occurred independent of the alleged act or omission, the cause in fact has not been established; second, if a given risk could not have been reasonably anticipated, the alleged act cannot be considered as the proximate cause of an injury. In summary, *legal causation* is mainly a question of "foreseeability." An actor is liable for the foreseeable but not the unforeseeable consequences of his or her act. The workers' compensation systems vary from state to state in terms of their *causation* and work-related rules.

Maximum Medical Improvement Determination (eSlide 5.11)

The physician examiner is required to provide a final statement that includes an estimate of when MMI occurred or is expected to occur. From a rehabilitative perspective, a claimant should not be considered for MMI as long as expectations for continuing functional improvement are being met by demonstrable and ongoing performance gains. When functional progress is no longer evident or tenable and a sufficient (typically 6 months) healing period has transpired, MMI is generally thought to have occurred. Deterioration that might normally be expected with the passage of time does not preclude MMI determination. The physician should also address issues of future medical management and follow-up anticipated to be necessary to maintain MMI for a given condition.

Disability as Return-to-Work Restrictions (eSlides 5.12, 5.13, and 5.14)

The PM&R physicians can be asked to provide a patient status report and return-to-work/fitness-for-duty form. If treatment is ongoing and transitional work is available, the physician might recommend modified duty in terms of restrictions on the allowed number of hours of work and the permissible activities in terms of frequency or degree of material handling tolerated during the healing period. If no modified duty options are available or applicable, the physician may be required to render a temporary total disability determination until MMI is reached. Because the probability of returning to work decreases precipitously as time out of work increases, the physician should make every effort to return the claimant safely to a transitional work setting as soon as possible. In cases when transitional return-to-work options are not available, work conditioning and work hardening may be preferable and viable alternatives to forced inactivity and should be considered whenever feasible and medically necessary. At the point of MMI, the physician must also render a final opinion on permanent restrictions applicable in going forward. The functional capacity evaluation can be used to help establish a performance baseline and treatment goals for the injured worker to monitor recovery and establish a new performance baseline when treatment has been completed. A job description can provide a useful list of the essential functions of the job in question; a job site evaluation can validate the essential functions listed in the job description with respect to critical physical demands and relative amounts of time spent performing specific activities within each function. Ergonomic analysis can help quantify the job's physical demands and enable accommodation in terms of job redesign or workplace modification. Finally, employer and claimant willingness and ability to comply with recommended accommodations can also be addressed. Physician examiners should avail themselves of these assessment tools to ensure that the prognostic inferences derived and sanctions imposed are founded on valid, empirical, and functionally based data to the fullest extent possible.

• LEGAL AND ETHICAL CONSIDERATIONS

Expert Witness Testimony (eSlide 5.15)

The opinions set forth in an IME and the resulting formal report comprise expert witness testimony that must validate or refute the presence and severity of injury toward, and resulting in disability to, any claimant. This occurs within a legal infrastructure from which the claimant maintains certain legal rights and entitlements and may derive significant monetary gain.

Physiatrists and other practitioners in the field of disability medicine performing IMEs and giving expert testimony should be aware of not only the legal liabilities in the overall practice of their subspecialty but also the additional malpractices and civil liabilities entailed with exposure to the practice constraints under which IMEs and expert witness work is performed. Physicians attracted to disability assessment and inclined to serve as independent medical examiners are encouraged to attend several of the high-quality training programs offered in the United States for independent medical examiners and expert witnesses, with the goal of empowering them with greater knowledge, skills, and abilities necessary to practice as an independent medical examiner or expert witness in the field of disability medicine. IME physicians or expert witnesses can be successful despite these challenges if they remember several key principles, including intellectual honesty, professionalism, and respect for the judicial process at all times. An ethical and objective examiner who performs a thorough evaluation, deals with the plaintiff (or claimant) in an empathetic, unbiased manner, and avoids advocacy has a lesser risk of getting entangled in the allegations of wrongdoing.

• CONCLUSION AND ETHICAL CONSIDERATIONS

The PM&R physician must remain committed to preserving patient autonomy as a member of the treatment team and also maximizing functional recovery and reducing or eliminating dependency to the fullest extent possible on the treating system and caregivers, including the disability system itself. The patient, as a claimant, may otherwise choose to behave in a manner that is counterproductive to these goals and thereby appear noncompliant.

The physician must also remain cognizant of the paradox of compensable injury—that financial compensation can discourage return to work and thereby promote disability. Undue prolongation of an open claim might further serve to legitimize disability in the claimant's mind and can inhibit the likelihood of functional recovery and return to work.

Clinical Pearls

Physiatrists appear uniquely qualified among medical specialists to perform impairment ratings and disability evaluations because of their special focus on human functioning.

The *ICF* offers a conceptual platform for identifying the disabling consequences of impairment in an individual with a health condition, while taking into account the modifying influences of environmental and personal factors.

The impairment rating represents the keystone to any disability determination, and a source of data for all major current disability systems designed with the intent to compensate individuals financially for losses due to their qualifying disablement.

The PM&R specialist performing an IME is expected to provide the specific diagnosis for each and all allowed conditions relevant to a specific claim and to help determine both *medical* and *legal causation.*

While performing an IME, the PM&R physician must remain committed to preserving patient autonomy as a member of the treatment team and also to maximizing functional recovery and reducing or eliminating dependency to the fullest extent possible on the treating system and caregivers, including the disability system itself.

BIBLIOGRAPHY

The complete bibliography is available on ExpertConsult.com.

6 Employment of People with Disabilities

Renald Peter Ty Ramiro

Disability ranks as the largest public health problem in the United States. An interdisciplinary approach to treat the multifaceted implications of disability is needed to address concerns such as personal care, work and finances, social integration, and leisure (eSlide 6.1). Strategies include restoration of functional capacity, prevention of deterioration in function, maintenance and improvement of quality of life (QOL), physical rehabilitation, and prevention of secondary complications (eSlide 6.2).

According to Howard Rusk, "a rehabilitation program is designed to take a disabled person from his bed back to his job, fitting him for the best life possible commensurate with his disability and more importantly with his ability" (eSlide 6.3).

Return-to-work addresses the following issues: discuss the concept of disability, economic assistance, and vocational rehabilitation strategies; review national data on disability and employment and policies supporting employment of people with disabilities (PWDs); consider the economic impact of disability; enumerate the incentives and disincentives for returning to work; and postulate that vocational rehabilitation serves as a rehabilitation treatment and disability prevention strategy for PWDs (eSlide 6.4).

• CONCEPT OF DISABILITY

The World Health Organization provides a global common health language on disability known as the International Classification of Functioning, Disability, and Health (formerly the International Classification of Impairments, Disabilities, and Handicaps). This reflects the biopsychosocial model of disablement, with dynamic interactions between health conditions and conceptual factors. Dimensions of dysfunction are defined as follows: *impairment* is the loss or abnormality of body structure or of a physiologic or psychological function; *activity* is the nature and extent of functioning at the level of the person; and *participation* is the nature and extent of a person's involvement in life situations in relation to impairment, activities, health conditions, and contextual factors; it can be restricted in nature, duration, and quality (eSlide 6.5).

• DATA: IMPAIRMENT AND DISABILITY

eSlides 6.6 and 6.7 show the 15 conditions with the highest prevalence of functional compromise or disability as well as the ranking of percentage of people with functional limitations for specific conditions.

• SOCIOECONOMIC EFFECT OF DISABILITY

Work disability or work participation restriction affect direct expenditures (medical and personal care, architectural modification, assistive technology, institutional care, and income support), which lead to impoverishment, with a higher incidence of disabled people being below the poverty level. Employment and earnings data show disparities in salaries based on disability (eSlide 6.8). Governments within the United States have responded by developing disability-related programs, such as Social Security Disability Insurance (SSDI), Supplemental Security Income (SSI), Medicare, and Medicaid (eSlide 6.9).

• TREATMENT OF THE INJURED WORKER

Workers' Compensation Medicine

Workers' compensation medicine involves models that promote a safe return to work through functional capacity evaluation (FCE), work hardening programs (WHPs), functional restoration programs (FRPs), and treatment. An FCE tests the physical and cognitive demands of moderately or heavily strenuous work, such as perception, range of motion, strength, endurance, coordination, the ability to lift and assume certain postures, and the ability to tolerate standing, walking, and climbing. A WHP is a multidisciplinary "work-oriented treatment program" that consists of work tolerance screening and work capacity evaluation components with job simulation activities, psychological treatment, and an interdisciplinary pain program. An FRP restores the patient's physical, psychosocial, and socioeconomic situation through a physician-driven interdisciplinary program that emphasizes the importance of function over pain elimination, pain acceptance, pain management, and proactive coping strategies. The sessions include intensive exercise program, cognitive-behavioral therapy, and ergonomic therapy.

• DISABILITY-RELATED PROGRAMS AND POLICIES

Programs

Disability-related programs can be characterized as ameliorative or corrective. Ameliorative programs provide payment for income support and medical care. Corrective programs facilitate the individual's ability to return to work and reduce or remove the disablement. Disability-related programs can be categorized into three basic types: cash transfers, medical care programs, and direct service programs.

Public Disability Policies

eSlide 6.10 reviews the prominent federal disability laws that mandate that housing and transportation be accessible, education for children with disabilities be appropriate, and employment practices be nondiscriminatory.

Three legislative actions deserve to be highlighted: (1) the Rehabilitation Act of 1973 extended civil rights protection to PWDs, including antidiscrimination and affirmative action in employment; (2) the Rehabilitation Act Amendments of 1978 broadened the responsibility of the Rehabilitation Services Administration to include independent living programs and created the National Council of the Handicapped; and (3) the Americans with Disabilities Act (ADA) of 1990 established a clear and comprehensive prohibition of discrimination based on disability.

Vocational Rehabilitation

TRADITIONAL APPROACHES TO VOCATIONAL REHABILITATION

eSlide 6.11 shows the traditional approach, based on referral to a vocational rehabilitation counselor for diagnosis, evaluation, and adjustment training. Obtaining
an employment history and performing vocational testing are important components of this approach.

Alternative Approaches to Vocational Rehabilitation (eSlide 6.12)

SHELTERED WORKSHOPS

A sheltered workshop is a "public nonprofit organization certified by the U.S.
Department of Labor to pay 'subminimum' wages to persons with diminished
earning capacity." This form of employment serves people with severe disabilities,
including limited vision, mental illness, mental retardation, and alcoholism.

DAY PROGRAMS

Day programs provide supervised vocational activity for people with severe disabilities, usually those with mental retardation or mental illness.

HOME-BASED PROGRAMS

Home-based programs include training in a variety of jobs, including telephone
solicitation, typing, or computer-assisted occupations such as graphic designing,
accounting, or drafting.

PROJECTS WITH INDUSTRY

Projects With Industry is a federally sponsored collaborative program established
by the Vocational Rehabilitation Act to enable competitive employment by providing specific job skills training.

TRANSITIONAL AND SUPPORTED EMPLOYMENT

Two newer strategies for returning PWDs to competitive, integrated, and gainful employment are transitional and supported employment. Transitional employment consists of providing job placement, training, and support services necessary
to help people move into independent or supported employment. Supported
employment requires ongoing support after placement, including counseling for
the employee and co-workers, and assistance with transportation, housing, and
other non–work-related activities.

INDEPENDENT LIVING CENTERS

The independent living centers movement involves a combination of vocational
and nonvocational services, such as housing, independent living skills, advocacy,
and peer counseling, for PWDs.

Disincentives for Vocational Rehabilitation

Despite growing acceptance in the public and political arenas through better policies and attitudes, there are still a number of disincentives for vocational rehabilitation, a few examples of which include (1) "red tape" in getting cash and medical
benefits from SSI and SSDI; (2) the risk of losing benefits once the PWDs are
employed; (3) the pervasive stereotype of PWDs being unproductive, leading to the
attitude that it is easier to give them a disability check than to implement the ADA;

(4) employers' negative attitudes toward employees with disabilities and ignorance of their vocational needs; and (5) the tendency of physiatrists and other physicians to label an individual as "totally and permanently disabled" or restrict their activities.

Incentives for Vocational Rehabilitation

In an effort to overcome disincentives, government policymakers have created incentives for PWDs and potential employers (eSlide 6.13).

Incentives for Individuals

Incentives for the individuals include trial work period, substantial gainful activity, extended period of eligibility, impairment-related work expenses, "blind" work expenses, and plans for achieving self-support.

Incentives for Industry

Government policymakers have made various attempts to offer tax incentives to businesses and industries to make the workplace accessible. Examples include deductible expenses for barrier removal, Targeted Jobs Tax Credit, and the Work Incentives Improvement Act of 1999.

Disability Prevention

The public health model defines three categories of disability prevention: primary, secondary, and tertiary (eSlide 6.14). Primary prevention is intended for healthy people to avoid the onset of a pathologic condition and for people with disabilities to prevent worsening of their impairments. Secondary prevention is aimed at early identification and treatment of a pathologic condition. Provision of assistive technology can be considered secondary prevention. Tertiary prevention focuses on arresting the progression of a pathologic condition and limiting disablement. Environmental modifications, changes in social attitudes, and reforms in legislation and policies are tertiary prevention strategies. Medical rehabilitation is traditionally considered a tertiary prevention strategy.

• CONCLUSION

Holistic management is the key in the comprehensive rehabilitation of disablement. This approach maximizes physical, mental, social, and economic functions of individuals with disabilities through various interventions directed at human functioning. The physiatrist, as a team leader, collaborates with professionals outside the traditional medical rehabilitation team, such as those involved in vocational rehabilitation. This eventually improves QOL and function, which greatly affect the individuals and society in terms of significant socioeconomic consequences (eSlide 6.15).

Clinical Pearls

1. Holistic management is the key in the comprehensive rehabilitation of disablement, which maximizes the physical, mental, social, and economic functions of people with disabilities through various interventions directed at human functioning.
2. Disability, being the largest public health concern in the United States, should encourage physiatrists to take the lead in its therapeutic and public health management through prevention strategies, including collaboration with professionals outside the traditional medical rehabilitation team, such as those involved in vocational rehabilitation.
3. The prevention strategies for people with disabilities are the following:
   • Primary prevention: preventing the worsening of impairments.
   • Secondary prevention: providing ameliorative and corrective programs including vocational rehabilitation, to reduce activity limitation and increase employment.
   • Tertiary prevention: limiting the restriction of a person's participation by the provision of a facilitator or the removal of a barrier.
4. Vocational rehabilitation is an integral component in the holistic approach to disability management, improving QOL and function, with eventual significant socioeconomic consequences.

BIBLIOGRAPHY
The complete bibliography is available on ExpertConsult.com.

Quality and Outcome Measures for Medical Rehabilitation

7

Elizabeth J. Halmai

Health care quality can be defined as safe and effective care that improves outcome, optimizes health, and results in high patient satisfaction and quality of life. In the current environment of health care reform in the United States, the focus has shifted from the fee-for-service model, in which the volume of health care services rendered was rewarded, to emphasis on quality, safety, and outcome as top priorities. This chapter discusses health care quality, evidence-based medicine (EBM), clinical practice guidelines (CPGs), outcome and performance measures, practice improvement, patient safety, and accreditation.

Access, affordability, and high quality in health care are the main objectives of the Patient Protection and Affordable Care Act of 2010. To accomplish these goals, the U.S. Department of Health and Human Services (HHS) has outlined a National Quality Strategy (NQS) that was developed through a collaborative and participatory process, including input from a wide variety of stakeholders from all over the health care industry (eSlide 7.1).

Quality of care is a measure of performance in the six specified health care aims of the Institute of Medicine (IOM): safety, timeliness, effectiveness, equity, efficiency, and patient centeredness. On the basis of performance metrics, providers, individuals, organizations, and health plans are incentivized to improve quality through accountability (eSlide 7.2). The ultimate objective is to deliver high-quality health care and rehabilitation and improve the health of the population we serve (eSlide 7.3).

OUTCOME MEASURES

In health care, an outcome is the health consequence that results from the health care provided. An outcome measure is the assessment of clinical outcomes by qualitative or quantitative means.

Types of Outcome Measures

In 1966, Donabedian conceptualized how the information regarding health care quality may be gathered and modeled three dimensions of health care: structure, process, and outcome (eSlide 7.4). Because attribution of outcomes to particular processes is challenging, many providers and hospitals prefer to measure processes instead of outcomes. When selecting a process measure, it is important to determine that there is strong scientific evidence that links the process to the outcome. One must adjust for risk factors or stratify the population when using outcome measures because it is challenging to account for all factors that may influence health outcomes.

International Classification of Functioning, Disability, and Health

The physical medicine and rehabilitation (PM&R) community is well versed in outcome measurement, especially as it relates to functional outcome and pain reduction. The International Classification of Functioning, Disability and Health (ICF) was released in 2001 as an update by the World Health Organization to their International Classification of Impairments, Disabilities, and Handicaps. In the ICF, function occurs at three levels: (1) level of the body part or system, (2) level of the person (activities), and (3) level of the person in society (participation). Functional outcomes can be measured at each of the levels described in the ICF, and interventions may be geared at any one or more of these levels.

Functional Independence Measure

The aggregation of individual patient outcome measurements allows providers and hospitals to benchmark and helps identify areas for improvement in health care delivery. Most inpatient rehabilitation programs submit their patients' Functional Independence Measure (FIM) scores to the Uniform Data System (UDS) (eSlide 7.5). Tracking functional progress is a key activity in inpatient rehabilitation, and aggregate data can speak volumes about what the facility and providers are doing to promote function. The UDS provides report cards that detail FIM change (discharge FIM–admission FIM) and FIM efficiency (FIM change/length of stay) for patients by impairment grouping. It also tracks the percentage of patients successfully discharged to home.

Choosing Outcome Measures

Several factors must be considered when choosing an outcome measure to use (eSlide 7.6). The Rehabilitation Measures Database has numerous measures listed that can be used to track outcomes in a patient population of interest. This database intends to provide clinicians with a list of instruments that can be used to screen and monitor patient progress (eSlide 7.7).

• EVIDENCE AND GUIDELINES

Definitions of Evidence-Based Medicine

In 1992, the Evidence-Based Medicine Working Group published a treatise on EBM, calling it a "new paradigm for medical practice." EBM has been defined as "the integration of best research evidence with clinical expertise and patient values." Using EBM, physicians can address clinical questions by assessing the quality of evidence in medical information available in both basic science and clinical research.

Assessing, Evaluating, and Applying Evidence

Sackett et al. recommend the application of EBM with a simple and straightforward approach to answer any clinical question: (1) define a clinical question, (2) find the evidence that will help answer the question, (3) assess whether this evidence is valid and important, and (4) apply the evidence to the patient (eSlide 7.8).

In general, the level of evidence provided by a published article can be determined from the level of evidence hierarchy (eSlide 7.9). One can also appraise the level of evidence of a research article using evidence tables such as the one produced by The Oxford Center for Evidence-Based Medicine or the criteria adopted by the American Academy of Physical Medicine and Rehabilitation (AAPMR). Other potentially useful EBM concepts are the "evidence-based triad" discussed by Glasziou et al. (eSlide 7.10) and patient-oriented evidence that matters (POEM).

Clinical Practice Guidelines

CPGs are systematically developed written statements, made after a systematic evaluation of available evidence, and are intended to assist practitioners and patients in making appropriate decisions about health care in specific conditions or circumstances (eSlide 7.11). The IOM's eight standards for developing CPGs are considered the "gold standard" that every CPG aims to achieve (eSlide 7.12). The National Guideline Clearinghouse is a useful website to find relevant CPGs to suit one's needs. It is a public resource that is published online by the Agency for Healthcare Research and Quality.

PERFORMANCE MEASURES AND METRICS

Performance measurement is a way to compute whether and how often the health care system does what it should. The result of a measure is a ratio or percentage that helps to compare providers and benchmark local and national performances. Development of performance metrics helps in transforming health care quality by measuring sustained gains obtained with improvement methodologies to create data-driven processes in organizations. Stakeholders who support and drive this change by reporting on quality and patient safety culture in hospitals include local and regional purchasers, payers, consumer representatives, and communities.

Measure Development

Development of performance metrics needs finance, labor, technology, education, and a learning environment over long timelines to reduce variation in care delivery across the United States. Because of the increase in people born with disabilities and those who acquire disabilities, particularly in the context of multiple chronic conditions and disparities in care, there is a continuous need to develop methods to measure performance toward the NQS. In addition, the Centers for Medicare and Medicaid Services (CMS) uses different criteria, such as lack of applicability across specialties, to remove measures, further compelling the development of new performance metrics.

Challenges in Measure Development

DESIRABLE ATTRIBUTES OF A MEASURE ARE COMPLEX

By consensus from the American Medical Association (AMA), The Joint Commission (TJC), and the National Committee for Quality Assurance (NCQA), a performance measure must have the following characteristics: (1) address a topic area that is of high priority to maximize the health of people or populations, be financially important, and demonstrate a variation in care and/or potential improvement; (2) be useful in improving patient outcomes based on established clinical recommendations and be potentially actionable, meaningful to, and interpretable by the user; and (3) have a measure design with well-defined specifications and documented reliability and validity and allow risk adjustment while being feasible, confidential, and publicly available.

MEASURE TESTING THAT IS CRITICAL TO THE PROCESS OF ITS DEVELOP-MENT IS ELABORATE

Measure testing requires the involvement of all stakeholders, patients, and providers, including insurers, technology providers, individual or groups of clinicians, and health care organizations.

MEASURES ARE TESTED BY DIFFERENT AGENCIES BEFORE BEING VETTED

The AMA's Physician Consortium for Performance Improvement (PCPI) is one agency that recommends that performance measures must be tested in the areas of needs assessment, feasibility and implementation, reliability, validity, unintended consequences, and applications.

MEASURE DEVELOPMENT INVOLVES EXTENSIVE COSTS THROUGH THE LIFE CYCLE OF THE MEASURE

For example, the life cycle of a measure endorsed by the National Quality Forum (NQF), which sets priorities for performance measurement, entails the following: (1) studying evidence-based data on disease prevalence, (2) using an assessment tool to study disease severity, (3) applying a local initiative to measure improvement with the process, (4) leading change toward improvement locally, (5) public reporting on local performance, (6) endorsing the measure as a national consensus standard, (7) retooling the measure for use in electronic health care records, and (8) including the meaningful use program of CMS so that measure adoption is widespread and leads to better patient care.

RISK ADJUSTMENT

Risk factors are patient characteristics associated with a statistically significant level of variance to allow valid comparisons across providers and organizations.

PRIVACY, SECURITY, AND DATABASES

Because public reporting is done with multiple systems and methods for transparency, with measures collected in databases or registries, training and monitoring of providers are required to keep patient information secure from external threats (particularly in this era of transition to electronic health care records across providers).

Strategically Improving Health Care Quality With Performance Measurement

Despite the various challenges, performance measurement is imperative because it helps provide quality at a lower cost. Performance measurement aligns providers to the six priorities of the NQS (eSlide 7.13).

• SAFETY AND ACCREDITATION

Health plan accreditation standards are used to ensure that plans are performing on par with industry standards by measuring their performance with respect to quality. Consumers use these data to compare plans. Other purchasers, such as employers and state and federal regulators, also use these metrics to pay for performance. The NCQA, Utilization Review Accreditation Commission, and TJC are examples of such agencies.

Public reporting by the CMS on nursing homes and measuring the performance of home-based and community-based services with financial incentives are steps that have been taken toward improving health care quality in the long term and in postacute care arenas. In addition, physician performance metrics are gathered using the Physician Quality Reporting System, which are coupled to financial incentives and penalties. Public reporting of performance metrics is a driver of health care quality because it encourages transparency and accountability.

MAINTENANCE OF CERTIFICATION AND QUALITY IMPROVEMENT

The American Board of Physical Medicine and Rehabilitation's (ABPMR) Maintenance of Certification (MOC) program is designed to verify a diplomate's credentials, licensure, professional standing, and practice performance. ABPMR diplomates demonstrate the ability to investigate and evaluate the care of patients, appraise and assimilate scientific evidence, and continuously improve patient care based on constant self-evaluation and lifelong learning through the practice improvement project (PIP) requirement (eSlide 7.14).

SUMMARY

We are in a state of turbulent transition from volume-based health care to value-based health care. The two main drivers of this change are increasing costs and decreasing or stagnant quality. For this transition to succeed and eventually lead to efficient, safe, effective, and valuable health care, all rehabilitation professionals, including physiatrists, must work together with a unified focus on better quality and outcomes for our patients. Practicing safe medicine and EBM, with unchanging focus on values and outcomes, can help us get there. A fair, transparent, valid, and objective measurement of quality and safety can be embraced by everyone. Together, we can evolve as an accessible, affordable, and high-quality health care system that can be valuable and sustainable over the long term.

Clinical Pearls

- The IOM report "To Err Is Human: Building a Safer Health System" was considered "the tipping point" after which patients and payers began demanding a higher standard of care.
- In 2008, more than 45 million Americans were uninsured.
- The AMA's PCPI is a group involved in the development of performance measures.
- NQF is involved in measure endorsement.
- CMS is involved in performance measure implementation.
- The FIM tool is designed to track patient progress during inpatient rehabilitation.
- Medicare Part A requires the completion of the Inpatient Rehabilitation Facility–Patient Assessment Instrument for payment.
- The medical reason for admission to inpatient rehabilitation (impairment group) must be clearly documented by the physiatrist.
- Under the prospective payment system, a facility receives the same payment regardless of length of stay.
- Changes in FIM scores from admission to discharge, length of stay, and discharge destination are currently used to evaluate efficiency or effectiveness of an inpatient rehabilitation program.

BIBLIOGRAPHY
The complete bibliography is available on ExpertConsult.com.

8 Electrodiagnostic Medicine

Chein-Wei Chang

Electrodiagnostic medicine is a specific area of medical practice in which a physician uses information obtained from clinical history, physical examination, and the techniques of electrophysiologic study to diagnose and treat neuromuscular disorders (eSlide 8.1). Electrodiagnosis is a basic tool for physiatrists and is commonly used for diagnosis and differentiation in many neuromuscular diseases. The roles of electrodiagnosis (eSlide 8.2) include determining the localization and distribution of a lesion and severity of a disease, characterizing the evolution of a disease, estimating prognosis, differentiating neuropathy and myopathy, and monitoring the response to a treatment. Electrodiagnosis requires a logical approach during every step of testing, enabling examiners to refine their rationale during the examination, followed by a series of proper data analyses and clinical correlations.

• CONVENTIONAL ELECTRODIAGNOSIS (eSlide 8.3)

1. Strength-duration curve (SDC) and nerve excitability tests: An SDC study may show the earliest objective sign of denervation. It reveals an abnormality when a nerve is injured for more than 72 hours. If reinnervation occurs, it can be characterized by a shift of the curve to the left, with a fall in the chronaxie and the appearance of a plateau. The earliest evidence of nerve degeneration after injury is the failure to respond to electrical stimulation. In addition, abnormal nerve excitability presents 3-5 days after a nerve lesion.
2. Nerve conduction studies (NCSs): Nerve conduction velocity (NCV) is the propagation speed of an action potential along nerve fibers. It is often affected by myelination of the nerve. Besides the conduction velocity itself, the amplitude of the compound muscle action potential (CMAP) and sensory nerve action potential (SNAP) reflects the axonal numbers of the tested nerve. The reducing amplitude of CMAP or SNAP observed during NCSs always represents a neuropathy associated with axonal degeneration. The NCS mainly contributes in the assessment of peripheral neuropathy, entrapment neuropathy, and peripheral nerve injury. It is the most common method of objective and quantitative testing of neural functions.
3. Repetitive nerve stimulation test (Jolly test): This test is frequently used in screening of neuromuscular junction diseases. The function of the neuromuscular junction can be indirectly assessed by repetitive stimulation of a motor nerve with a recording electrode placed over the appropriate muscle. It is helpful in diagnosing neuromuscular junction disorders such as myasthenia gravis, myasthenic syndrome (Lambert-Eaton syndrome), and botulism. The significant decremental response at lower rate (2–10 Hz) stimulation in myasthenia gravis is more than 10%. The significant incremental response at a higher rate (20–50 Hz) stimulation in myasthenic syndrome is more than 50%.

4. Long latency reflex studies: Long latency reflex studies include those of Hoffmann (H) reflexes, which are considered to originate from spinal reflexes and are induced by both electrical stimulation of afferent nerve (Aα) fibers in the mixed nerve to the muscle and activation of motor neurons to the muscle through a monosynaptic connection in the spinal cord. These reflexes often appear in the S1 spinal nerve pathway and are commonly used in the diagnosis of S1 radiculopathy. The F wave is a compound action potential that is evoked intermittently from a muscle by a supramaximal electrical stimulus to the nerve. It is induced by antidromic activation of motor neurons. During the test, the F wave always requires 10-20 stimuli and is selected by minimal or mean conduction latency. Blink reflexes are compound muscle action potentials that are evoked from the orbicularis oculi muscles and that present as a result of brief electrical or mechanical stimuli to the cutaneous area, innervated by the supraorbital branch of the trigeminal nerve. They always require bilateral muscle recordings and present as an ipsilateral monosynaptic R1 wave response and a multisynaptic R2 wave response, accompanied by a contralateral R2 wave. Deep tendon reflexes are reflexes that occur in response to a muscle tendon being tapped briskly. Much like a stretch reflex, a tendon reflex is the contraction of a muscle in response to the stretching of muscle spindles, which triggers the receptors that lie parallel to extrafusal muscle fibers.

5. Electromyography (EMG): By inserting a needle electrode into the muscle under examination, muscular activities and motor unit action potentials (MUAPs) can be identified in an oscilloscope as different diagnostic patterns. Four steps should always be observed during an EMG examination:

   a. Insertion of the needle electrode: Prolonged insertional activities are frequently encountered in denervation, myositis, and myotonia, whereas shortened activities are seen in areas of muscle atrophy, fatty degeneration, and myofibrosis.

   b. Muscle at rest: Normal muscle will exhibit electrical silence during this step. Abnormal conditions include spontaneous activities, such as fibrillation, positive sharp waves, fasciculation, myokymia, myotonic discharges, and complex repetitive discharges (CRDs).

   c. Muscle during volitional contraction: This step may show the shape and figure of individual MUAPs. The parameters of an MUAP, such as amplitude, phase, turn, and duration, can be measured. This is important for the determination of acute or chronic neuropathy and the measurement of disease progression and treatment outcomes.

   d. Muscle during maximal contraction: This step reveals interference or recruitment in muscle activation and reflects both the quantity and firing rate of neurons. It is an important test for differentiating between neuropathy and myopathy.

6. Evoked potential (EP) studies: These studies include somatosensory evoked potentials (SSEPs), visual evoked potentials (VEPs), brainstem auditory evoked potentials (BAEPs), and event-related potentials (ERPs). They are recorded at the scalp over the cortices or at various sites along sensory pathways and are elicited by stimulating the corresponding receptors, which could be the skin, eye, ear, or nerves themselves. EP studies show the physiologic integrity of sensory pathways and are able to detect abnormalities that may not be clinically obvious. Motor evoked potential (MEP) studies, developed in recent decades, have been used to assess the physiologic integrity of motor pathways in the

central nervous system by stimulating the motor cortex beneath the scalp. Clinically, EP studies are useful in determining central nerve conduction status and monitoring patients during surgery.

• ADVANCED ELECTRODIAGNOSIS (eSlide 8.4)

New advances that have been brought to electrodiagnosis include advanced EMG, different techniques of NCS, magnetoencephalography (MEG), and transcranial direct current stimulation (tDCS). Needle EMG is invasive. However, it is essential and irreplaceable in the diagnosis of neuromuscular diseases. Surface EMG (eSlide 8.5) is noninvasive and has been widely used in various aspects of rehabilitation medicine, including rhythmic and involuntary movement monitoring, muscle reeducation, motor control, biofeedback, gait and motion analysis, and kinematic measurement. Although single fiber EMG has been in use for almost half a century, it remains the most sensitive clinical method for studying the stability of neuromuscular transmission and functional integrity of peripheral nerves. Stimulated single fiber EMG (eSlides 8.6 and 8.7) has been modified for use in testing paralyzed muscles, unconscious patients, uncooperative patients, pediatric patients, and patients with involuntary movements. Other advanced electrodiagnostic methods, such as quantitative EMG, refractory period studies, decomposition EMG, quantitative sensory tests, and power spectrum analysis, have been in use for years for special purposes.

• TRANSCRANIAL MAGNETIC STIMULATION (eSlide 8.8)

MEP with transcranial magnetic stimulation (TMS) and deep brain stimulation are the most commonly used electrodiagnosis methods in recent years. TMS is a noninvasive method that excites neurons in the brain. A weak current is induced in the tissue by rapidly changing magnetic fields, through a process called electromagnetic induction. For diagnostic purposes, clinical uses of MEP with TMS may serve as a tool for the evaluation of central motor pathways using measurements of central motor conduction time and estimates of spinal cord motor conduction velocity (eSlide 8.9). For therapeutic purposes, MEP with TMS can be used as a prognostic indicator for motor recovery of central nervous system diseases, such as stroke, traumatic brain injury, or aphasia. It can also be used in the measurement of functional integrity and as potential treatment for many neurologic and psychological conditions, such as migraines, Parkinson disease, dystonia, tinnitus, neurogenic pain, drug addiction, schizophrenia, obsessive–compulsive disorder, Tourette syndrome, autism, bipolar disorder, and major depressive disorder (eSlide 8.10). Among MEP applications, TMS is commonly used because of its advantages of noninvasiveness, with painless but deep penetration of nerve tissues. The magnetic pulse can easily pass through highly electroresistant tissues, such as the skull. It can also be applied in the study of deep-seated peripheral nerves.

• MAGNETOENCEPHALOGRAPHY (eSlide 8.11)

MEG is a noninvasive technique for investigating human brain activity. It allows the measurements of ongoing brain activity on a millisecond basis and shows where the brain activity is produced. MEG signals are obtained directly from neuronal electrical activity and are able to show absolute neuronal activity, whereas functional magnetic resonance imaging (MRI) signals show only relative neuronal activity. MEG can also electrophysiologically provide a more accurate spatial location of neural activities than electroencephalography (EEG). Current equipment, which includes up to several hundreds of whole-head channels, may accurately detect cortical and subcortical activities. Apart from evaluating physiologic activity, MEG may also be used for assessing many conditions, such as epilepsy, dementia, movement disorders, stroke, and learning disabilities, as well as in fetal studies and precise cortical delimitation prior to tumor or lesion resection. It has been a great advance in the diagnostic approaches in neurosciences.

• FUTURE PROSPECTIVE OF ELECTRODIAGNOSIS (eSlide 8.12)

Electrodiagnosis has become increasingly important in rehabilitation medicine and in many applications, including clinical and biomedical diagnosis, neuroprosthetics or rehabilitation devices, brain-computer interfaces, and neuromodulations. The future of electrodiagnosis requires more neurotechnological assistance to develop new equipment and techniques for the tests and methods to apply them in clinical diagnosis and therapeutic medicine.

Clinical Pearls

Electrodiagnostic medicine is used for diagnosis and differentiation in many neuromuscular diseases encountered in rehabilitation medicine.

BIBLIOGRAPHY
The complete bibliography is available on ExpertConsult.com.

TREATMENT TECHNIQUES AND SPECIAL EQUIPMENT

Rehabilitation and Prosthetic Restoration in Upper Limb Amputation

9

Joseph Burris

Amputation is associated with diabetes, peripheral vascular disease, trauma, infection, and malignancy. Upper limb loss is commonly associated with trauma. Manual control systems remain the primary prosthetic management, although advances are being made in myoelectric, bionic, and replantation or transplantation technologies. Early interdisciplinary team involvement for education and early prosthetic fitting are keys to successful prosthetic upper limb amputation outcomes.

DEMOGRAPHICS, INCIDENCE, AND PREVALENCE

In the United States, an estimated 185,000 people undergo amputation of the upper or lower limb each year. In 2008, it was estimated that 1.9 million people were living with limb loss in the United States. Approximately 500,000 people had minor (fingers or hands) upper limb loss, and 41,000 people were living with major upper limb amputations. Trauma accounts for 90% of all upper limb amputations. Finger amputations represent the highest percentage (78%). Excluding finger amputation, the most common upper limb amputations are located at the level of the forearm (transradial) and humerus (transhumeral). One-fifth of all combat-related major amputations involve the upper limb. Two-thirds of amputations that result from trauma occur among adolescents and adults younger than 45 years. Males account for greater than 75% of people with upper limb loss.

An estimated 4.1 per 10,000 babies are born each year with a limb difference. Congenital deficiencies are more common in the upper limb (58%) than in the lower limb, and they occur slightly more often in boys than in girls. The most common congenital amputation is at the left short transradial level. Teratogenic agents and amniotic band syndrome are two causes. The International Society for Prosthetics and Orthotics (ISPO) provides the current classification system for congenital limb difference. A child with a *transverse deficiency* has no distal remaining parts. In *longitudinal deficiencies*, distal portions are present but with a partial or total absence of a specific bone.

NOMENCLATURE AND FUNCTIONAL LEVELS OF AMPUTATIONS (eSlides 9.1 and 9.2)

The *residual limb* refers to the remaining part of the amputated limb. Digit amputations may or may not benefit from prosthetic restoration, primarily depending on the need for prehension. *Wrist disarticulation/transradial amputation, elbow disarticulation/transhumeral amputation,* and *shoulder disarticulation/forequarter amputation* are the major upper limb amputation levels. Further categorizations can be made, such as short, medium, or long, to define the *residual limb* into approximate thirds.

Wrist disarticulation preserves maximum pronation and supination. *Transradial amputation* results in a reduction of forearm pronation and supination. *Elbow disarticulation* creates prosthetic fit difficulties that are related to suspension and elbow joint placement. With *transhumeral amputation,* the more humeral length preserved, the more optimal the prosthetic restoration. *Shoulder disarticulation* and *forequarter amputation* are usually related to malignancy or severe trauma, and prosthetic acceptance is low.

PRINCIPLES OF LIMB SALVAGE AND AMPUTATION SURGERY

Limb-sparing procedures have become possible because of advances in imaging, reconstructive surgery, microsurgery, and cancer treatment. The best decision is one formed by the consensus of experienced trauma, oncology, and rehabilitation specialists.

The *mangled extremity syndrome* is defined as a significant injury to at least three of the four tissue groups (skin or soft tissue, nerve, vessel, and bone). The *mangled extremity scoring systems* have been shown to be poor predictors of amputation or salvage for functional outcome.

Once it has been decided that amputation is more appropriate than limb salvage, the team must determine the most distal level possible on the basis of the principles of wound healing and functional prosthetic fitting. Remnant muscles may be retained by *myodesis,* in which the deep layers are sutured directly to the periosteum, or by *myoplasty,* in which the superficial antagonistic muscles are sutured together and to deeper muscle layers.

Neuroma formation is a normal and expected consequence of amputation. Nerves should be withdrawn from the wound, sharply divided, and allowed to retract under the cover of soft tissue.

MANAGEMENT: PREAMPUTATION, PREPROSTHETIC, AND PROSTHETIC REHABILITATION (eSlide 9.3)

The *team approach to amputee rehabilitation* ideally begins in the preamputation phase whenever possible. The surgical and rehabilitation teams educate and counsel each other and the patient. It is important to include family members and other supporting individuals in the counseling. Important discussions need to be held with the patient about the planned surgical outcome and postsurgical period. This should also include a discussion about the different types of pain that might occur, the prevention of possible complications, and a preview of potential functional outcomes. An amputee peer visitor may be helpful. The Amputee Coalition of America has an array of resources to assist with this process.

The focus of immediate postamputation period is to control pain and edema, promote healing, prevent contractures, initiate mobilization, and continue counseling and education.

Pain control requires an early aggressive approach that considers multiple potential pain generators in the postsurgical period. Patient-controlled analgesia is transitioned to regularly scheduled long-acting and short-acting oral opioids. Understanding the characteristics of postsurgical residual limb pain (RLP) and phantom limb pain (PLP) allows the clinical team to wisely choose pain interventions. RLP is located in the remaining limb and is generated from soft tissue and musculoskeletal components. PLP is pain in the absent limb and is considered neuropathic. PLP is typically more intense at night and is characterized as burning, stabbing, or numbness/tingling. Phantom sensations occur in more than 70% of amputees and do not have to be treated unless painful and disruptive. Medications known for controlling neuropathic pain include anticonvulsants, such as gabapentin and pregabalin, and antidepressants, such as tricyclic antidepressants and serotonin-norepinephrine reuptake inhibitors.

The new amputee should be taught how to change dressings and use desensitization techniques. Counseling and mirror therapy may be helpful with pain control.

Edema control is important for limb shaping and protection, and it may reduce pain. An *immediate postoperative rigid dressing* (IPORD) can be placed in the operating room. Elastic shrinkers, gel liner sleeves, or low-tension figure-of-eight ace wraps may also assist in this process and are more commonly used. Proper tension and donning technique reduce complications associated with excess skin pressure or abnormal shaping for prosthetic fitting. Ideally, the *residual limb* will have a cylindrical appearance before prosthetic fitting. Soft tissue defects, including scarring and grafting, are common challenges. Early prosthetic fitting is important because prosthetic acceptance declines if fitting is delayed beyond the third postoperative month.

Activities of daily living (ADL) are mastered with one hand and with the use of adaptive equipment. Because balance is often disrupted in a new amputee, goals should include strengthening of the trunk and lower limbs using isometric exercise and aerobic training. Motor training with neuromuscular reeducation is conducted to increase muscle activity at potential myoelectric control sites.

• PROSTHETIC TRAINING

The prosthetic training phase begins with the delivery of the prosthesis. Initial focus is on donning and doffing as well as on wearing the prosthesis for short periods, with close monitoring of the *residual limb* skin. ADL are then incorporated, followed by higher-level homemaking skills and community reentry activities such as driving, work, and recreation.

• UPPER LIMB PROSTHESES

Prosthetic fitting options include the *passive system, body-powered system, externally powered system,* and *hybrid system.* Each patient's functional and vocational goals, geographic locations, anticipated environmental exposures, access to a prosthetist for maintenance, and financial resources need to be considered.

A *passive system* is in part cosmetic but also functions as a stabilizer. It is fabricated if the patient does not have enough strength or movement to control a prosthesis or accomplishes tasks without device movements. Sometimes, young children initially use *passive* upper limb prostheses for balance and crawling. A *body-powered system* prosthesis uses the patient's own residual limb or body strength and range of movement (ROM) to control the prosthesis. An *externally powered system* uses an outside power source, such as a battery, to operate the prosthesis. A *hybrid system* uses components of both types of controls.

Socket, Suspension, and Control Systems (eSlides 9.4 to 9.10)

Upper limb sockets are typically double walled. They may also contain an inner flexible thermoplastic liner to allow for growth and other fluctuations in size. Donning sleeves may be employed to don a socket. Gel liners with external sleeves, lanyards, seal-in rings, and locking pins may be used for the limb-to-device interface and suspension of devices. Prosthetic sock ply may be used to adjust fit for changes in limb volume. An elevated vacuum system with one-way air valves may also improve suspension of devices. The shorter the *residual limb* or the heavier the anticipated workload, the more necessary the proximal anchoring of the prosthesis with single or polycentric hinges and shoulder harness systems. Flexible hinges allow for some pronation and supination.

A *figure-of-eight* or *figure-of-nine harness* is used for control and suspension. Shoulder flexion and biscapular protraction increase the excursion of the cabling system and control the terminal device, elbow joint, or both. If amputees are given training regarding both *myoelectric* and *body-powered prostheses*, they will self-select their primary choice, although they may use either for different activities. *Body-powered* or *manual-controlled prostheses* use forces generated by body movements, which are transmitted through cables, to operate joints and terminal devices. *Body-powered prostheses* give higher sensory feedback and are more durable, less expensive, and lighter than *externally controlled prostheses*.

Externally powered prostheses use muscle contractions (myoelectric controlled) or manual switches to activate the prosthesis. Prostheses powered by electric motors can provide more proximal function and greater grip strength, along with improved cosmesis.

Externally powered prostheses require a control system. With myoelectric control, muscle contractions are detected by surface electrodes, and these surface electromyographic signals are transmitted to prosthetic motors. The patient uses antagonist muscle contractions or contractions of different strengths to differentiate between flexion and extension of the prosthesis.

Switch-controlled externally powered prostheses use small switches to operate the electric motors. These switches are typically enclosed inside the socket or incorporated into the suspension harness of the prosthesis, such as the "nudge," which is operated by the chin depressing the switch on a chest strap. A *hybrid system* incorporates both power options.

Shoulder disarticulation has two commonly used socket designs. The *complete enclosure shoulder socket* encases the shoulder and may be poorly tolerated because of its weight. The *X-frame socket* uses very rigid materials to maintain a shape that will lock into the wedge-shaped anatomy of the upper torso to provide a secure suspension.

Terminal Devices, Wrist Units, and Elbow Controls (eSlides 9.11 to 9.14)

Multitudes of terminal devices are available for upper limb amputees, although the functionality of these devices is limited. Terminal devices are generally grouped into one of two categories: *passive* or *active*. *Passive terminal devices* may provide some function and cosmesis. Examples of functional *passive terminal devices* include the child mitt frequently used on an infant's first prosthesis to facilitate crawling and the ball handling terminal devices used by older children and adults for ball sports.

Active terminal devices most commonly involve *hooks* and *artificial hands.* These may be operated with a manual or external control. External control for heavy-duty prehensile activities may be performed using the Greifer terminal device. Cable-operated terminal devices (hooks or hands) can be of a *voluntary opening design* (most commonly used) or a *voluntary closing design.* With a *voluntary opening mechanism,* the terminal device is closed at rest. The patient uses the control cable motion to open the terminal device against the resistive force of rubber bands (hook) or internal springs or cables (hand). With a *voluntary closing mechanism,* the terminal device is open at rest. The patient uses the control cable motion to close the terminal device, grasping the desired object.

In general, hook-style terminal devices provide the equivalent of an active lateral pinch grip, whereas active hands provide a tripod or *three-point chuck* grip. Many different options are available for terminal devices that address vocational and avocational hobbies or sports.

With myoelectric control, it is possible to initiate palmar fingertip grasp by contracting residual forearm flexors and to initiate release by contracting residual extensors. Various types of electronic hands and terminal devices are available. In addition to tripod and lateral tip pinch grips, newer myoelectric devices may offer precision, hook power, and spherical grip patterns. The most advanced prosthetic upper limbs commercially available are the i-Limb, BeBionic, Contineo, and Michelangelo hand. The advent of self-powered digits also makes it possible to replace as many fingers as necessary for a partial hand amputee.

The *wrist unit* can be positioned manually or with external power (myoelectric or switch). It is held in place by a friction or mechanical lock. Options include a quick disconnect unit and a flexion unit.

Manual *elbow systems* include single, polycentric, or flexible hinges for below-elbow amputees, and cable-controlled or spring-loaded systems for above-elbow amputees. External controlled systems include myoelectric and switch-operated devices.

ADVANCES IN TECHNOLOGY

Osseointegration is an emerging surgical technique for direct skeletal attachment of the prosthesis. It entails the use of a metal spike that is inserted into the terminal end of the bone, which is eventually connected to the prosthesis after completion of a multistage surgical procedure. Benefits include improved suspension, control, and proprioception, whereas risks include infection and device loosening. *Targeted muscle reinnervation* (TMR) rewires the nerves that no longer have innervation points to the pectoral muscle. Wireless and brain electrodes have been developed that can be implanted into muscle and sense nerve impulses, respectively. Signal technology, known as advance pattern recognition (APR), can provide prosthetic control input. The United States Defense Advanced Research Projects Agency (DARPA) funds research to advance prosthetic technology.

HAND REPLANTATION AND TRANSPLANTATION

Hand replantation (HR) of traumatically amputated limbs is now possible. All indications for replantation must consider the patient's general health; the limb ischemia time; and the level, type, and extent of tissue damage. HR requires prolonged recovery time, multiple procedures, and motivated patients. Because nerves transected in the proximal arm must regenerate over a considerable length, only limited motor return is typically seen in the forearm and hand, particularly the intrinsic muscles of the hand. Useful functions of the wrist and hand are unusual and limited at best. *Hand transplantation* (HT) is now performed on a limited basis in the United States. Selection of the appropriate patient, detailed preoperative planning, and precise surgical technique are of paramount importance. Following HR or HT, active and passive exercises to improve ROM, grip strengthening exercises, and sensory reeducation are required over several years.

• CONCLUSION AND FOLLOW-UP (eSlide 9.15)

Lifelong follow-up by the rehabilitation team, including the physiatrist, improves outcomes. After discharge from the therapy program, the amputee should be regularly monitored in an outpatient clinic by the rehabilitation team. Follow-up may be the most important aspect of prosthetic rehabilitation and yet is often neglected. Issues such as pain, depression, skin irritation, limb size change, and activity change are all more easily addressed early and thoroughly by the team to encourage continued prosthesis use. Many aspects of upper limb prosthetic rehabilitation cannot be addressed until the patient has had time to become acclimated to the amputation.

The successful long-term use of an upper limb prosthesis depends primarily on its comfort and perceived value to the amputee. Careful attention to follow-up adjustments and prescription revisions on the basis of the amputee's changing needs are essential factors for successful prosthetic rehabilitation.

Clinical Pearls

- Trauma accounts for 90% of all upper limb amputations.
- Finger amputation is the most common level of upper limb amputation.
- Males account for greater than 75% of people with upper limb amputation.
- Congenital deficiencies are more common in the upper versus the lower limb.
- The most common congenital amputation is at the left short transradial level.
- A transverse deficiency has no distal remaining anatomic parts.
- A longitudinal deficiency has distal anatomic parts present but with partial or total absence of a specific bone.
- The percentage of remaining pronation and supination in transradial amputation is directly correlated with the preserved percentage of residual limb length.
- The mangled extremity scoring system (MESS) is a poor predictor of amputation or salvage for functional outcome.
- The stages of amputation rehabilitation include preamputation, preprosthetic, and prosthetic phases.
- Postamputation pain control ideally involves pharmacologic and nonpharmacologic interventions.
- Upper limb prosthetic devices include passive, body-powered, externally powered, and hybrid-powered systems.
- Osseointegration, targeted muscle reinnervation, replantation, and transplantation represent advanced and emerging techniques in the treatment of upper limb amputation.
- Lifelong follow-up with a rehabilitation team, including a physiatrist, with attention to indicated adjustments for the patient's needs, improves outcomes in prosthetic use in patients with upper limb amputation.

BIBLIOGRAPHY

The complete bibliography is available on ExpertConsult.com.

Lower Limb Amputation and Gait

10

Matthew J. McLaughlin

The rate of lower limb amputations secondary to vascular injuries is increasing, and the need for physiatric providers to improve the quality of life of these patients remains paramount. Physiatrists need to maintain knowledge about the changing technologies in prosthetics, understand gait and its analysis, and know the complications encountered by prosthetic users. By improving function of these patients, their quality of life can be altered in a positive way.

• EPIDEMIOLOGY

The number of patients with limb loss has continued to increase because of several factors, thereby requiring more rehabilitation intervention. An aging population, an increase in the number of dysvascular cases for amputation, and an increase in the frequency of osteomyelitis contribute to these increases. Studies predict a doubling of the elderly dysvascular amputation population by 2030 and a doubling of the overall amputation population prevalence by 2050. The majority (82%) of people with lower limb amputations undergo amputation as a result of disease processes, such as diabetes mellitus (DM) or peripheral vascular disease. Other causes include trauma (16%), malignancy (1%), or congenital abnormality (1%). DM increases the risk for amputation to a greater degree than either smoking or hypertension. DM is reported to contribute to 67% of all amputations, and cigarette use is associated with a reamputation risk 25 times greater than that of nonsmokers. Individuals with amputation at an earlier age require a longer continuum of care.

The most frequent amputation level in the lower extremity varies according to the etiology. Toe amputations are the most common level overall when considering both major and minor amputations. With advances in limb salvage techniques, the number of partial foot amputation procedures has shown a significant increase over the past 10-15 years. The transtibial level is the most common major amputation level in the lower extremity, with transfemoral being the second most common.

• AMPUTATION TERMINOLOGY

The International Organization for Standardization (ISO) terminology for the description of both acquired amputations and congenital limb deficiencies has been widely accepted and increasingly used.

REHABILITATION IMPLICATIONS OF AMPUTATION LEVEL AND SURGICAL TECHNIQUE

The main goal of surgery is to remove diseased or damaged tissue to allow healing. Without healing, prosthetic training cannot begin. The large numbers of muscles within the leg complicate surgery (eSlide 10.1). The amputation level and surgical healing affect outcomes following amputation. In general, preservation of limb length with accommodations for future prosthetic fitting improves outcomes. Presurgical planning allows for consultation with the physiatrist and aids in discussion about the amputation level and future prosthetic fitting. Myodesis (suturing muscle attachment to bone) and myoplasty (suturing muscle fibers to fascia) are commonly performed surgical closures.

Postoperative healing, daily skin care, and residual limb shaping are of increased importance after amputation. Shrinkers or figure-of-8 wraps should be used to maintain limb shape when not wearing the prosthesis. To prevent loss of the contralateral limb, daily skin care and inspection should also be performed on this limb. Inadequate socket pressure on the distal end of the residual limb leads to verrucous hyperplasia. Shrinker socks and modification of the socket to apply appropriate pressure on the distal end help resolve this problem. Hyperhidrosis is a common symptom in amputee patients. Topical antiperspirants and botulinum toxin type B have been used in this population.

Heterotopic ossification can occur secondary to osteoblast activity. This can lead to range of movement (ROM) issues, problems with ambulation, or neurologic or vascular compromise. Diagnosis can be made on the basis of increased alkaline phosphatase levels and radiographs when suspicion of heterotopic ossification is high.

PAIN MANAGEMENT

Residual limb pain (RLP), phantom limb pain (PLP), and phantom limb sensation (PLS) are frequent findings after an acquired limb amputation. RLP is confined to the affected limb; PLP is pain in an area that is no longer present. PLS is prevalent in the immediate postoperative period and improves with prosthetic use and desensitization strategies. PLP varies and is described as dull, squeezing, cramping, electric shock-like, shooting, or sharp. Medications for PLP include N-methyl-D-aspartate receptor antagonists, opioids, anticonvulsants, antidepressants, local anesthetics, and calcitonin. Mirror therapy and transcutaneous electrical nerve stimulation have also been used for PLP.

PSYCHOLOGICAL SUPPORT

Undergoing amputation is a traumatic physical and psychological experience. Amputees may go through several stages of recovery: shock and confusion, mourning, and ultimately, adjustment and self-worth. Family support, goal-directedness, patient attitude, and spirituality are indicative of positive psychological predictors. Return-to-work is correlated with better prosthetic fitting, fewer medical conditions, amputation level, and premorbid career.

PROSTHETIC FITTING TIMELINE AND REHABILITATION CONSIDERATIONS

Preprosthetic fitting begins before surgery and continues until prosthetic training is initiated. Positioning and shaping of the limb and ROM exercises are important aspects of this phase. Wound healing, pain management, and edema control limit progression to prosthetic fitting in this phase. Preambulatory therapy and awareness of a changed center of mass after amputation are characteristics of therapy concerns during this phase.

During initial prosthetic training, standing, balancing, and simple stepping exercises predominate. Pregait activities, involving dynamic weight-shifting exercises, occur after mastery of the basics. Gait deviations are frequently seen, which require modifications from prosthetists during this phase. Fit, sock management, and donning and doffing of the prosthetic safely and effectively improve long-term use. Limb size and shape change during this phase as fluid shifts occur. Residual limb changes occur during this time, necessitating socket modifications. Skin redness or irritation indicates prosthetic fit issues. Time in the prosthesis should be gradually increased.

• FUNCTIONAL CLASSIFICATION AND PROSTHETIC PRESCRIPTION

The Centers for Medicare and Medicaid Services have published a functional classification system that guides prosthetic limb prescription. Five levels (termed K-levels) assist providers in selecting appropriate devices, based on anticipated goals and medical comorbidities. With the prosthetic prescription, the emphasis should be on identifying the class of prosthetic components best suited to achieve the patient's functional goals. Design of the prosthesis is a team decision that includes input from the patient, physiatrist, physical therapist, and prosthetist.

Socket Designs

Prosthetic sockets serve as the connection between the limb and patient, and they occasionally provide support. Transtibial sockets (patellar tendon bearing, patellar tendon bearing with supracondylar suspension, or full contact) and transfemoral sockets (quadrilateral and ischial containment) accommodate patients with differing residual limb lengths. Each socket type provides different benefits to the user. In patients with transtibial amputations, the patellar tendon-bearing socket is most frequently used and provides pressure relief in soft tissue areas that are able to resist forces during walking. The ischial containment socket for transfemoral amputees has gained popularity over the quadrilateral socket because it incorporates a more anatomic approach to fitting by "containing" the ischium within the trim line.

Prosthetic Limb Suspension

Suspension holds the socket and prosthesis onto the residual limb. Suspension is extremely important when considering the safety and use of prosthesis. Suction systems create a negative pressure within the socket to maintain suspension. Complications arise when the distal contact between the residual limb and prosthesis is lost. Pin-locking suspensions require a gel liner worn by the patient, with a threaded pin that engages the prosthesis. This can be used in transtibial or transfemoral amputees. The audible click heard when engaging the prosthesis provides feedback to ensure proper suspension. Lanyard suspensions are also used in transfemoral amputees to aid in prosthetic wearing. Higher-level amputations, such as shorter transfemoral amputations with short residual limbs, may require Silesian belt suspensions or a combination approach with a mixture of suspension types.

Patients with short transtibial amputations may need supracondylar suspension or cuff suspension mechanisms.

Recently developed prosthetic liners provide protection against shearing forces with softer materials such as Pelite, gel, urethane, and silicone. Unfortunately, there are some issues with durability and wear and tear, and thus occasional replacing is required.

Prosthetic Limb Frame Options (Endoskeletal or Exoskeletal)

Prosthetic frame options include endoskeletal or exoskeletal designs. Exoskeletal sockets use rigid exterior lamination, which helps with heavier patients or cosmesis under clothing. Endoskeletal devices, on the other hand, are more commonly used and require a pylon system to connect the socket to the foot, as in the case of a transtibial amputee. This also allows for customization of prosthetic height.

Prosthetic Feet

Prosthetic feet are available in many different materials and designs. Each has some benefit or potential drawback, depending on the function of the individual wearing the prosthesis. Solid ankle cushion heel (SACH; eSlide 10.2) feet are used for K1 level amputees; they have no moving parts, allowing for a lightweight, durable, and inexpensive design. A stationary attachment flexible endoskeleton (SAFE) prosthetic foot is similar to the SACH foot in that it has no joint articulations and is durable and inexpensive. The SAFE foot is primarily indicated for K1 and low-level K2 ambulators. Neither the SACH nor SAFE foot is an articulated design.

Articulated feet provide an advantage of increased movement in higher-functioning prosthetic users. Single axis feet (for K1 and K2 level ambulators; eSlide 10.3) allow controlled dorsiflexion and plantar flexion, with bumpers to limit any excessive motion. Multiaxial feet (K2 and K3) allow movement in multiple planes as the foot interacts with the ground (eSlide 10.4). Some feet allow energy storage and return in the gait cycle, improving efficiency. Energy-storing feet allow active patients to have spring-like ground effects that propel them into the next push-off phase in gait or provide cushioning (e-Slides 10.5 and 10.6). This type of foot is indicated for K3 and K4 level ambulators. Microprocessor-controlled feet are commercially available and provide improvements when walking over varying ground, but they are not always covered by insurance companies, which limit their accessibility (eSlide 10.7). Specialized feet are available for higher-level prosthetic users (eSlide 10.8).

Prosthetic Knees

Prosthetic knees used by transfemoral amputees are classified with respect to use and functional levels. Prosthetic users with increased functional abilities may use increasingly complex knee units that respond quickly to changes in gait, stride length, or cadence. Manual locking knees are for K1 level patients; they are either hinged and freely mobile or locked in place (such as in extension while standing). These are inexpensive and durable knees but provide poor gait mechanics compared with higher-level knee units. Single axis knee units (for K1 level ambulators) have a spring-assisted extension for quicker swing of the foot through the gait cycle. However, proximal muscle control is needed to prevent falling. Weight-activated stance control knee units (indicated for K1 and K2 level ambulators) are single axis knee units, but the knee locks when weight is applied through the prosthesis in the stance phase. When the weight is shifted off the prosthesis, the locking mechanism disengages, allowing for flexion in the swing phase. Polycentric knee units provide stability because of their construction and points of rotation, which are aligned to improve stability and knee flexion compared with single axis knee units (eSlide 10.9). Hydraulic knee units improve the ability to control the distal prosthetic limb using either fluid-filled or air-filled devices. These knees are indicated for K3 level ambulators as they allow for varied cadences and are adjustable. Microprocessor knee units provide increased feedback with a processor analyzing information at 50-1000 times per second to account for knee resistance forces (eSlide 10.10). One limitation is the inability to use these in areas that are at a risk of being exposed to water. They are for high-functioning K2 or K3 level amputees.

Additional Componentry Considerations

Torque absorbers are needed to automatically return the prosthetic to its original position. This is worthwhile in K3 level patients who would be able to torque a knee unit when walking or performing tasks. Diagnostic test sockets are frequently ordered before constructing a final socket to ensure fit before costly materials are used. Prosthetic socks, ranging from 1-ply to 5-ply, allow a user to adjust the fit quickly and precisely. When a patient starts to wear 10-ply socks, the general rule is to consider replacing the socket. Certain cosmetic covers can be added to allow the affected limb to appear more similar to the contralateral side.

Prosthetic Prescription for Partial Foot Amputations

There are many levels of partial foot amputations, which are treated in different ways. Any prosthetic design should reduce shear forces and pressure points. With an ankle disarticulation (Syme) amputation, patients can actually bear weight on the residual limb; however, the limb length does not allow for most energy-storing feet to be used. The liner is typically a gel liner with padding such as Pelite. Prosthetic foot options include a low-profile Syme SACH foot or a carbon composite foot. The carbon foot allows some energy storage and also provides better accommodation over uneven surfaces.

Prosthetic Prescription Algorithms for Transtibial Amputees

The choice of components for transtibial prosthetic prescriptions depends on the individual's current or potential functional abilities and the patient's goals for prosthetic use. The following recommendations for each functional level are for general consideration; it is important to develop a prescription that is individualized to a specific individual. The essential elements for transtibial prosthesis that need to be included for every functional level are socket, interface, suspension, pylon or frame, and type of foot and ankle. Items included in all prescriptions for prosthesis are a clear diagnostic socket and socks (single-ply and multiple-ply, six of each). The patient can select a custom-shaped cover, a prosthetic skin, or both to help address cosmetic concerns.

FUNCTIONAL LEVEL ONE (K1)

Patients in this functional category have the ability to use a prosthesis for transfers or to ambulate over level surfaces for short household distances. Safety is the greatest priority for this population. The socket design should be a total contact style, with special considerations for comfort during sitting. The type of interface and suspension system used should consider the patient's ability to don and doff the prosthesis and manage his or her hygiene independently. The frame should be lightweight and endoskeletal (with or without alignment ability) in design. Recommended foot and ankle components include a nonarticulated foot, such as the SACH or SAFE foot, or a simple articulated foot, such as the single axis foot. Also included in this prescription will be a clear diagnostic socket, prosthetic socks, and a cosmetic cover.

FUNCTIONAL LEVEL TWO (K2)

Patients in this functional category have the ability to perform limited community distance ambulation and traverse some environmental barriers. The major changes in the prosthetic prescription will be that the components should be alignable and the prosthetic foot should be a multiaxial or flexible keel-type foot to allow for accommodation over uneven terrain. Suspension for this group can use a pin lock, sleeve or suction suspension with a sleeve, and one-way expulsion valve in the socket.

FUNCTIONAL LEVEL THREE (K3)

Functional K3-level amputees are community distance ambulators who have the ability to traverse most environmental barriers and ambulate with variable cadence. Special consideration for this group will be the type of prosthetic foot. This will be some type of energy-storing (dynamic response) foot, and depending on the activities they are performing, it can include a dynamic pylon or feature that allows greater accommodation over uneven terrain. Foot and ankle components that incorporate hydraulic units, with or without microprocessor control, can also be considered in this population. A foot and ankle component with both microprocessor control and internal power may also be indicated for these patients. An additional consideration for prosthetic suspension is the use of an elevated vacuum technology.

FUNCTIONAL LEVEL FOUR (K4)

Patients in this classification level have the ability or potential ability for ambulation that exceeds normal requirements. This may include sports or recreational activities that require high impact, high stress, or high energy levels, which are typical of the prosthetic demands of a child, high-activity adult, or athlete. At this level, specialty components are running feet, waterproof foot and ankle components, and components with heel height adjustability. Suspension is also a key for this group to avoid catastrophic disruption of the prosthetic connection during activity. This may include use of a backup or secondary suspension method. Special considerations are also needed for the pediatric population because of growth and the wearing out of components secondary to high usage.

Knee Disarticulation

A knee disarticulation amputation level leaves the femur intact and creates a distal weight-bearing surface with retained thigh musculature. This long lever provides potentially better control of the prosthetic limb and maintains the distal growth plate of the femur, which is important for individuals who are skeletally immature at the time of amputation. The disadvantages of this amputation level are the discrepancies between the height of the prosthetic knee center and contralateral anatomic knee, as well as the worse cosmetic appearance. As with the ankle disarticulation level, the prosthesis proximal trim line will depend on the patient's ability to bear weight on the distal end of the residual limb. If full weight bearing occurs,

TABLE 10.1 Medicare Functional Classification Level (MFCL) Descriptions and Prosthetic Component Recommendations for Each Level

Functional Index Level	Description	Recommended Prosthetic Components
K0	No ability or potential to ambulate or transfer with use of a prosthesis, and prosthesis does not enhance the quality of life	None for function Potential for cosmetic prosthesis
K1	Ability or potential to transfer or ambulate with a prosthesis for household distances on level surfaces at a fixed cadence	Feet: solid ankle cushion heel, single axis Knees: manual locking, weight-activated stance control
K2	Ability or potential to ambulate limited community distances and traverse low-level environmental barriers. Ambulation at a fixed cadence	Feet: multiaxial and flexible keel feet Knees: weight-activated stance control
K3	Ability or potential to ambulate unlimited community distances and traverse most environmental barriers. Ambulation with variable cadence	Feet: multiaxial, energy storing Knees: hydraulic, pneumatic, and microprocessor-controlled
K4	Ability or potential to exceed normal ambulation activities and use a prosthesis for activities exhibiting high impact, high stress, or high energy levels	Feet: energy storing or other specialty feet Knees: no specific limitations

then the proximal trim can be lowered to the subischial level. If there is no distal end weight bearing, then the residual limb is treated as a transfemoral amputation with use of a more traditional ischial containment socket.

PRESCRIPTION CRITERIA
Socket design for this level typically includes an anatomically shaped socket with a flexible inner socket. The proximal trim lines of the socket will be determined based on distal weight-bearing tolerance as noted earlier. Interface and suspension options are generally the same as those for the transfemoral level, but there is also the possibility of creating suspension of the prosthesis with use of femoral condyles. Polycentric knee units are commonly recommended to reduce the difference in knee centers between the prosthetic limb side and the intact limb side. Depending on the functional goals of the patient, additional features, such as a hydraulic mechanism, may be indicated and beneficial.

Prosthetic Prescription Algorithms for Transfemoral Amputees
The prosthetic prescription for transfemoral amputees is based on current and potential functional abilities when considering medical comorbidities and social situations. Table 10.1 summarizes traditional prosthetic prescription parts for each K-level. In patients with transfemoral amputations, considerations about the knee unit and alternative methods of suspension are needed for safety purposes.

Prosthetic Limb Fitting and Replacement Considerations
Initially, basic components are used to allow for initial pregait and ambulation activities. This is subsequently replaced with a more definitive prosthesis every 3–5

years, depending on wear and use. Factors such as socket replacement versus modifications need to be weighed when considering replacement of a full prosthesis.

ENERGY CONSUMPTION

Gait in amputee patients is not as efficient as in people without an amputation. The increase in energy consumption for a given distance (metabolic cost) for a traumatic transtibial amputee walking with prosthesis is around 25% and for a transfemoral amputee is 63%. Values for dysvascular amputees at the same levels are 40% and 120%, respectively. Compared with using crutches with a swing-through gait, higher energy expenditures are seen with crutches than with prosthesis.

In general, dysvascular amputees have a slower walking speed and higher oxygen consumption rate. Preservation of knee function in transtibial amputees leads to improved energy expenditure. Bilateral amputees have higher energy expenditures than unilateral amputees. Dysvascular amputees have increased energy requirements compared with traumatic amputees.

Bilateral Amputee Considerations

Bilateral amputees, whether dysvascular or traumatic, face additional challenges. Up to 50% of unilateral dysvascular amputees will become bilateral amputees over a 5-year period. Successful transition from a unilateral amputee to a bilateral amputee occurs if a patient was initially successful as a unilateral amputee. Bilateral amputees have an increased need for cardiac capacity, and because of the lack of proprioceptive feedback, they will have slower selected walking speeds and wider bases of gait. The same selection of components is used for bilateral and unilateral amputees.

• PEDIATRIC LOWER LIMB LOSS

In contrast to the adult population, pediatric lower limb loss is usually congenital (21 per 10,000 births) and less frequently traumatic. Health-related quality of life remains high in pediatric patients with limb differences compared with children having other medical conditions. Both longitudinal and transverse limb differences occur, requiring different treatments, but they can generally be classified using the same ISO system. A challenging aspect of the pediatric patient is the growth of the residual limb, which sometimes necessitates surgery. In addition, in acquired amputation, terminal overgrowth (spiking) can occur, which complicates prosthetic fitting. Because of continued growth in pediatric patients, preservation of growth plates is beneficial. Leg length discrepancies occur frequently; therefore, knee disarticulations are more frequently performed in children than in adult populations. Proximal focal femoral deficiency with a shortened femur may require a Van Ness rotationplasty, in which the ankle is surgically attached to the femur to serve as a knee unit. Prosthetic fitting can occur after this surgery.

• NORMAL HUMAN GAIT

Normal human gait is a complex process that requires an understanding of the kinematics through multiple joints. Walking has double-limb support for approximately 20% of the gait cycle. Saunders and Inman described the six determinants of gait to obtain the most efficient pattern with a consistent center of gravity. These six determinants can be described as pelvic rotation in the horizontal plane, pelvic tilt in the frontal plane, lateral displacement of the pelvis, early knee flexion, foot and ankle mechanisms, and late knee flexion. eSlide 10.11 shows the normal human gait cycle, and eSlide 10.12 shows the axis of the ground force reactions. Different muscles are active or inactive during the various gait phases (eSlide 10.13), and each joint goes through a reciprocal process of flexion and extension during gait (eSlide 10.14).

Prosthetic Gait Deviations

Alignment of the prosthesis is a challenging and dynamic process. Each aspect of the prosthetic device can cause issues. Shortened stride length can be seen in patients who lack confidence in a prosthetic because of training issues, difficulties with fit, or knee mechanism problems. Asymmetric step length is seen when the prosthetic side is a different length than the contralateral limb. Vaulting or circumduction is seen with prosthesis that is too long. Visible pistoning occurs with a poor socket fit, which can occur with limb volume changes. Excessive lumbar lordosis may occur in compensation for a tightened hip flexor muscle. Medial or lateral "heel whips" occur during clearance when the knee is either internally or externally rotated.

Clinical Pearls

- Pain, improper fit or prosthetic alignment issues may contribute to abnormal gait deviations. Evaluating each individually helps providers determine primary and compensatory mechanisms affecting gait.
- By correctly classifying functional K-levels, providers are able to select more appropriate prosthetic components.
- Inappropriate surgical healing, prolonged immobilization, or poor preprosthetic care may contribute to negative outcomes. The residual limb shaping can be improved with a shrinker sock or figure-8 dressing to improve future prosthetic fit.
- In general, residual limb size changes drastically between surgery and 1 year after prosthetic fitting. Maintaining good socket fit is imperative for continued improvement in gait training after receiving a prosthesis.
- Continual evaluation of the skin integrity is paramount for long-term prosthetic use.
- Understanding basic human kinematics allows for interpretations of deviations, which can occur because of patient issues or prosthetic issues.

BIBLIOGRAPHY
The complete bibliography is available on ExpertConsult.com.

11 Upper Limb Orthoses

Chih-Kuang Chen

An orthosis is an externally applied device used to modify structural and functional characteristics of the neuromuscular skeletal system. Upper limb orthoses are commonly used in patients with upper limb disorders; thus members of the rehabilitation team should be familiar with the principles and applications of common upper limb orthoses.

• PRINCIPLES AND INDICATIONS

The objectives of upper limb orthotic applications can be classified into three major areas:

- *Protection:* Orthoses can provide compressive forces and traction in a controlled manner to protect the impaired joint or body part. Restricting or preventing joint motion may correct alignment and prevent progressive deformity. Protective orthoses can also stabilize unstable bony components and promote healing of soft tissues and bones.
- *Correction:* Orthoses help in correcting joint contractures and subluxation of joints or tendons. They assist in the prevention and reduction of joint deformities.
- *Assistance with function:* Orthoses can assist function by compensating for deformity, muscle weakness, or increased muscle tone.

• CLASSIFICATION AND NOMENCLATURE

Many different terms are used to describe upper limb orthoses. They are named by the joint(s) they cross, function they provide, or condition they treat. Some are named by their appearance, and still others bear the name of the person who designed them. To date, however, no single naming system has been universally accepted and used. The terms *orthotic device* and *splint* will be used interchangeably in this chapter, although the terms *splint* and *brace* are less preferred now because they imply only immobilization and do not suggest either improved function or restoration of mobility.

• BIOMECHANICAL AND ANATOMIC CONSIDERATIONS (eSlide 11.1)

- The wrist acts as the base for hand positioning and splinting, except isolated digital splinting. The weight of the immobile hand, gravity, and resting muscle tension tend to pull the wrist into flexion. This increases tension in the extrinsic extensor tendons, pulling the metacarpophalangeal (MCP) joints into hyperextension. Concurrently, the tension of the extrinsic flexor tendons is maintained and forces the interphalangeal (IP) joints [which include the proximal interphalangeal (PIP) and distal interphalangeal (DIP) joints] into flexion. The metacarpal arch of the hand flattens, and the thumb falls into adduction, resulting in a "claw hand" that is not functional. Prevention of this deformity is one of the goals of hand splinting.

- Bone configuration of the hand and tension of the muscles and ligaments in this region contribute to the creation of an arch system composed of the proximal transverse and longitudinal distal metacarpal arches. This arch system is vital for positioning the hand for normal function related to grasp and prehension. Incorporating these arches within the orthosis is essential to allow maximum function and comfort.

- The MCP joint is the key for finger function. When MCP joints are hyperextended, the IP joints flex because of the tension of the flexors and the delicate balance between the finger extensors and flexors. Extension stability of the wrist is important for optimal function of the hand. The wrist should be placed in slight extension to maintain flexor tendon length and to improve hand function. This position will place the MCP collateral ligaments in maximum stretch, preserve the anatomic arches of the hand, and thus oppose the development of a "claw hand" deformity. This position is also referred to as the "safe" or "intrinsic plus" position. It facilitates the weaker intrinsic motions of MCP flexion and IP extension, which are difficult to obtain.

- The hand is used during functional activities through basic prehension patterns: to pinch, grasp, or hook objects. There are two basic types of hand grips: power and precision. For the power grip, the wrist is held in extension with the fingers wrapped around an object held in the palm. The spherical grip is useful for holding a ball. The hook pattern is useful for carrying heavy objects. For the precision grip, the thumb is held against the tip of the index and middle fingers. Functional hand splinting is typically aimed at improving pinch. There are three types of pinch: (1) oppositional pinch (three-jaw chuck), (2) precision pinch, and (3) lateral key pinch. It is best to splint the hand toward an oppositional pinch. This allows the best compromise between the fine precision pinch and strong lateral pinch. No practical orthosis can substitute for or improve thumb adduction. When making a splint, the therapist should fabricate it in a position that enhances prehension and does not force the thumb into a position of extension and radial abduction. This position causes the rest of the arm to compensate for poor thumb positioning.

- When increasing joint range of movement (ROM) with splinting, the angle of pull needs to be perpendicular to the bony axis that is being mobilized. Otherwise, the forces on the skin and underlying structures may cause injury through excessive pressure on the skin and deforming stresses on the underlying healing structures.

- The improvement in ROM is directly proportional to the length of time a joint is held at its end range. This is known as the total end range time principle and is used with static progressive splinting. The load should be low and the application time long. The clinically safe degree of force covers a very narrow range.

DIAGNOSTIC CATEGORIES AND SPLINT EXAMPLES

There are many common clinical conditions for which orthotic intervention is appropriate. This section gives a brief overview of the features of specific diagnoses and the corresponding type of splint that is commonly indicated.

Musculoskeletal Conditions

TENDONITIS, TENOSYNOVITIS, AND ENTHESOPATHY (eSlide 11.2)

Tendonitis, tenosynovitis, and enthesopathy can all result from excessive repetitive movements or external stressors. The upper limb tendons most commonly involved are wrist extensors and the abductor pollicis longus and extensor pollicis brevis muscles of the thumb. The goal of splinting for these conditions is to immobilize the affected structures to facilitate healing and decrease inflammation. For example, the forearm-based thumb spica splint used for de Quervain stenosing tenosynovitis immobilizes the wrist, carpometacarpal (CMC) joint, and MCP joint of the thumb. The IP joint of the thumb needs no fixation because the affected tendons do not move this joint.

Lateral epicondylitis is a common enthesopathy of the upper limb, which can be treated with a tennis elbow orthosis. This is a forearm band that changes the lever arm against which the wrist extensors pull. In essence, it puts the origin of the extensor muscles at rest and decreases the microtrauma from overuse. This orthotic device is a firm strap against which the extensors press when contracting; it is placed approximately 2 fingerbreadths distal to the lateral epicondyle. A similar orthosis is used for medial epicondylitis.

Trigger finger causes a snapping sensation in the volar surface of the digits on release of the grasp. It is usually a result of trauma to the flexor tendon sheath of the fingers or thumb, producing thickened tendinous sheaths and restriction of motion. In advanced trigger finger, the digit can become "locked" in flexion. The goal of trigger finger treatment is to temporarily halt the repetitive motion to allow the sheath to heal. Functional use of the hand should be maintained, although the affected digit is immobilized. The splint for trigger finger covers the proximal phalanx and MCP joint of the involved digit. It decreases the tendinous excursion through the first annular pulley at the base of the MCP joint and allows the inflamed structures to rest.

SPRAINS (eSlide 11.3)

Sprains are defined as momentary subluxations with spontaneous reduction that result in torn ligamentous structures. Sprains require joint immobilization in a position of function to allow for healing as well as functional use. Common sprains include dislocation of the IP and MCP joints caused by hyperextension and are often seen in sports injuries.

Splints commonly used for digital sprains are finger extension splints that hold the PIP joint in extension but allow flexion of the DIP joint. This position keeps the oblique retinacular ligament and terminal extensor tendon lengthened, preventing boutonnière deformities during the healing phase. Ulnar collateral ligamentous injuries at the MCP joint of the thumb are treated with a hand-based thumb spica splint to immobilize the joint during the healing phase. Wrist splints that place the wrist in slight extension are used for wrist sprains. For mild sprains, splints with no spline (metal bar insert) permit some motion and avoid creating significant stiffness. They also limit available range to approximately 40 degrees of total motion. Elbow neoprene sleeves are helpful for mild sprains in the elbow because they limit the extremes of ROM but allow some functional movement.

FRACTURES (eSlide 11.4)

Most major fractures need total immobilization by casting, surgical intervention, or both. Some fractures, however, do not need total limb immobilization and can be treated with orthotic devices. These devices should immobilize the body part or the joint sufficiently to promote healing while also optimizing function. A gutter splint is used primarily for phalangeal and metacarpal fractures. These splints extend from the proximal forearm to beyond the DIP joint and can be radial (immobilizing the index and long fingers) or ulnar (immobilizing the ring and little fingers; also called a boxer splint). The splint should be wide enough to surround both fingers and the wrist. Other examples include traction-type splints that allow for very controlled motion during the healing phase of intraarticular finger fractures treated with pinning. Joint movement has been credited with enhancing cartilage nutrition and preventing intraarticular adhesions.

ARTHRITIS (eSlide 11.5)

Joint diseases of the hand and wrist have the most significant impact on function. Orthotic devices can provide functional positioning to prevent further deformity and loss of use in arthritic diseases, as well as to protect the joints from further injury.

Rheumatoid arthritis is a chronic inflammatory disease that primarily affects synovial joints. The most frequently affected joints in the upper limb are the wrists, MCP joints, and PIP joints. Deformities include subluxation and ulnar deviation at the MCP joints, subluxation and radial deviation at the wrist, and swan neck and boutonnière deformities of the fingers. These deformities usually progress, especially if no attempt is made to rest and protect the affected joints from overuse. Several options are available for splinting the rheumatoid hand. Ulnar deviation splints that pull the MCP joints toward radial deviation and increase the functional use of the hand are now lightweight and permit full MCP joint motion in flexion and extension. Wrist splints that provide light support for the wrist are usually well tolerated. Swan neck and boutonnière splints can be made from thermoplastics but are often bulky and cosmetically unpleasing. The swan neck splint allows for flexion of the digit but blocks hyperextension. The boutonnière splint holds the DIP or PIP joint in extension.

Osteoarthritis most commonly involves the CMC joint of the thumb. A hand-based or forearm-based thumb spica splint can be prescribed for CMC joint *osteoarthritis*. By limiting motion at the base of the thumb, the splint decreases pain, especially with pinching-type activities.

Neuromuscular Conditions
NERVE INJURIES (eSlides 11.6 and 11.7)

When a peripheral nerve is injured, the level and completeness of the injury determines the extent of the deficit incurred. For example, in a distal median nerve injury, a simian hand deformity may occur, and the functions most affected are thumb palmar abduction and opposition. The goal of an orthotic device is to help restore this function. The splint usually has a spring coil design that holds the MCP joints in slight flexion but permits MCP extension. This splint also has a portion to position the thumb in palmar abduction.

Radial nerve injuries distal to the humeral spiral groove commonly present with wrist drop and finger drop. The goal in these cases is to enhance wrist and finger extension. A radial nerve palsy orthosis is based on the forearm, with an outrigger holding the wrist, fingers, and thumb in extension and allowing flexion of the digits.

With a proximal ulnar nerve injury, the patient has a "benediction hand," characterized by hyperextension of the fourth and fifth MCP joints and flexion of the PIP joints because of the loss of balance between the extrinsic and intrinsic hand muscles. Here the goal is to prevent fixed deformity of the fourth and fifth MCP joints and improve function. An ulnar nerve palsy orthosis holds the MCP joints of the fourth and fifth fingers in slight flexion by a spring coil or figure-of-eight splint design. The spring coil design assists MCP flexion and permits extension of the MCP joints but blocks hyperextension. This can also be accomplished with a static splint that uses a "lumbrical bar" to prevent hyperextension of the MCP joints of the fourth and fifth digits. Thumb position is most often compromised in low median and ulnar nerve injuries, which leave the patient with no or a weakened ability to place the thumb in opposition and palmar abduction.

Incomplete nerve injuries can be caused by compression without producing complete paralysis (for example, in median nerve injury from carpal tunnel syndrome). The purpose of the splint is to immobilize the wrist to minimize swelling from overuse of the tendons. Complete resolution of carpal tunnel syndrome can occur if wrist orthoses are applied early, when symptoms first appear. The splint is molded to the patient from a thermoplastic that offers excellent conformity to hold the wrist in 0-5 degrees of extension. The splint's commonly used name, *wrist cock-up splint*, is misleading and should be avoided because it implies that the wrist should be placed in extension. The patient should be instructed to reduce activities that stress the wrist and to wear the splint all night.

A word of caution is in order regarding prefabricated wrist splints for carpal tunnel syndrome. Many of these splints have an angled metal bar to hold the wrist in 45 degrees of extension. This angle far exceeds the recommended 0-5 degrees of extension needed to decrease pressure in the carpal tunnel. Patients need to be instructed to remove the metal spline, flatten it, and then replace it in the fabric sleeve. Usually, this splint should be worn for 4-6 weeks, with gradual weaning from the splint and return to activity with workstation modifications.

Cubital tunnel syndrome (compression of the ulnar nerve at the elbow) can be treated with long arm splints that hold the elbow in 45 degrees of flexion, the forearm in neutral position, and the wrist in 0-5 degrees of extension, leaving the thumb and fingers free.

BRAIN INJURY AND STROKE (eSlide 11.8)

Depending on the area of brain injury and ensuing deficits, particularly if there is a change in muscle tone, orthotic devices should be designed to prevent deformities and help adjust muscle tone. Resting and positioning orthotic devices are also necessary to help prevent complications, such as distal edema, joint subluxation, and contracture formation. In upper limb paralysis, a resting hand splint is commonly used to position the wrist in slight extension, the MCP joints in slight flexion, and the IP joints in extension. The thumb is supported in a position between palmar and radial abduction. Full support of the first CMC joint prevents ligamentous stresses on the thumb, especially in the insensate hand. This thumb position uses a reflex-inhibiting posture to decrease tone in the hand. The antispasticity ball splint places the fingers and hand in a reflex-inhibiting position and serves to reduce tone.

A mobile arm support can be used to enhance function for patients with proximal upper limb weakness, especially when the weakness is profound and the outlook for recovery is guarded. A mobile arm support is particularly helpful when activities of daily living, such as eating and grooming, are performed. When attached to a wheelchair with a swivel joint, the mobile arm support is often called a balanced forearm orthosis.

Many types of slings are available for patients with decreased tone in the upper limb. Decreased tone can result in shoulder subluxation, and a sling can decrease this deformity. These slings restrict active motion of the shoulder by keeping the humerus in adduction and internal rotation and placing the elbow in flexion. They are designed to unload the weight of the arm on the shoulder, but they do not approximate the humeral head back into the glenoid fossa. Slings or half-arm trays do not completely correct shoulder subluxation. The arm trough or half-lap board is often preferred because it does not restrict use of the limb and places the humerus in a position that is more naturally approximated into the glenoid fossa.

SPINAL CORD INJURY (eSlides 11.9 and 11.10)

In patients with spinal cord injury, orthotic devices are needed to enhance function, help with positioning, or both. The type of device depends on the level of injury and the extent of neurologic compromise. With spinal cord injury at the C1-C3 level, the goals are to prevent contractures and hold the wrist and digits in a position of function with a resting hand splint. In a C4-level injury, the goal is to use the available shoulder strength by providing mobile arm support to enhance function, as previously described. In a C5-level injury, the goal is to statically position the wrist in extension with a ratchet-type hinged orthotic device to hold devices and use the shoulder musculature for function. An orthotic device for a C6 tetraplegia patient can enhance finger flexion with a tenodesis flexion effect from wrist extension. For example, a Rehabilitation Institute of Chicago tenodesis splint, molded from thermoplastic materials, has several positioning components. A thumb post component positions the thumb in palmar abduction. A dorsal finger piece component, which is attached with a static line to a volar forearm component, holds the PIP joints of the index and long fingers in slight flexion. When the patient extends the wrist, the static line pulls the fingers toward the thumb post. This produces a three-point pinch, allowing the patient to grasp an object. When the patient relaxes the wrist, the fingers extend passively, releasing the object. The degree of pinch varies depending on the strength of the wrist extensors and the degree of finger flexion, extension, and opposition. This custom-made thermoplastic tenodesis device is mainly used in training and practice. If a patient finds the device useful, a light metal custom-made tenodesis orthosis achieves better functional restoration. An adaptive or functional use orthosis promotes functional use of an upper limb that is impaired because of weakness, paralysis, or loss of a body part. An example is the universal cuff, which encompasses the hand and holds various small items, such as a fork, pen, or toothbrush, to enhance independence.

Orthoses for Other Injuries

POSTSURGICAL AND POSTINJURY ORTHOSES (eSlides 11.11, 11.12, and 11.13)

Many types of splints have been developed to help regain motion in stiff joints. Examples of such splints include dynamic elbow flexion and extension splints after upper arm or elbow fracture, dynamic wrist flexion and extension splints after a Colles fracture, and dynamic finger flexion and extension splints for stiffness after crush injuries to the hand. Similar splints can be fabricated with a static progressive approach. Joints that have a soft end feel do well with dynamic splints. Those with a rigid end feel typically respond better to a static progressive approach that will maintain a constant joint position while the tissue gently accommodates to the tension, without the influence of gravity or motion. Examples of static progressive splints are the Joint Jack or cinch straps and splints for PIP and DIP joint contractures with the MERiT components. Selection of forearm-based or hand-based splints is determined by the need for stabilization. In general, the goal is to immobilize as few joints as feasible. Forearm pronation–supination splints with both dynamic and static features are very helpful in regaining motion after fractures of the radius and ulna.

Several splint designs are currently used after repair of tendon injuries. The type of surgical procedure or injury level often dictates the type of splint used so that the splints cannot be used interchangeably. After flexor tendon repair, Kleinert and Duran splints are commonly used. The Kleinert splint features dynamic traction into flexion but allows active digit extension within the constraints of the splint. The Duran splint statically positions the wrist and MCP joints in flexion and IP joints in extension. The Indiana Protocol splint can also be used. This splint adds a tenodesis-type action splint to the Kleinert componentry for specific, active-assisted ROM exercises. It can be used only if a specific surgical suture technique has been used.

The type of extensor tendon repair splint depends on the level of injury. A mallet finger injury requires only a Stax splint, which is a static splint holding the DIP joint in full extension. A more proximal injury, however, needs a splint that holds the wrist statically in extension, with dynamic extension of the MCP and IP joints. Such a splint permits active flexion of the MCP joints within the constraints of the splint to an angle of approximately 30 degrees. Injuries to the thumb flexor or extensor tendons require more specific splinting that depends on the level of the injury.

Postoperative joint replacements for the PIP, DIP, or MCP joints of the hand require specific splints that promote healing or encapsulation of the joints while preserving ROM during the healing phases.

ORTHOSES FOR BURNS (eSlide 11.14)

After burn injuries, body parts should be repositioned to prevent the development of expected deformities. For example, in burns of the dorsal surface of the hand, the wrist is placed in 15-20 degrees of extension, the MCP joints in 60-70 degrees of flexion, the PIP and DIP joints in full extension, and the thumb between radial and palmar abduction. If tendons are exposed, flexion of the MCP joints should be decreased to 30-40 degrees to keep some slack in the tendons until there is wound closure. Palmar hand burns require maximum stretching to counteract the contracting forces of the healing burn. The antideformity position of a palmar burn consists of 15-20 degrees of wrist extension, extension of the MCP and IP joints, digital abduction, and thumb abduction and extension. This has been referred to as an "open palm" or "pancake" position. For prevention of shoulder adduction deformity after axillary burns, the shoulder should be held in abduction with an airplane splint. The tendency toward hypertrophic scarring after a burn is addressed with a selection of compression garments, elastomer molds, facial splints, gel shell splints, and silicone gel sheeting.

• PEDIATRIC APPLICATIONS (eSlide 11.15)

Major reasons for the use of orthoses in the pediatric patients include functional positioning, normalizing muscle tone, postoperative protection, and positioning after surgery for a congenital deformity. Orthotic management of the child must consider the child's age, developmental status, growth, and functional status. Orthoses are expected to last at least a year, so the material must accommodate some growth, as well as be durable and safe (especially when used in young children who have a tendency to chew on their hand braces). Parents should be educated on how to apply the orthosis and watch for any skin injury related to the orthosis.

Children with abnormal tone or progressive neuromuscular disorders are at higher risk for contracture development. A major rationale for controlling the degree of contracture development is to minimize the adverse effects of contractures on function. It is important to acknowledge that static positioning of the limbs in patients with weak musculature is the most important cause of contracture development. Upper limb contractures may not negatively affect function if they are mild. Stretching and ROM exercises are the mainstays in preserving function.

SPECIAL CONSIDERATIONS

Splints can be perfectly designed and skillfully fabricated but are useless if not worn. The more choice and input patients have in splint design, the more compliant they are with splint wear. The wearing schedule depends on the goals for the splint and the patient's tolerance for wearing it. For example, a patient with a brain injury who is "storming" (i.e., sweating excessively and posturing) may tolerate a resting hand splint for positioning for just 30 minutes on and 3 hours off. In contrast, a patient with stroke and mild spasticity could wear a resting hand splint for 2 hours on and 2 hours off during the day and keep it on all night. Static progressive splint wear depends on the tissue response to gentle stretching. The stretch should be perceived as mild, and it should never awaken the patient at night. In a patient with both flexion and extension splinting needs, the flexion splint can be worn 1 hour on and 2 hours off during the day and the extension splint can be worn at night.

Blueness or redness of the digits when wearing a splint tells the observer that an overly aggressive stretch is being applied to the shortened neurovascular bundles. These structures sometimes shorten because of joint contractures, in which case the splint tension must be decreased and the contracture stretch should be less aggressive. Skin checks should be performed after a splint is removed. More frequent checks should be done, especially if the splint is new or has been recently changed. Complaints of pain or tenderness may signal where to focus the examination. The skin is examined for abrasions and erythema. A blanchable lesion will lose its redness when pressed and is not as serious as a nonblanchable lesion, which reflects underlying tissue injury.

ORTHOTIC MATERIALS

Most splinting materials are low-temperature thermoplastics. Many are known by their trademark names, such as Orthoplast, Aquaplast, and Orfit. Low-temperature thermoplastics become soft and pliable when exposed to relatively low temperatures and can be shaped in a water bath at 150° F to 180° F (66° C–82° C). High-temperature thermoplastics are more durable but require oven heating (up to 350° F, or 177° C) and placement over a mold to achieve the desired shape.

Clinical Pearls

- For an orthosis to be fabricated, a sound understanding of the anatomy, biomechanics, and the tissue physiology of the upper limb is required.
- People prescribing upper limb orthotic devices should have a thorough knowledge of the musculoskeletal and neurological conditions amenable to treatment by orthoses.
- The clinicians must understand other avenues of treatment, such as exercise therapy, and be aware of the indications of surgery.

BIBLIOGRAPHY
The complete bibliography is available on ExpertConsult.com.

Lower Limb Orthoses

12

Tze Yang Chung

Lower limb orthoses are commonly used in physical medicine for a wide range of conditions. Therefore, a sound understanding of the different types of orthoses and their biomechanical properties and indications is essential for proper prescription.

• PRINCIPLES OF LOWER LIMB ORTHOSES (eSlide 12.1)

An orthosis is defined as a device attached or applied to the external surface of the body to improve function, restrict or enforce motion, or support a body segment. Lower limb orthoses are indicated to assist gait, reduce pain, decrease weight bearing, control movement, and minimize progression of a deformity.

• TERMINOLOGY FOR LOWER LIMB ORTHOSES

Often, the terminologies for orthoses themselves are not uniform and can be sources of confusion. The most common nomenclature uses the first letter of each joint the orthosis crosses, from proximal to distal. For example, KAFO refers to a knee-ankle-foot orthosis. Other added descriptions may include the material used [e.g., plastic ankle-foot orthosis (AFO)], function performed [e.g., reciprocating gait orthosis (RGO)], or even an eponym (e.g., Scott-Craig orthosis). An orthosis is not put on and taken off but is rather donned and doffed.

• SHOES

Proper shoe fitting is important. The sole should be pliable, and the index finger should fit between the tip of the great toe and toe box. The presence of calluses from friction indicates a poor fit.

Shoe Parts (eSlide 12.2)

Two types of dress shoes are commonly worn: the Blucher and the Balmoral. A Blucher shoe has an open throat and is recommended for patients requiring an orthosis because there is more room to don and doff the shoe or orthosis. One should be familiar with the parts of the shoe, such as shank, vamp, and toe box. The heel counter is the back of the shoe, which controls the rearfoot. A strong heel counter is critical to control the entire foot.

• FOOT ORTHOSES (eSlide 12.3)

Foot orthoses range from over-the-counter arch supports to customized fabricated orthoses. They can affect ground reaction forces that act on proximal joints and rotational components during gait. Customized orthoses are usually available in soft, semi-rigid, and rigid types, depending on the needs for shock absorbency and degree of control for the specific deformity. For a custom foot orthosis, the fabrication process involves taking a cast of the foot to create a negative mold from which a positive mold is obtained. It is the positive mold that is modified and over which the final orthosis is formed. It is important that the subtalar joint be casted in a neutral position to minimize abnormal foot and ankle rotation.

Common Foot Conditions

PES PLANUS (FLAT FOOT) (eSlide 12.3)

Pes planus can be due to abnormalities such as excessive internal torsion of the tibia (which results in pronation of the foot) or malalignment of the calcaneus. Pronation of the foot can be defined as a rotation of the foot in the longitudinal axis that results in the lowering of the medial aspect of the foot. Pronation occurs at the subtalar joint; therefore the key to controlling excess pronation is to control the calcaneus to maintain the subtalar joint in a neutral position. The orthosis should cup and elevate the anteromedial calcaneus, exerting an upward thrust against the sustentaculum tali to prevent pronation. It should also extend beyond the metatarsal heads to provide better leverage. A custom-made foot orthosis designed to prevent hyperpronation is also referred to as a UCBL orthosis (or UCB), denoting the University of California Biomechanics Laboratory.

Some cases of pes planus are because of ligamentous laxity within the foot for which medial longitudinal arch supports can be helpful. Because the foot develops a tolerance for the inlay, the height of the arch can be increased as required. A Thomas heel (provides increased medial length to the heel) can also offer medial support, particularly for heavier individuals. Runners having hyperpronation or pes planus require running shoes with a firm medial heel counter and a wide shank.

PES CAVUS (HIGH-ARCHED FOOT)

Pes cavus leads to excess pressure along the heel and metatarsal head areas, causing pain. Increasing the height of the longitudinal support to fill in the space between the shank of the shoe and arch of the foot, as well as extending the lift to the metatarsal heads, will evenly redistribute the weight. The high point of the arch should be located at the talonavicular joint.

If excess supination is caused by an externally rotated tibia, the foot orthosis must be molded with the subtalar joint in a neutral position to prevent excess supination.

FOREFOOT PAIN (METATARSALGIA)

The aim is to redistribute the weight-bearing forces to an area proximal to the metatarsal heads. A metatarsal pad (cookie) can be placed inside the shoe just proximal to the second, third, and fourth metatarsal heads; proximal to the lateral aspects of the first metatarsal; and medial to the fifth metatarsal head. A metatarsal bar can be externally placed on the sole proximal to the metatarsal heads. A rocker bottom can also be used. Patients should avoid shoes with high heels or pointed toes.

HEEL PAIN

Again, the aim is to redistribute the weight to reduce pain. Rubber heel pads can be placed inside the shoe. A calcaneal bar is externally placed distal to the painful area to prevent the calcaneus from full weight bearing. Other modifications include shoes that have a spring for the heel set on the anterior calcaneus or a rocker bottom shoe. They place the heel strike anteriorly and the ground reaction force anterior to the painful calcaneus.

Plantar fasciitis is another common source of heel pain. For plantar fasciitis associated with hyperpronation, recommendations are similar to those for pes planus, such as an orthosis with the subtalar joint in neutral position and shoes with a firm medial heel counter and wide shank. If pes cavus is present, an elevated medial arch support or a heel well can be used. Commercially, a plantar fascia night splint, which is a prefabricated AFO that is placed in a few degrees of dorsiflexion, can provide the plantar fascia and plantar flexors with a therapeutic stretch during sleep hours.

Heel lifts help relieve some causes of Achilles pain by decreasing the amount of stretch placed on the Achilles tendon. They are only used for weeks, not months, to prevent the development of a plantar flexion contracture. They can also be helpful for treating plantar flexion spasticity or contracture.

TOE PAIN
Common conditions associated with toe pain include hallux rigidus, gout, and arthritis. The aim here is to decrease pain by immobilization. A full-length carbon insert can be placed along the sole of the shoe to reduce the mobility of distal joints.

LEG LENGTH DISCREPANCY
Proper limb length measurements are essential. Leg length discrepancies less than 0.5 inch do not need correction. The total discrepancy is never corrected. At most, 75% of the leg length discrepancy should be corrected. The first 0.5 inch of the discrepancy can be managed with a heel pad. Additional correction requires the heel and sole to be externally built up.

OSTEOARTHRITIS OF THE KNEE
When medial compartment narrowing is present, lateral heel wedges of 0.25-inch thickness can be used for conservative treatment of osteoarthritis by unloading the medial compartment. Therefore these wedges may also be helpful for medial meniscus injuries.

PEDIATRIC SHOES
Pediatric shoes should have a simple design without a heel; the soles should be soft. High-quarter or three-quarter shoes are preferred during the first few years of life. Flat feet are common in infants and children and improve over time; therefore not all flat feet need to be treated in children, especially if there are no symptoms.

• ANKLE-FOOT ORTHOSES
AFOs are the most commonly prescribed lower limb orthoses. Controlling dorsiflexion and plantar flexion, mediolateral stability, and subtalar joint motion (rotation at the subtalar joint is accompanied by rotation of the tibia) should be considered. AFOs can also stabilize the knee during gait. Remember that plantar flexion creates a knee extension moment, and dorsiflexion creates a knee flexion moment.

Metal Ankle-Foot Orthoses (eSlide 12.4)
Metal AFOs are now much less common than the plastic type, although metal joints are frequently used in combination with plastic orthoses. However, older

patients accustomed to metal AFOs may still want to continue with this type of AFO, and morbidly obese patients may require extra durability and stability. Ankle joint motion is controlled by pins or springs inserted into channels (anterior or posterior).

A solid stirrup is a U-shaped metal piece that is permanently attached to the shoe. Its two ends are bent upward to articulate with the medial and lateral ankle joints. The sole plate can be extended beyond the metatarsal head area for conditions requiring a longer lever arm for better control of plantar flexion.

A split stirrup has a sole plate with two flat channels for insertion of the uprights. The two uprights are now called calipers because they can open and close distally to allow donning and doffing of the AFO. A split stirrup allows removal of the uprights from the shoes so that the AFO can be worn with other shoes. The split stirrup is not as stable as the solid stirrup.

ANKLE STOPS AND ASSISTS

The ankle joint can be positioned in a neutral, dorsiflexed, or plantar flexed position. It is set by placement of pins and screws into the two channels of the ankle joint.

Plantar Stop (Posterior Stop). The plantar stop is used to control plantar spasticity or help incrementally stretch plantar contractures. It is commonly set at 90 degrees. A pin is inserted into the posterior channel of the ankle joint. An AFO at 90 degrees produces a flexion moment at the knee during heel strike and may lead to an unstable gait via buckling. The opposite occurs at toe-off, with an extension moment created at the knee. A cushioned heel acts like a shock absorber at heel strike and is able to partially substitute for the dorsiflexors, which cannot be eccentrically activated when an AFO is set at 90 degrees. This helps move the ground reactive force more anteriorly at the foot and knee, stabilizing the knee. In contrast, a firm heel promotes a knee flexion moment and can be used with an AFO for a patient with genu recurvatum.

Dorsiflexion Stop (Anterior Stop). A pin is inserted into the anterior channel of the ankle joint. It is used in conditions with weak calf muscles (gastrocnemius or soleus complex) or quadriceps and is usually set at 5 degrees of dorsiflexion. The anterior stop assists with push-off and assists the knee joint into extension. It should be used in combination with a stirrup and the sole extended to the metatarsal heads. The earlier the dorsiflexion stop occurs during the stance phase, the greater the extension moment at the knee, which substitutes weak quadriceps. A balance should be obtained such that the extension at the knee is sufficient for stability yet prevents genu recurvatum.

Dorsiflexion Assist (Posterior Spring). A posterior spring substitutes for concentric contraction of dorsiflexors to prevent flaccid foot drop after toe-off, and it also substitutes (albeit inadequately) for the eccentric activation of the dorsiflexors after heel strike. The posterior spring prevents rapid plantar flexion at heel strike during its compression in the posterior channel. The spring is again compressed during plantar flexion in the late stance before toe-off. It provides a downward thrust posterior to the ankle joint at toe-off, which results in dorsiflexion anterior to the ankle joint, helping in toe clearance during the swing phase.

Metal Ankle-Foot Orthosis Varus-Valgus Control (eSlide 12.4). Varus and valgus deformities are associated with rotation at the subtalar joint. A T strap is attached along the side of the shoe distal to the subtalar joint to help minimize the deformity. T straps may be placed medially or laterally. A lateral T strap is used to control a varus deformity and vice versa.

Plastic Ankle-Foot Orthoses (eSlide 12.5)

Plastic AFOs are now the most commonly used AFOs because of their cost, cosmesis, light weight, interchangeability with shoes, ability to control varus or valgus deformities, and provision of better foot support.

PLASTIC ANKLE-FOOT ORTHOSIS COMPONENTS

The footplate can be extended beyond the toes to reduce spasticity aggravated by toe flexion.

The strength of the AFO should be matched to the patient's weight and activity level. The ankle and subtalar joints can be made more stable by the following: (1) extending the trim line (anterior border of the plastic AFO) more anteriorly at the ankle level, (2) making the plastic material thicker, (3) placing carbon inserts along the medial and lateral aspects of the ankle joint, or (4) incorporating corrugations within the posterior leaf of the AFO.

Plastic AFOs can also be hinged at the ankle, permitting a more natural gait. Plastic ankle joints are light and are a good choice for children. Metal ankle joints are preferred for adults, particularly heavy adults. Newer designs have a single midline posterior pin/spring mechanism. *Hinging an AFO adds mediolateral stability.* The leg component should encompass three-quarters of the leg and should be padded along its internal surface. The proximal extent should end 1 inch below the fibular neck to prevent compressive common peroneal nerve palsy.

Solid Plastic Ankle-Foot Orthoses. The term *solid* refers to an AFO that is made of a single piece of plastic. It does not have ankle joints. However, the trim line of the AFO will determine the level of flexibility and control at the ankle. Anterior trim lines (anterior to the medial malleolus) are the most rigid (but still flexible enough to allow some ankle motion), whereas posterior trim lines (behind the medial malleolus) provide some flexibility (with little or no mediolateral control).

Solid AFOs set at 90 degrees are commonly used for foot drop. The AFO can be fixed in a few degrees of plantar flexion to provide stability at the knee during the stance phase of gait. Genu recurvatum can also be treated with a solid AFO. The more rigid the AFO, the greater the flexion moment at the knee at heel strike. The flexion moment at the knee becomes even greater during midstance if the ankle is placed in a few degrees of dorsiflexion.

Plastic Ankle-Foot Orthoses Varus-Valgus Control (eSlide 12.6). A three-point system is used to provide the counterforces necessary to oppose the forces of the deformity. An equinovarus (or inversion) deformity is controlled by applying forces medially at the metatarsal head area and calcaneus. The third force is applied more proximally along the lateral aspect of the distal fibula. A more proximal medial tibial force is applied to stabilize the leg portion of the plastic AFO by providing an opposing force to the fibular area. It is reversed for valgus control.

PATELLAR TENDON–BEARING ANKLE-FOOT ORTHOSES (eSlide 12.7)

A patellar tendon–bearing (PTB) AFO uses the patellar tendon and tibial condyles to partially relieve weight-bearing stress on skeletal structures distally, with more weight bearing distributed along the medial tibial condyle. PTB is actually a misnomer because only approximately 10% of the weight is distributed along the patellar tendon and medial tibial condyle. Most of the weight bearing is distributed throughout the soft tissues of the leg that are compressed by an appropriately fitted orthosis. PTB AFOs are often prescribed for diabetic ulcerations of the foot, tibial fractures, painful heel conditions (such as calcaneal fractures), ankle fusions in the postoperative period, Charcot joint, and avascular necrosis of the foot or ankle.

CHARCOT RESTRAINT ORTHOTIC WALKER BOOT (eSlide 12.7)

The Charcot restraint orthotic walker (CROW) boot is a custom-molded bivalve plastic AFO that accommodates the entire foot and leg up to the knee for the purpose of off-loading a plantar ulcer or stabilizing the progressive deformity from the Charcot joint of the foot and ankle. The device has a rocker bottom and rubber sole for indoor and outdoor ambulation.

PRESSURE RELIEF ANKLE-FOOT ORTHOSES

A pressure relief AFO (PRAFO) serves the following two purposes: pressure relief (avoiding pressures at the heel and malleoli) and contracture prevention at the immobilized or motionless lower limb.

Common Ankle-Foot Orthosis Prescriptions (see eSlide 12.5)

The most common AFO prescription for foot drop is a posterior leaf spring AFO, but for associated significant subtalar joint instability, a hinged plastic AFO with metal double-action ankle joints with springs in the posterior channels or a hinged, spring-loaded midline posterior stop AFO may be a better option.

For plantar spasticity, common prescriptions include either a hinged custom plastic AFO with a single midline posterior stop or a hinged custom plastic AFO with pins in the posterior channels to provide a plantar stop at 90 degrees. Permitting dorsiflexion allows a more normalized gait and provides a therapeutic stretch to the plantar flexors. Prefabricated carbon fiber AFOs are also available. The advantages of carbon fiber AFOs are lighter weight, lower profile footplate, and ability to provide some dynamic response or propulsion to substitute for weak plantar flexors.

For lumbar spinal cord injury, the typical AFO prescription is a bilateral custom plastic ground reaction (anterior tibial shell closing) AFO that is fixed in 10 degrees of plantar flexion. The plantar flexion creates knee extension moments with weight bearing to add stability to the knees during ambulation.

Checkout

The patient should be examined after fitting and using the orthosis to verify gait improvement and ease of donning and doffing. When the orthosis is off, the skin should be carefully observed for areas of breakdown.

• KNEE-ANKLE-FOOT ORTHOSES

The components of KAFOs include knee joints, knee locks, thigh uprights, and proximal thigh bands. KAFOs are used in patients with severe knee extensor and hamstring weakness, structural knee instability, or knee flexion spasticity.

Knee Joints (eSlides 12.8 and 12.9)

There are three basic types of knee joints. The straight set knee joint provides rotation about a single axis. It allows free flexion but prevents hyperextension. It is often used in combination with a drop lock. The polycentric knee joint uses a double-axis system to simulate the flexion-extension movements of the femur and tibia at the knee joint. It also adds bulk to the orthosis. It is most frequently used in sport knee orthoses. The third type of knee joint is the posterior offset knee joint. It is prescribed for patients with weak knee extensors and some hip extensor strength. It helps keep the orthotic ground reactive force in front of the knee axis during stance. If additional knee stability is needed, the ankle component of the KAFO can also be set at 10–15 degrees of plantar flexion.

Knee Locks (eSlide 12.10)

There are four common types of knee locks. The ratchet lock has recently become the most commonly prescribed knee lock. It has a catching mechanism that operates in 12-degree increments. It has an element of safety because it keeps the gains made toward extension as the user rises from a seated to standing position. Knee flexion is achieved either by pressing down on a release lever or by sliding the locking mechanism. The drop lock (ring lock) is commonly used in both the medial and lateral uprights of the KAFO. Its advantage is simplicity of design without bulk. However, fine motor coordination skills are needed to lock and unlock the knee in complete extension. The bail lock (also known as the Swiss, French, Schweitzer, or pawl lock) provides the easiest method of simultaneously unlocking the medial and lateral knee joints of a KAFO. Two hands can be used for two bail locks. The locking mechanism is spring loaded to assist locking the knee in extension.

The dial lock (formerly known as a turn buckle) is used to stabilize the knee in varying amounts of flexion. It can be adjusted in 6-degree increments and is more precise for management of a knee with a flexion contracture than a KAFO with ratchet locks. Its uses include preventing progression of a flexion contracture or assisting with gradual reduction of a flexion contracture.

Thigh and Calf Components of a Knee-Ankle-Foot Orthosis

The thigh and calf bands can consist of either padded metal bands or molded plastics, but they need to be wide enough to adequately distribute the pressure for comfort.

Scott-Craig Orthosis

The Scott-Craig orthosis was designed for patients with paraplegia who have a complete lesion at L1 or higher. The orthotic design consists of an offset knee joint with a bail lock and an ankle with a dorsiflexion stop and a posterior stop set at 90 degrees.

Stance Control Orthosis

The stance control KAFO is designed to lock the knee in the stance phase and allow knee flexion in the swing phase of gait. This category of KAFOs is still evolving, but currently, there are several orthotic manufacturers that offer stance control knee joints in centrally fabricated KAFOs.

• KNEE ORTHOSES (eSlide 12.11)

Swedish Knee Cage

The knee orthosis (KO) known as a Swedish knee cage is used to control minor to moderate genu recurvatum. The Swedish knee cage uses a classic three-point orthotic system. Severe genu recurvatum might need to be controlled with longer lever arms, such as those offered by a KAFO.

Osteoarthritis Knee Orthoses

Osteoarthritis KOs are commonly used in patients with medial compartment narrowing. The three-point system distribution is achieved by a strap that is applied across the knee joint. The foot orthosis with a lateral buildup is considered to be the preferred first-line orthotic treatment for osteoarthritis of the knee.

Sport Knee Orthoses

Sport KOs can be divided into prophylactic, rehabilitative, and functional categories. Prophylactic knee bracing attempts to prevent or reduce the severity of knee injuries. Rehabilitative knee bracing is used to allow protected motion within defined limits. It is useful for postoperative and conservative management of knee injuries, such as anterior cruciate ligament–reconstructed knees and patellofemoral pain syndrome. Functional knee bracing is designed to assist or provide stability for the unstable knee and most commonly to stabilize a laterally subluxing patella or an anterior cruciate ligament–deficient knee.

• PEDIATRIC ORTHOSES (eSlide 12.12)

Caster Cart

The caster cart is used for children with a developmental delay in ambulatory skills. It serves as an initial mobility aid and is most often prescribed for children with spina bifida.

Standing Frame

The age range for initial use of the standing frame is usually 8–15 months. Children who pull themselves up along furniture are typically ready for a standing frame. The standing frame helps balance the body in space and allows free use of the upper limbs for participation in activities.

Parapodium/Swivel Orthosis

A parapodium is an appropriate prescription for children who are unlikely to become functional walkers because of the severity of their impairment. It often complements wheelchair use. It is most commonly prescribed for children between 2.5 and 5 years of age. Ambulation occurs by the child pivoting the hips to swivel one side of the oval-based stand forward and then repeating the same action for the other side. A parapodium is similar to the standing frame, but it has hip and knee joints that can be unlocked to permit sitting.

Reciprocating Gait Orthosis

The purpose of the RGO is to provide contralateral hip extension with ipsilateral hip flexion. The RGO is appropriate for children who have used the standing frame, developed good trunk control and coordination, can safely stand, and are mentally prepared for ambulation. Good upper limb strength, trunk balance, and active hip flexion are important positive variables for ambulation. Spinal cord injury level is not a very reliable predictor of ambulation capability in children. The RGO is prescribed most commonly for children aged 3–6 years.

• AMBULATION AIDS (eSlide 12.13)

The purpose of using ambulation aids is to increase the area of support. Their proper use requires adequate upper limb strength and coordination. The type of aid needed depends on how much balance and weight-bearing assistance are required. The body weight transmission for a unilateral cane opposite the affected side is 20%–25%. It is 40%–50% with the use of a forearm or arm cane. Body weight transmission with bilateral crutches is estimated to be up to 80%.

Aids include canes such as C canes and quad canes. Canes are used on the side opposite the supporting lower limb. A walker provides maximum support for the patient but also necessitates a slow gait. A crutch is defined as a device that provides support from the axilla to the floor. Nonaxillary crutches include the Lofstrand forearm orthosis, Kenny stick, Everett or Warm Springs crutch, Canadian crutch, platform forearm orthosis.

• PRESCRIPTION (Box 12.1)

A medical diagnosis with delineation of the impairment and any resulting disability should be made before an orthotic prescription is written. The orthotic goals should be documented for the orthotist.

Summary Reference for Prescription Pad

BOX 12.1

FOOT ORTHOSIS
- University of California Biomechanics Laboratory: Hyperpronating "flat" foot
- Metatarsal pad: Temporary mild to moderate metatarsalgia
- Metatarsal bar to shoe: Severe metatarsalgia (cannot stand in shoe) or permanent metatarsalgia (e.g., arthritis)
- Heel lift: Temporary use for Achilles tendinitis or plantar fasciitis
- Heel cup: Fat pad syndrome (heel bruise)
- Lateral heel wedge: Osteoarthritis with medial compartment narrowing

ANKLE-FOOT ORTHOSIS
- *Over-the-counter:* For a trial basis only
- *Custom:* For long-term use
- *Plastic:* For almost everyone
- *Metal:* For patients weighing >250 lb with a hinged ankle-foot orthosis

Common Types
- Custom solid (flexible) ankle-foot orthosis set at 90 degrees: Foot drop
- Custom solid (rigid) ankle-foot orthosis set at 90 degrees: Plantar spasticity

Hinge Indications
- Significant mediolateral instability at subtalar joint but patient with ankle dorsiflexion and plantar flexion (rare).
- Tight plantar flexors in patients with spasticity and improving lower limb function (they can take advantage of a more "normal" gait via dorsiflexion from midstance to toe-off, and plantar stretching is therapeutic over this part of the gait cycle).
- An active patient with foot drop or plantar flexor spasticity can take advantage of the hinged feature during stair climbing, rising from sit to stand, frequent walking, etc.

KNEE-ANKLE-FOOT ORTHOSIS

Knee Type
- *Straight set:* Most common; always used unless posterior offset is indicated

Continued

Summary Reference for Prescription Pad—cont'd

- *Posterior offset:* Patient with weak knee extensor triad (quadriceps, plantar flexors, and hamstrings)
- *Polycentric:* A two-joint system that theoretically simulates femur-tibia translation
  - Standard on most sport orthoses for the above marketing purpose
  - No clear-cut indications

Knee Locks
- *Ratchet lock:* Most common
- *Drop lock:* Can be difficult to pull up after "settling in" from walking
- *Bail lock:* Bulkier and less desirable than drop locks for most patients but necessary for those without fine hand control
- *Dial lock:* Used to lock an unstable knee in extension but adjusted to account for knee flexion contractures

Hip Joints (common to prescribe one of each of the following)
- *Standard:* Allows flexion and extension
- *Abduction:* Permits flexion and extension but also permits abduction to allow self-catheterization of the urinary bladder and seating in a hip-flexed and abducted position

• SUMMARY

An appropriate lower limb orthotic prescription requires a thorough biomechanical analysis of gait and knowledge of the available orthotic components available to treat specific conditions. The prescribing physician should maintain a close working relationship with the certified orthotist to ensure that the patient is receiving the best orthotic option available.

Clinical Pearls

1. Control of the subtalar joint in a neutral position is important in most foot orthoses.
2. Rotation at the subtalar joint is also accompanied by rotation of the tibia (i.e., foot pronation is accompanied by tibial internal rotation and vice versa).
3. In an AFO, ankle plantar flexion creates a knee extension moment and ankle dorsiflexion creates a knee flexion moment.
4. A cushioned heel in an AFO can add stability to the knee immediately after heel strike by moving the ground reaction force anteriorly.
5. KAFO often complements the use of wheelchairs in functional and therapeutic walking.
6. Spinal cord injury level is not a very reliable predictor of ambulation capability in children.

BIBLIOGRAPHY
The complete bibliography is available on ExpertConsult.com.

Spinal Orthoses

13

Wai-Keung Lee

The primary goals of spinal orthoses are to aid a weakened muscle group, correct a deformed body part, and maintain the stability of a fractured spine. The orthosis can protect a body part from further injury or can correct the position of a body part. Technology has revamped the field of orthotics, with newer orthoses that are stronger and lighter.

• HISTORY OF SPINAL ORTHOTIC MANAGEMENT (eSlide 13.1)

The first evidence of the use of spinal orthoses can be traced back to Galen (c. AD 131–201). Primitive orthotic devices were made of items that were readily available during this period.

• TERMINOLOGY OF SPINAL ORTHOSES (eSlide 13.2)

The most standard way to name an orthosis is by the joints that it encompasses and the motion it controls.

• PREFABRICATED OR CUSTOM ORTHOSES

Orthoses can be prefabricated to fit a large variety of patients of various sizes and can be fitted to patients often with little or no adjustment. Orthoses that are custom molded to a specific patient provide a more comfortable fit with a higher degree of control and can be designed to accommodate a patient's unique body shape or deformities.

• ORTHOTIC PRESCRIPTION

Orthotic prescription should include the following items: patient identifiers, date, date the orthosis is needed, diagnosis, functional goal, orthosis description, and precautions. Prescriptions should include a justification for the orthosis, such as to correct alignment, decrease pain, or improve function. Established acronyms are acceptable [e.g., TLSO (thoracolumbosacral orthosis)]. Detailed descriptions of the orthoses, joints involved, and functional goals are important. Before the prescription is finalized, inputs from the patient, physician, therapist, and orthotist are needed. It is especially important for physicians to review the use or lack of use of past orthoses because this will help in writing the new prescription. It enables improved communication among clinicians and serves as a justification for funding the orthosis.

• SPINAL ANATOMY

The vertebral column not only bears the weight of the body but also allows motion between body parts and serves to protect the spinal cord from injury.

The three-column stability concept includes (1) the anterior column consisting of the anterior longitudinal ligament, annulus fibrosus, and anterior half of the vertebral body; (2) the middle column consisting of the posterior longitudinal ligament, annulus fibrosus, and posterior half of the vertebral body; and (3) the posterior column consisting of the interspinous and supraspinous ligaments, facet joints, laminas, pedicles, and spinous processes. It reveals that if the middle column and either the anterior or posterior column are compromised, the spine may be unstable. This concept helps to ensure that a proper orthosis is prescribed.

Spine motion can be classified with reference to the horizontal, frontal, and sagittal planes (eSlide 13.3).

In the cervical spine, extension occurs predominantly at the occipital-C1 junction. Lateral bending mainly occurs at the C3-C4 and C4-C5 levels. Axial rotation occurs mostly at the C1-C2 level. In the thoracic spine, flexion and extension occur primarily at the T11-T12 and T12-L1 levels. Lateral bending is fairly evenly distributed throughout the thoracic levels. Axial rotation occurs mostly at the T1-T2 level, with a gradual decrease toward the lumbar spine. In the lumbar spinal segment, movement in the sagittal plane occurs more at the distal segment, with lateral bending predominantly at the L3-L4 level. There is insignificant axial rotation in the lumbar spinal segments. Range of motion helps in understanding how the various cervical orthoses can limit that range (eSlide 13.4).

Soft collars provide very little restriction in any plane. The Philadelphia collar mostly limits flexion and extension. The four-poster brace has better restriction, especially for flexion-extension and rotation. The halo brace and Minerva body jacket have the most restriction in all planes of motion.

The coupling phenomenon that is related to movement in the spine occurs during motion. If the movement along one axis is consistently associated with movement around another axis, coupling occurs (eSlide 13.5).

• DESCRIPTION OF ORTHOSES

Head Cervicothoracic Orthoses
TYPE: HALO ORTHOSIS (eSlide 13.6)
Biomechanics. This orthosis provides flexion, extension, and rotational control of the cervical region. Pressure systems are used for control of motion, as well as to provide slight distraction for immobilization of the cervical spine.

Design and Fabrication. The halo orthosis consists of prefabricated components, such as halo rings, pins, uprights (or superstructures), and vests. The design is used to effectively immobilize the cervical spine. It provides maximum restriction of motion of all the cervical orthoses. A halo is used for approximately 3 months (10-12 weeks) to ensure healing of a fracture or spinal fusion. All pins on the halo ring should be checked to ensure tightness 24–48 hours after application and retorqued if necessary.

Cervical Orthoses
TYPE: PHILADELPHIA, MIAMI J, AND ASPEN COLLARS (eSlide 13.6)
Biomechanics. These orthoses provide some control of flexion, extension, and lateral bending, as well as minimal rotational control of the cervical region. Pressure

systems are used for control of motion, as well as to provide slight distraction for immobilization of the cervical spine. Circumferential pressure is also intended to provide warmth and act as a kinesthetic reminder for the patient.

Design and Fabrication. These orthoses are prefabricated and consist of one or two pieces that are usually attached with Velcro straps. The anterior aspect supports the mandible and rests on the superior edge of the sternum. The posterior aspect of the collar supports the head at the occipital level.

TYPE: SOFT CERVICAL COLLAR
The soft collar is usually used as a kinesthetic reminder for patients to limit their neck motion. It does not provide any mechanical restriction to the head motion. It can provide some warmth and comfort for patients with muscle strain.

Cervicothoracic Orthoses
TYPE: STERNAL OCCIPITAL MANDIBULAR IMMOBILIZER (eSlide 13.7)
Biomechanics. The sternal occipital mandibular immobilizer (SOMI) provides control of flexion, extension, lateral bending, and rotation of the cervical spine. Pressure systems are used for control of motion, as well as to provide slight distraction for immobilization of the spine. It can be donned while the patient is in the supine position (which is useful for patients who are restricted to bed) because there are no posterior rods to interfere with the comfort of the patient. A headband can be added so that the chin piece can be removed. This maintains stability but improves accessibility for daily hygiene and eating.

Design and Fabrication. The SOMI is prefabricated and consists of a cervical portion with a removable chin piece and bars that curve over the shoulders. The anterior section supports the mandible and rests on the superior edge of the sternum, with the inferior anterior edge terminating at the level of the xiphoid. The posterior aspect of the orthosis supports the head at the occipital level.

FOUR-POSTER ORTHOSIS
This is a rigid cervical orthosis with anterior and posterior sections that consist of pads that lie on the chest and are connected by leather straps. The struts on the anterior and posterior sections are adjustable in height. Straps are used to connect the occipital and mandibular support pieces by over-the-shoulder method.

Cervicothoracolumbosacral Orthoses
TYPE: MILWAUKEE ORTHOSIS
Biomechanics. The Milwaukee orthosis provides control of flexion, extension, and lateral bending of the cervical, thoracic, and lumbar spine. It also provides some rotational control of the thoracic and lumbar spine. Pressure systems are used for control of motion, as well as to provide correction of the spine. It is a good choice for patients who need correction in the higher thoracic region of the spine.

Design and Fabrication. This orthosis is custom-made and consists of a cervical portion with the option of a removable cervical ring. There is also a thoracolumbar section, which helps achieve the correction of the lower thoracic and lumbar spine regions.

Indications. The Milwaukee orthosis is used primarily for scoliosis management of the higher thoracic curves along with thoracic and lumbar curves of the spine.

Contraindications. This orthosis is not indicated for lower thoracic and lumbar curves. With lower thoracic and lumbar curves, a thoracolumbar orthosis could be used, without using a cervical component.

Thoracolumbosacral Orthoses

TYPE: THORACOLUMBOSACRAL ORTHOSIS (PREFABRICATED) (eSlide 13.8)

Biomechanics. Prefabricated TLSO provides control of flexion, extension, lateral bending, and rotation using a three-point pressure system and circumferential compression.

Design and Fabrication. These orthoses can be designed in modular forms, with anterior and posterior sections connected by padded lateral panels and fastened with Velcro straps or pulley systems. Many of these orthoses are covered in breathable fabric and have varieties of different shapes and options, such as sternal pads or shoulder straps.

TYPE: THORACOLUMBOSACRAL ORTHOSIS (CUSTOM-FABRICATED BODY JACKET) (eSlide 13.8)

Biomechanics. This type of TLSO provides control of flexion, extension, lateral bending, and rotation using the three-point pressure system and circumferential compression.

Design and Fabrication. This orthosis is molded to fit the patient and designed as per the patient's needs. Anterior and posterior trim lines are adjusted during fitting to allow patients to sit comfortably and use their arms as much as possible without compromising the function of the orthosis.

TYPE: CRUCIFORM ANTERIOR SPINAL HYPEREXTENSION THORACOLUMBOSACRAL ORTHOSIS (eSlide 13.9)

Biomechanics. The cruciform anterior spinal hyperextension (CASH) TLSO provides flexion control for the lower thoracic and lumbar regions via the three-point pressure system. The system consists of posteriorly directed forces through sternal and suprapubic pads and an anteriorly directed force applied through a thoracolumbar pad attached to a strap that extends to the horizontal anterior bar.

Design and Fabrication. This orthosis is prefabricated and consists of an anterior frame in the form of a cross, from which pads are attached laterally on a horizontal bar and at the sternal and suprapubic areas. When properly fitted, the sternal pad is 0.5 inch below the sternal notch, and the suprapubic pad is 0.5 inch above the symphysis pubis.

TYPE: JEWETT HYPEREXTENSION THORACOLUMBOSACRAL ORTHOSIS (eSlide 13.10)

Biomechanics. This type of TLSO provides flexion control for the lower thoracic and lumbar regions via the three-point pressure system that consists of posteriorly directed forces through sternal and suprapubic pads and an anteriorly directed force applied through a thoracolumbar pad attached to a strap that extends to the lateral uprights.

Design and Fabrication. This orthosis is prefabricated and consists of an anterior and lateral frame to which the pads are attached laterally on and at the sternal and suprapubic areas. The Jewett TLSO has more lateral support than the CASH TLSO.

TYPE: TAYLOR AND KNIGHT-TAYLOR THORACOLUMBOSACRAL ORTHOSES

Biomechanics. These TLSOs provide control of flexion, extension, and a minimal amount of axial rotation by means of the three-point pressure system for each direction of motion. For example, flexion is controlled by the posteriorly directed forces applied through the axillary straps and abdominal apron and an anteriorly directed force through the paraspinal uprights.

Design and Fabrication. The design of the Taylor orthosis consists of two paraspinal uprights extending to the spine of the scapula and a series of straps from the paraspinal to pelvic regions. A posterior pelvic band extends past the midsagittal plane and across the sacral area. This band provides additional lateral support and motion control to the trunk.

Indications. These orthoses are used for postsurgical support of traumatic fractures, spondylolisthesis, scoliosis, spinal stenosis, herniated disks, and disk infections.

Contraindications. They are contraindicated for unstable fractures that require maximum stabilization.

Special Considerations. The pressure per square inch is high for these orthoses because of the width of the bands and uprights.

Lumbosacral Orthoses
TYPE: LUMBOSACRAL CORSET (eSlide 13.11)
Biomechanics. The lumbosacral corset provides anterior and lateral trunk containment and assists in elevating intraabdominal pressure. Restriction of flexion and extension can be achieved with the addition of steel straps posteriorly.

Design and Fabrication. This orthosis is usually made from a cloth that wraps around the torso and hips. Adjustments are made with laces on the sides, back, or front. Custom corsets can be fabricated on the basis of careful measurements of the individual patient.

TYPE: LUMBOSACRAL CHAIRBACK ORTHOSES (eSlide 13.12)
Biomechanics. These orthoses provide limitation of flexion, extension, and lateral flexion. They also provide elevation of intraabdominal pressure.

Design and Fabrication. These types of orthoses have pelvic and thoracic bands that are connected by two paraspinal uprights posteriorly and a lateral upright on each side at the midsagittal line. They can be fabricated from a traditional aluminum frame that is covered in leather or thermoplastic material molded into the same shape.

Sacroiliac Orthoses
TYPE: SACROILIAC ORTHOSIS OR SACRAL ORTHOSIS
Biomechanics. This type of orthosis provides anterior and lateral trunk containment and assists in restriction of some pelvic flexion and extension. It also aids in

compression of the pelvis.

Design and Fabrication. This orthosis is usually made from a cloth that wraps around the pelvis and hips. Custom orthoses can be fabricated based on careful measurements of the individual patient.

Indications. This orthosis is most frequently prescribed as a support for patients with pelvic fractures or symphysis pubis fractures or strains. It is useful to control motion and pain.

Contraindications. This type of orthosis should not be used for unstable fractures and for fractures or other conditions in the lumbar region.

• SCOLIOSIS

Patients with idiopathic scoliosis, the most common form of scoliosis, should be evaluated to ensure that they do not have anomalous vertebrae, spinal tumors, or other neurologic abnormalities. Progressive curves need to be treated; nutritional supplementation, exercise, or chiropractic treatment may be appropriate. There is strong evidence to indicate that an orthosis can slow the progression of idiopathic scoliosis, and therefore use of an orthosis is the nonoperative treatment of choice. Juvenile idiopathic scoliosis is more likely to be associated with adult cor pulmonale and death. Treatment should begin when curves reach approximately 25 degrees. Because thoracic curves predominate, a Milwaukee brace, which has the pelvic section in close contact with the iliac crest and lumbar spine, might be more effective than a TLSO. Three uprights (one anterior and two posterior) typically connect to a neck ring, throat mold, and occipital pad. The Boston brace uses symmetric standardized modules, eliminating the need for casting. It extends from below the breast to the beginning of the pelvic area and below the scapulae posteriorly. It maintains flexion of the lumbar area by increasing pressure on the abdomen and is a popular TLSO brace. Adolescent idiopathic scoliosis is the most common type of scoliosis for which an orthosis is indicated, usually for curves between 25 and 45 degrees. Curves with an apex at T9 or lower can be managed with a TLSO. Curves with a higher apex require a Milwaukee brace. Single lumbar curves are treated with a lumbosacral orthosis.

Type: Thoracolumbosacral Low-Profile Scoliosis Orthoses (eSlide 13.13)

BOSTON BRACE, MIAMI ORTHOSIS, AND WILMINGTON BRACE
Biomechanics. These orthoses provide dynamic action using three principles (end-point control, transverse loading, and curve correction) to prevent curve progression and stabilize the spine.

Design and Fabrication. The main use of these orthoses or other devices is to halt the curve progression of structural scoliosis. The Milwaukee orthosis is the most popular orthosis for scoliosis. The effectiveness of any orthotic system depends on compliance with the wearing schedule. Most patients should wear the orthosis 23–24 hours per day for it to be effective.

• EMERGING TECHNOLOGY

Computer-Aided Design and Computer-Aided Manufacturing

Technology is available to help the practitioner improve efficiency in design and fabrication, as well as reduce the invasiveness of orthotic measurements of patients. The BioScanner BioSculptor, one of the computer-aided design (CAD)/computer-aided manufacturing (CAM) systems (eSlide 13.14), enables accurate measurement and detailed surface information, which is often not provided with a cast or mechanical digitizer. The digital scans may be easily recalled or modified for rapid refitting, and medical justification of new devices can be given by showing volumetric changes.

Bone Stimulation (eSlide 13.15)

The CMF SpinaLogic bone growth stimulator is a portable, battery-powered, micro-controlled, noninvasive bone growth stimulator indicated for adjunct electromagnetic treatment after primary lumbar spinal fusion surgery at one or two levels.

Three-Dimensional Clinical Ultrasound

Recent advances in three-dimensional clinical ultrasound have allowed estimation of the spinous process angle (SPA) in patients with adolescent idiopathic scoliosis. This in turn has been able to provide orthotists with a fast and safe method to assess the SPA in real time and determine the optimal placement of pressure pads to maximize the effectiveness of the orthosis in correcting the spinal deformity.

• SUMMARY

Proper prescription, construction, and fitting of a spinal orthosis are complicated processes that require consideration of biomechanics, designs and fabrications, indications, and contraindications. A complete, clear, and agreed plan of care should be constructed. The patient and experienced, knowledgeable providers (including the orthotist, rehabilitation physician, and therapist) working in a team approach provide the maximum likelihood that an orthosis will contribute to the overall therapeutic goals for the patient. Advanced technology is available to help practitioners improve the efficiency of orthosis design and fabrication.

Clinical Pearls

Spinal orthoses can stabilize the spine after fracture (with or without neurologic deficit), limit spinal motion, prevent and protect susceptible areas, support posture, prevent deformity, assist and improve motion, and correct and align deformities. We need to know the indications and contraindications and special considerations of each type of spinal orthosis before prescription because they may interfere with the patient.

BIBLIOGRAPHY
The complete bibliography is available on ExpertConsult.com.

14 Wheelchairs and Seating Systems

Nazirah Hasnan

A team-based care approach that involves an interdisciplinary team of rehabilitation professionals, patients, and relevant family members or caregivers should be implemented to address issues such as assessment, prescription, training, product delivery, and functional outcomes of a wheelchair user.

• MEDICAL AND PHYSICAL ASSESSMENT

The physiatrist's role includes assessing, documenting, and sharing with the team the underlying medical conditions that require a prescription for a wheelchair. Factors to be considered include patient's age, disease prognosis, pain, obesity, cardiopulmonary or musculoskeletal problems, genitourinary or gastrointestinal problems, alterations in mental status, overall cognitive capacity, and risk for falls. Potential risks and secondary injuries, such as pressure ulcers, postural deformities, or upper limb repetitive strain injuries, associated with the use of equipment must also be assessed and considered. Comprehensive assessment includes physical-motor assessment of strength, range of movement, coordination, balance, posture, tone, contracture, endurance, sitting posture, trunk stability, cognition, perception, and use of external orthoses. Assessment of pelvic alignment is crucial because the pelvis serves as the base of all seating supports. Pelvic obliquities and spinal deformities need to be accommodated to facilitate sitting tolerance. The individual's preference for different seated postures, even if they do not appear to be technically correct, must be considered. Other crucial measurements include hip and knee range of movement, especially when seated.

Functional Assessment

Functional mobility assessments in the areas of self-care, reach, access to surfaces at various heights, transfer to various surfaces, and functional mobility in the user's natural environment should be incorporated in the overall assessment as the clinical setting is often very different from the natural or home setting.

Environmental Assessment

The user's role, interest, responsibility, and occupation in his or her environment need to be understood in the assessment and prescription process. Physical accessibilities within the home, work, school, or other areas of the community often have a major impact on the feasibility of wheelchair and seating system options. A thorough assessment and survey of the home, usability of the equipment in the occupational environment, and identification of barriers and facilitators is warranted when determining which mobility equipment options are most appropriate for the user.

• ASSESSMENT TOOLS

Anthropometrics

Rehabilitation professionals use calipers, rigid and soft tape measures, goniometers, scales, and digital cameras for comprehensive anthropometric measurements. These measurements are then translated into specific dimensions of the wheelchair and seating system.

Propulsion Analysis

Propulsion analysis is crucial for maintaining the long-term health of an individual by minimizing the likelihood for the development of upper limb pain and injury. Assessment tools include the wheelchair propulsion test using a stopwatch; tape measure; clinical observation; the SmartWheel protocol that uses force, torque, and distance-measuring pushrims; and clinical observation.

Pressure Analysis (eSlide 14.1)

Pressure analysis is used to set up the seating system, train individuals on proper pressure-relieving techniques (through biofeedback mechanisms), compare seating systems, and document the change in sitting tolerance over time. In addition to clinical observations and impressions, a pressure mapping system is used to provide a quantitative mechanism for measuring the pressure-relieving properties so that the likelihood of developing pressure ulcers and postural deformities is minimized.

Wheelchair Skills

The wheelchair skills test provides a quantitative method for assessing the ability of an individual to use a wheelchair in all domains of mobility and activities of daily living. Wheelchair skills assessment is important in determining the appropriate type of mobility, whether a person has the physical and cognitive capacity to use a wheelchair, and for training on the proper use of the wheelchair and seating system.

• WHEELED MOBILITY DEVICES

There is a wide range of wheeled mobility devices, which can be divided into manual, powered, hybrid, and scooter types. The key features, indications, contraindications for use, and the available technologies are described below and in the accompanying tables and eSlides.

Manual Wheelchairs (eSlide 14.2)

Manual wheelchairs for daily use are often categorized by their design features and costs. The standard wheelchair is designed for short-term hospital or institutional use and is not recommended as a primary mode of mobility. A "hemi" wheelchair enables lowering of the seat-to-floor height to allow people to propel their wheelchair with their feet. Lightweight wheelchairs are designed for long-term use by individuals who spend less than a couple of hours each day in a wheelchair. Pediatric wheelchairs may have adjustable frames or kits for accommodating the growth of the child. Active, full-time users with good upper limb function and endurance should use ultralight wheelchairs. Hybrid wheelchairs are available for people with impaired upper limb function or endurance or those who require frequent use of ramps or hilly terrain.

Basic Wheelchair Components and Anatomical Dimensions (eSlide 14.3)

Accurate anatomic measurement has a direct impact on the overall assessment and prescription of the wheelchair and seating support system. Maximizing the mobility of an individual while he or she is using the wheelchair and seating system is dependent on properly matching the anatomic dimensions of the person to the wheelchair dimensions. The seat should be high enough to accommodate enough space under the footrests to clear obstacles and should have enough knee clearance to fit under tables, counters and sinks, as well as have steering wheels or hand controls for those who drive. Adequate seat depth and width are needed to support the thighs and the widest part of the buttocks to prevent high sitting pressures and development of pressure ulcers behind the knees, calves, and pelvic bony prominences. The backrest should be low enough to provide adequate postural support but still allow the upper limbs to have good access to the pushrims for effective wheelchair propelling. Ideally, backrests should allow attachment of different types of back supports. Correct armrest height is important to allow good support to the upper limbs and shoulders, as well as provide good access to the pushrims.

Adjustments and Customization

The main advantage of using ultra-lightweight wheelchairs over other wheelchair types is their high degree of adjustability and customization, which results in optimization of wheelchair fit and propulsion biomechanics.

SEAT AND BACK ANGLE ADJUSTMENTS

Seat and back angle adjustments, separately or together, optimize the postural support and comfort for an individual. Adjusting the seat so that it slopes downward toward the rear of the wheelchair (seat dump) can assist people with limited trunk control by stabilizing their pelvis and spine, making it easier to propel the wheelchair. It can decrease extensor tone and posturing. However, excess seat dump increases pressure on the sacrum, increases the risk for skin breakdown, and makes it more difficult to transfer into and out of the wheelchair. An increased back angle or a reclined back might be needed when the person's hips do not flex well or gravity is needed to assist with balancing the trunk.

REAR WHEEL CAMBER (eSlide 14.4)

Camber is the angle the wheel makes from the vertical axis. Most wheelchairs generally do not have more than 8 degrees of camber.

REAR AXLE POSITION

The placement of rear wheels relative to an individual's upper limbs directly affects propulsion biomechanics and therefore the likelihood of upper limb pain and injury.

HORIZONTAL AND VERTICAL AXLE POSITIONS (eSlide 14.5)

A more forward axle position requires less muscle effort because rolling resistance is decreased when more weight is distributed over the larger rear wheels than over the smaller front casters. This position also facilitates performing a "wheelie," negotiating obstacles, and ascending or descending curbs. Because of the effects on stability, the axle should be moved forward incrementally with input from the wheelchair user. Adding weight to the chair can also affect stability and maneuverability of the wheelchair. Therefore packages or backpacks should ideally be located underneath the seat of the wheelchair. A lower seat position can improve propulsion biomechanics by increasing hand contact with the pushrims, thereby lowering stroke frequency and increasing mechanical efficiency and stability of the wheelchair. If the seat height is too low, however, the patient has to push with the shoulders abducted, which increases the risk for shoulder impingement.

AMPUTEE AXLE

People with lower limb amputations might need to have their axles adjusted farther back than those without amputations to increase the stability of the wheelchair. This is because of the loss of the counterbalancing weight of the lower limbs. However, a rearward axle position can have serious negative effects on shoulder biomechanics.

Power Wheelchairs (eSlides 14.6 and 14.7)

Power wheelchairs provide a flexible platform for mobility when a manual wheelchair or power-assist wheelchair no longer meets the unique characteristics of an individual (Table 14.1). Power wheelchairs can be grouped into four broad categories on the basis of their features and intended use. The power drive wheel location must be appropriate for the user's lifestyle and environment. The mobility of an individual is optimized by aligning his or her needs with the characteristics of each configuration.

Input Methods and Programmability (eSlide 14.8)

The most common input device is a joystick that is programmed for proportional control. If an individual cannot use a joystick, alternative controls include mechanical switches, pneumatic switches, fiber optic sensors, and proximity sensors, which are placed at the head, chin, or foot.

Wheelchair Performance (eSlide 14.9)

Wheelchairs that are less prone to failure are safer for the users. It is reported that component failures and engineering factors are responsible for 40%–60% of the injuries to power wheelchair users.

TABLE 14.1 Types of Power Wheelchairs

	Features	Indications	Disadvantages
Basic power wheelchairs	Simple electronics Standard proportional compact joystick For indoor use: small wheelchair footprint (i.e., area connecting the four wheels) for greater maneuverability in confined spaces	For light use on indoor surfaces Appropriate for limited indoor use for individuals with a short-term disability who have good trunk control and do not need specialized seating	Limited seating options Low quality
Folding and transport-able power wheelchairs	Designed for disassembling to facilitate transport	Typically used by individuals with reasonably good trunk and upper body control	Might not have the stability or power to negotiate obstacles outdoors

Continued

TABLE 14.1 Types of Power Wheelchairs—cont'd

	Features	Indications	Disadvantages
Combination indoor–outdoor power wheelchairs	Support simple to advanced controllers, a wide range of input devices (e.g., proportional and non-proportional), and power seating options (e.g., tilt, recline, leg rests) May incorporate drive wheel suspension to reduce road vibrations May be equipped with rehabilitation seating, which allows for the attachment of modular seating hardware (e.g., backrests, cushions, laterals, hip guides, and headrests)	For individuals with long-term disabilities Designed for use on indoor surfaces and finished surfaces (e.g., sidewalks and driveways) in the community	Bulky
All-terrain power wheelchairs	More powerful motors, drive wheel suspensions, large-diameter drive wheels with heavily treaded tires, or four-drive wheels for climbing obstacles and traversing rough terrains Capable of faster speeds and offer greater stability on steeper inclined surfaces	For use by people who live in communities without finished surfaces	Bulky Not suitable for indoor use

Power drive wheel location

Rear-wheel drive	Large drive wheels in the rear and small pivoting casters in the front Rear-wheel drive power wheelchairs steer and handle predictably and naturally track straight Most appropriate drive configuration for high-speed applications	In general, preferred by people who drive with special input devices (e.g., chin joystick and head array) or have reduced fine motor coordination because of its consistent tracking	Limited obstacle climbing by the small front casters Large turning radius
Mid-wheel drive	Drive wheels are located near the center of the power wheelchair Increased indoor maneuverability The most effective drive for both ascending and descending obstacles for skilled, practiced users More compact footprint and a tighter turning radius	For a more active wheelchair user who requires indoor and outdoor capability on uneven terrain	Possibility of getting "stuck" on the front or rear casters, which can suspend the drive wheel in midair with no contact to the ground

TABLE 14.1	Types of Power Wheelchairs—cont'd		
	Features	Indications	Disadvantages
Front-wheel drive	Large drive wheels in the front and small pivoting casters in the rear Very stable setup for uneven terrain and hills Best capability to climb forward over small obstacles Overall, turning radius is smaller than that of rear-wheel drive but larger than that of the mid-wheel drive power base	For a more active wheelchair user who requires out-door capability on an uneven terrain	Earlier models had a tendency for the back of the chair to wander side-to-side ("fishtailing"), especially with increased speeds

• SEATING PRINCIPLES

Proper positioning of the pelvis and trunk provides a stable base for the upper limbs to prevent upper limb overuse and injury. Without proper base positioning, the head and neck will not be well aligned with the spine. The pelvis should be stabilized on a cushion that provides postural support as well as optimal pressure distribution. The cushion should be mounted on a hard surface that maintains its position. The seating system needs to accommodate the pelvis and trunk in positions other than neutral. Proper positioning and support of the head and neck facilitate proper breathing and swallowing and can prevent excessive strain of the head and neck stabilizer muscles. Tilt and recline systems should always be equipped with a headrest to support the head when adjusting seat orientation and back angles. Additional seating considerations are needed for patients with sensory loss, paralysis or paresis, contractures, or spasticity and high tone.

Wheelchair Seating and Cushions (eSlide 14.10)

Wheelchairs are equipped with a solid seat pan or sling seat. A solid seat pan facilitates long-term performance of the seat cushion. Wheelchair cushions consist of various materials, such as foam, air, gel, and composites. They are divided into five categories: (1) general use cushions, (2) skin protection cushions, (3) positioning cushions, (4) skin protection and positioning cushions, and (5) custom-molded cushions. Comfort, stability, and pressure relief are important factors when selecting a cushion. As a result of tissue compression and circulation impairment, paralysis, loss of pain and pressure sensation, and the inability to relieve pressure increase the likelihood of developing pressure ulcers. Components such as adductor and abductor pads, hip guides, positioning belts, and transfer handles can be added to the wheelchair or cushion for increased postural support.

Back Supports (eSlide 14.11)

Manual chairs are equipped with sling backs, and most power chairs are equipped with seat canes for the attachment of back supports. There are four categories of back supports: (1) general use backs, (2) positioning backs, (3) skin protection and positioning backs, and (4) custom-molded backs. Back supports are typically planar, contour, or custom-made and are available in different varieties, such as foam and combinations of foam plus gel or foam plus air.

Seat Functions (eSlide 14.12)

Tilt and recline functions enable pressure distribution management. Seat elevators improve the reaching capability, increase independence, and enhance social interaction.

Other Wheelchair Essentials (eSlide 14.13)

Other wheelchair essentials that support the user's posture and comfort, ease of use, safety, and stability include armrests, headrests, laterals and harnesses, front riggers, wheels and tires, casters, wheel locks, pushrims, lever devices, and antitippers (Table 14.2). The ability to effectively propel the wheelchair depends on the physical capabilities of an individual; the weight, quality, and setup of the wheelchair; and the propulsion technique. The prescription of these essential items and that of optional and additional items should be discussed with the patient so that an informed decision is made on the basis of the patient's needs.

TABLE 14.2 Wheelchair Essentials

	Function	Type	Features
Armrests	Upper limb support Assist the user's stability	Full length • Allow greater surface for the forearm • Offer more assistance for sit-to-stand activities Desk length • Shorter than full-length armrest • One can get closer to tables	Can be standard leather, breathable materials, or gel pads Attachment points: Single post • Removable armrest Dual post • Swing-away armrest Cantilever armrest • Attached to the back of the chair and can swing behind the wheelchair
Laterals	Provide additional stability in conjunction with back supports	Laterals can be removed or swung away from the wheelchair • This allows the user to have minimal disruption during transfers	Come in various shapes, sizes, and contours
Shoulder harnesses	Designed to provide shoulder retraction and good head control and to correct shoulder rotation		Attach to the top of the wheelchair near the clavicle and at the bottom of the back support near the inferior/posterior aspect of the rib cage

TABLE 14.2   Wheelchair Essentials—cont'd

	Function	Type	Features
Chest harnesses	Provide more support than shoulder harnesses Offer increased support to the trunk Commonly used in driving for stability, but do not replace the occupant restraint system	Can be incorporated into the shoulder harness for full support or attached horizontally across the chest for stability	Single chest harnesses cover the lateral aspect of the chest
Headrests	Functions range from providing minimal head control when an individual tilts a wheelchair to providing maximal head control in all situations	Removable or swing away Removing a headrest is important for transfer and convenient if the headrest is not used at all times	Various shapes and sizes Important to ensure the headrest is providing support and not completely holding the head up
Front rigging: footrests, leg rests, footplates	Provide support for the legs and feet	Footrests can come in options that are removable, flip-up, or rigidly attached to the chair	Footrests and footplates support the feet and leg rests support the calves
Wheels and Tires	Indoor use: • Smooth to lightly treaded skinny tires Outdoor use: • Wider tires with medium knobby tread provide increased traction on rougher surfaces	Mag wheels • Heavier than spoke wheels • More durable, require less maintenance • Newer types can be lighter but are more costly Spoke wheels • Tendency to get out of alignment Pneumatic tires • Smoother ride for indoors or outdoors • Lower rolling resistance • Require more maintenance Solid tires • Plastic or foam • Require less maintenance • Heavier	Factors to consider when choosing the most suitable wheel and tire configuration: • Type of indoor and outdoor terrain • Activity level, maintenance, weight, and cost Most common rear tire diameters: 22, 24, and 26 inches The inner part of the tire or insert can either be air-filled (pneumatic) or solid
Caster wheels	Smaller casters provide for greater foot clearance and agility Larger casters provide the user with more security because they roll over changes in surface height more easily	Casters can be either pneumatic or solid (usually made of polyurethane) • Solid casters not as comfortable	Come in various sizes and configurations Smaller casters • Found on high-performance, ultralight, and sports wheelchairs • More apt to get stuck in cracks and at bumps, causing forward falls

Continued

TABLE 14.2 Wheelchair Essentials—cont'd

	Function	Type	Features
Wheel locks (brakes)	Wheel locks are essential for safety	Come in various styles but basically consist of two levers hinged together	Sometimes the levers are difficult for people to reach or manipulate • Wheel lock extensions can be added to lengthen the lever arm
Pushrims	For wheelchair propelling Accommodate people with limited gripping ability (e.g., low-level cervical injuries)	Larger diameter pushrims or a high-friction surface finish • Pushrims with vertical, horizontal, or angled projections	Pushrims are available in different sizes, shapes, and surface finishes
Lever drives	Propelling with levers versus pushrims has proven to be more mechanically efficient		Well-suited for people who frequently propel long distances and over outdoor terrain
Antitippers	Protect the user from tipping the wheelchair backward		Attach to the rear of the wheelchair frame and usually have adjustable length tubes with small wheels at the end

• SPECIAL CONSIDERATIONS

Wheelchairs for Sports and Recreation (eSlide 14.4)

Wheelchairs for sports and recreation are designed specifically for participating in athletic, fitness, and recreational activities, such as racing, cycling, rugby, tennis, and basketball. These wheelchairs are made of lightweight materials and usually have very aggressive axle positions and camber. Wheelchairs equipped with arm crank mechanisms (hand cycles) can help improve cardiovascular fitness. Arm cranking has been shown to be more efficient and less of a physical strain on the upper extremities than conventional wheelchair propulsion.

Stand-up Wheelchairs (eSlide 14.4)

Stand-up wheelchairs offer health, psychological, and functional benefits and thus should be considered. However, a thorough evaluation of upper body strength, joint flexibility, bone density, endurance, and cardiovascular health is warranted before using these wheelchairs.

Scooters (eSlide 14.7)

Scooters are designed to provide intermittent and alternative mobility support for individuals who have good arm function and truncal balance and those capable of independent transfers.

• WHEELCHAIR TRANSPORTATION

Wheelchair transportation involves entering and exiting the vehicle (which is most commonly accomplished via ramps and lift systems), securing the wheelchair using a stud and clamp locking system or four-point tie-down system, and securing the occupant using a three-point system. The combination of these systems ensures safe travel.

• CONSIDERATIONS FOR SELECT POPULATIONS
(eSlide 14.14)

It is important to recognize that special clinical populations have their own specific needs and wheelchair indications. A team-based assessment that involves users and caregivers or family members cannot be overemphasized.

Clinical Pearls

- Comprehensive assessment must include history taking and physical, functional and environmental assessments.
- Assessment tools must include measurable outcomes.
- The mobility of a wheelchair user can be maximized by accurately matching the anatomic dimensions of the user to the wheelchair. (Maximizing the mobility of a wheelchair user is dependent on accurate matching of the anatomic dimensions of the user to the wheelchair.)
- Individualized wheelchair positioning is crucial to achieve neutral pelvic positions and proper alignment not just to optimize function but to prevent complications, injuries, and long-term structural issues.
- A good understanding of the availability of the wide range of wheeled mobility devices and their indications is important.

BIBLIOGRAPHY
The complete bibliography is available on ExpertConsult.com.

15 Therapeutic Exercise

Rochelle Coleen Tan Dy

Maintaining cardiovascular fitness and regular physical activity are important components of a healthy lifestyle, which provide a number of health-related benefits. Proper exercise prescription is crucial, and it entails an understanding of exercise physiology, metabolic energy systems, and musculoskeletal and cardiorespiratory physiologies, with particular consideration for special populations.

• ENERGY SYSTEMS (eSlide 15.1)

The energy needed to fuel biologic processes is produced from the breakdown of adenosine triphosphate (ATP). There are limited stores of ATP in skeletal muscles, which can provide an immediate burst of high-intensity exercise for 5–10 seconds. After this, subsequent production of ATP may occur via three metabolic pathways: the ATP–creatine phosphate system, rapid glycolysis, and aerobic oxidation.

Adenosine Triphosphate–Creatine Phosphate System

The ATP–creatine phosphate system transfers a high-energy phosphate from creatine phosphate to adenosine diphosphate (ADP) to regenerate ATP. This anaerobic system can provide ATP for approximately 30 seconds for activities such as sprinting and weightlifting.

Rapid Glycolysis (Lactic Acid System)

Glycolysis uses carbohydrates, primarily muscle glycogen, as a fuel source. In the absence of oxygen, the anaerobic pathway is utilized, producing lactic acid. Anaerobic glycolysis begins and dominates for approximately 1.5–2 minutes to provide fuel for high-energy burst activities such as middle-distance sprints (400-, 600-, and 800-m runs) or weightlifting. Lactic acid accumulation limits physical activity as it leads to fatigue and diminished performance. However, under aerobic conditions, lactate serves as a metabolic intermediate, which is converted into pyruvic acid and subsequently into energy (ATP), or it can be used to produce glucose (hepatic gluconeogenesis) via the Cori cycle.

Aerobic Oxidation System

The final metabolic pathway for ATP production involves the Krebs cycle and electron transport chain. The mitochondrial aerobic oxidation system uses carbohydrates, fats, and small amounts of protein to produce ATP through oxidative phosphorylation, which provides energy after 2–3 minutes of activity and continues thereafter until limited by the amount of available fuel and oxygen. Short, intense activities rely on anaerobic systems, whereas longer and low-intensity activities use the aerobic system. Carbohydrates are primarily used at the onset of exercise, and there is a gradual shift to fat metabolism during prolonged exercise (lasting longer than 30 minutes).

• CARDIOVASCULAR EXERCISE

Cardiorespiratory Physiology

The cardiorespiratory system delivers oxygen and nutrients to the cells and removes metabolic waste products. The normal resting heart rate (HR) is 60–80 beats/min. The HR increases linearly in proportion to the relative workload and is affected by age, body position, fitness, type of activity, presence of heart disease, medications, blood volume, and certain environmental factors, such as temperature and humidity. The maximal HR (HR_{max}) decreases with age and can be estimated with the following formula: HR_{max} = 220 – age. Stroke volume (SV) is the amount of blood ejected from the left ventricle in a single heart beat and is equal to the difference between the left ventricular end-diastolic volume and left ventricular end-systolic volume. At rest, SV is 60–100 mL/beat and is generally higher in males than in females. During exercise, SV increases in a curvilinear relationship with the work rate but plateaus at approximately 50% of aerobic capacity because of reduced left ventricular filling time during diastole. Cardiac output (Q) is the volume of blood pumped by the heart each minute. Age, posture, body size, presence of cardiac disease, and physical conditioning can all affect the Q. During dynamic exercise, Q increases because of an increase in both the SV and HR. However, at 40%–50% of the maximal oxygen consumption ($\dot{V}_{O_{2max}}$), the increase is mainly because of an increase in HR. Blood pressure is the driving force behind blood flow. Systolic blood pressure (SBP) increases linearly with increasing work intensity, whereas diastolic blood pressure (DBP) remains unchanged or only slightly increased, regardless of body position. Failure of SBP to increase, decreased SBP with increasing work rate, or a significant increase in DBP are all abnormal responses to exercise. Arm work causes greater increases in HR, SBP, and DBP than leg work because a higher percentage of the available muscle mass is recruited to perform arm work.

Pulmonary ventilation ($\dot{V}e$) is the volume of air exchanged per minute. Increases in $\dot{V}e$ are generally directly proportional to an increase in oxygen consumption ($\dot{V}_{O_2}$) and carbon dioxide production ($\dot{V}_{CO_2}$) until the anaerobic threshold is reached, signifying the onset of metabolic acidosis. $\dot{V}_{O_{2max}}$ is widely used as a measure of cardiopulmonary fitness; it is defined as the highest rate of oxygen transport or use (i.e., consumption) that can be achieved at maximal physical exertion. Metabolic equivalents are used to quantify levels of energy expenditure and are considered the best index of physical work capacity. The physiologic effects of cardiovascular activity and other benefits of regular exercise training are summarized in eSlides 15.2 and 15.3.

These changes are lost after 4–8 weeks of detraining. Overtraining fatigue syndrome can occur and is characterized by premature fatigability, emotional and mood changes, lack of motivation, infections, and overuse injuries.

• EXERCISE PRESCRIPTIONS

Components of an exercise prescription include the mode, intensity, frequency, duration, and progression of an exercise. The prescription should be developed with careful consideration of the individual's health status, medications, risk factor profile, behavioral characteristics, personal goals, and exercise preferences. The recommendations for cardiorespiratory endurance training by the American College of Sports Medicine (ACSM) are summarized in eSlide 15.4.

• MEDICAL CLEARANCE AND PREEXERCISE EVALUATION

Exercise training may not be appropriate for everyone and is contraindicated in the settings of acute cardiac disease or other conditions in which exercise may exacerbate the disease. The preexercise screening and need for physician evaluation depend on the risk for the individual and the intensity of the planned physical activity. Exercise stress tests are warranted in patients with known or suspected coronary or valvular heart disease, documented cardiac rhythm disorders, multiple cardiac risk factors, or pulmonary limitations; healthy individuals in high-risk occupations, such as pilots, firefighters, law enforcement officers, and mass transit operators; and men older than 40 years and women older than 50 years who are sedentary and plan to start a vigorous exercise program.

• MUSCLE PHYSIOLOGY (eSlide 15.5)

Each skeletal muscle is made of many muscle fibers. The fibers contain hundreds to thousands of myofibrils that are suspended in a sarcoplasmic matrix containing potassium, magnesium, phosphate, enzymes, mitochondria, and the sarcoplasmic reticulum, which are essential for muscle contraction.

Physiology of Muscle Contraction

SLIDING FILAMENT MECHANISM (eSlide 15.6)
The sliding filament mechanism of muscle contraction is shown in eSlide 15.6. At the molecular level, as calcium is released from the sarcoplasmic reticulum, it binds to troponin C, uncovering active actin sites hidden by the troponin–tropomyosin complex, along with the release of ATP at the myosin heads, resulting in muscle contraction.

MUSCLE FIBER TYPES (eSlide 15.7)
Muscle fibers can be characterized on the basis of their speed of contraction or twitch. Type 1 (slow oxidative) fibers are best suited for endurance activities that require aerobic metabolism. Type 2 (fast twitch) fibers are most active during activities that require strength and speed. They are further categorized into type 2A (fast oxidative–glycolytic) and type 2B (fast glycolytic).

MUSCLE FIBER ORIENTATION
Muscle fibers are arranged parallel to the length of the muscle. This produces a greater range of movement (ROM) than similar-sized muscles with a pennate arrangement of fibers.

Types of Muscle Contraction and Factors Affecting Muscle Strength and Performance (eSlide 15.7)
Isometric contractions cause no change in muscle length and no joint or limb motion. Isotonic contractions result in muscle length changes, producing limb motion. Concentric contractions result in muscle shortening, whereas eccentric

contractions produce muscle lengthening. In general, more fast-twitch fibers are recruited during eccentric contractions than during concentric contractions. Isokinetic contractions are performed at a constant velocity.

LENGTH–TENSION RELATIONSHIP
The maximum force of contraction occurs when a muscle is at its normal resting muscle length, which corresponds to about the midrange of joint motion or slightly longer; it is the length at which tension just begins to exceed zero. If a muscle is stretched beyond its resting length before contraction, resting tension develops and active tension (the increase in tension during contraction) decreases. The most efficient work occurs at approximately 30% of the maximum velocity of muscle contraction.

TORQUE–VELOCITY RELATIONSHIP
A muscle generates the greatest amount of force during fast eccentric (lengthening) contractions, followed by isometric contractions and slow concentric contractions. The least force is produced during fast concentric (shortening) contractions.

Effects of Resistance Training (eSlide 15.8)
The specific adaptations to imposed demands (SAID) principle states that a muscle adapts to the specific demands imposed on it, enabling it to handle a greater load. Observed strength gains within the first few weeks of a weightlifting program are mostly because of neuromuscular adaptations. Muscle hypertrophy is the enlargement of total muscle mass and cross-sectional area. It occurs after 6–7 weeks of resistance training and is more prominent in fast-twitch muscles than in slow-twitch muscles.

Exercise Prescription
Advancements in a training program can include increasing the amount of weight lifted (progressive resistive exercise), number of repetitions, or rate of exercise. One repetition maximum (RM) is the maximum weight that can be lifted at a time and is commonly used as a measure of one's current strength and a basis for establishing strength training programs and goals. Exercising to the point of fatigue can be critical for developing muscle strength. Using higher weights to the point of fatigue is more effective; however, low weight–high repetitions can be more appropriate, especially when training after an injury.

PROGRESSIVE RESISTANCE EXERCISE PROTOCOLS
Examples of progressive resistance exercise protocols are as follows:
1. The DeLorme (progressive resistive) method: three sets of 10 repetitions. The weight for the first set is 50% of the 10-RM, the second set is 75%, and the third set is 100%.
2. The Oxford (regressive resistive) technique: 10 repetitions at 100% of the 10-RM, followed by 10 repetitions at 75% and 10 repetitions at 50%.
3. Daily adjusted progressive resistance exercise (DAPRE) method: four sets of exercise per muscle group. The first set in DAPRE involves 10 repetitions at 50% of the individual's 6-RM, second set involves six repetitions at 75%, and the third set involves as many repetitions as possible at the individual's 6-RM. The number of repetitions performed in the third set determines the resistance for the fourth set.

Plyometrics

Plyometric exercises are brief explosive maneuvers that consist of an eccentric muscle contraction followed immediately by a concentric contraction. This more advanced type of stretch–shortening cycle is analogous to a spring coiling and uncoiling. It involves a more neural feedback that influences muscle length and tension and is primarily used in athletic training.

Proprioception

Proprioceptive organs, including muscles (particularly intrafusal spindle fibers), skin, ligaments, and joint capsules, generate afferent information crucial to the effective and safe performance of motor tasks. Impaired proprioception increases the risk for injury and may influence progressive joint deterioration associated with osteoarthritis, rheumatoid arthritis, and Charcot disease.

The tilt or wobble board is commonly used as part of proprioceptive training after ankle ligamentous injuries.

• NEUROFACILITATION TECHNIQUES

Neurofacilitation techniques may be applied in patients with central nervous system (CNS) dysfunction. The following are commonly used in a more eclectic manner to provide compensatory techniques during the course of recovery, with the goal of improving function.

Proprioceptive Neuromuscular Facilitation

Proprioceptive neuromuscular facilitation (PNF) uses spiral or diagonal movement patterns to indirectly facilitate movement, with the therapist providing maximal resistance to the stronger motor components, thereby facilitating the weaker components of the patterns. PNF techniques are best used in patients with hypotonia of supraspinal origin and are not recommended for spastic patients because they may increase tone.

Brunnstrom Techniques

These techniques use resistance and primitive postural reactions to facilitate gross synergistic movement patterns and increase muscle tone during early recovery from CNS injury. They are useful in patients with flaccid hemiplegia.

Bobath Techniques

These are neurodevelopmental techniques that use reflex inhibitory movement patterns to decrease hypertonia. These inhibitory patterns are generally antagonistic to the primitive synergistic patterns performed without resistance. Neurodevelopmental techniques also incorporate advanced postural reactions to stimulate recovery.

• FLEXIBILITY (eSlide 15.9)

Flexibility is the ROM present in a joint or group of joints that allows normal and unimpaired function. Although it varies innately with gender (females have more flexibility than males) and ethnicity, improved flexibility can be acquired through stretch training. Flexibility is greatest during infancy and early childhood and decreases with age. It is an important component of therapeutic exercise that prevents injury, reduces muscle soreness, enhances skill and performance, and provides muscle relaxation. Excessive flexibility may be a detriment to performance if it produces instability. In general, stiff structures benefit from stretching, whereas hypermobile structures require stabilization rather than additional mobilization.

Determinants of Flexibility

The muscle–tendon unit is the primary target of flexibility training, given that muscle has the largest capacity for lengthening. Dynamic factors include neuromuscular variables, such as the muscle tension feedback control system composed of intrafusal fibers (muscle spindles) and Golgi tendon organs (musculotendinous unit) that act via their segmental input at the spinal cord, as well as external factors, such as pain associated with an injury. Flexibility is generally assessed in terms of limb joint ROM with the use of a goniometer or similar device. The Schober test and fingertip-to-floor measurements can be used to assess trunk flexibility.

Methods of Stretching

BALLISTIC
This method uses the repetitive rapid application of force in a bouncing or jerking maneuver. Ballistic stretching is not recommended as it increases the risk for injury because of muscle guarding caused by overstretching.

PASSIVE
This method is performed by a partner or therapist who applies a stretch to a relaxed joint or extremity. It requires excellent communication and slow and sensitive application of force.

STATIC
This method involves the application of a steady force for a period of 15–60 seconds. It is the easiest and safest type of stretching and is particularly helpful for any form of therapeutic or recreational exercise, including athletic activity. It is also associated with decreased muscle soreness after exercise.

NEUROMUSCULAR FACILITATION
This is most frequently used in hold–relax and contract–relax techniques, wherein isometric or concentric contraction of the musculotendinous unit follows a passive or static stretch. The prestretch contraction facilitates relaxation and flexibility via the muscle length–tension thermostat discussed previously in this chapter.

ACSM's Guidelines for Exercise Prescriptions for Strength Training and Musculoskeletal Flexibility (eSlide 15.10)
Please refer to eSlide 15.10 for the recommended guidelines.

• EXERCISE FOR SPECIAL POPULATIONS

Physical Inactivity and Obesity
Physical inactivity is associated with increased fat and visceral adipose tissue accumulation, which increases the risk for diabetes, heart disease, and stroke. Body mass index (BMI) greater than 23 kg/m^2 and 25 kg/m^2 in middle-aged women and men, respectively, increases the risk for coronary heart disease. Treatment of obesity should be tailored according to its severity and the presence of comorbidities.

EXERCISE FOR FAT REDUCTION (see eSlide 15.15)

Successful weight loss requires a combination of diet and exercise. Caloric restriction should accompany moderate-intensity, land-based activity of 30–60 minutes per day at least twice a week, with a regimen aiming to reach 60%–85% of resting HR during exercise and activating all major muscle groups (in the chest, abdomen, back, and all extremities). Medications may be considered as an adjunct among people with BMI greater than 30 kg/m^2 or those with obesity-related disorders.

Pregnancy (eSlide 15.11)

The acute physiologic responses to exercise are generally increased during pregnancy.

Pregnant women can continue to do aerobic exercise at mild-to-moderate intensity (30 minutes at least three times a week) and undergo strength-training program that incorporates all major muscle groups and permits multiple repetitions. However, pregnant women should avoid exercising in the supine position after the first trimester (because of decreased Q in that position), isometric exercises and Valsalva maneuvers, prolonged periods of motionless standing, and recreational activities with a high risk for falling or abdominal trauma. Adequate hydration and nutrition (e.g., an additional 300 kcal/day) should be ensured, and exercise should be continued only to the point of fatigue and not exhaustion. Exercise is contraindicated in the presence of vaginal bleeding, dyspnea before exertion, dizziness, headache, chest pain, muscle weakness, calf pain or swelling, preterm labor, decreased fetal movement, and amniotic fluid leakage. If calf pain and swelling are present, thrombophlebitis should be ruled out. Exercise may be resumed 4–6 weeks postpartum.

Children (eSlide 15.12)

Healthy children should be encouraged to engage in physical activity on a regular basis, especially in light of the increasing rates of childhood obesity and comorbidities. However, given their immature anatomy and physiology, the design of any exercise program should consider their increased risk for overuse injuries, the possibility of damage to epiphyseal growth plates, and their tendency toward hypothermia or hyperthermia (because of less efficient thermoregulation).

Activity for Older Adults (eSlide 15.13)

The loss of strength and stamina, attributed to aging, is partly caused by reduced physical activity. Loss of muscle mass (known as sarcopenia) results from disuse of the muscle, with an associated decrease in growth factors and functional motor units. $\dot{V}O_{2max}$ decreases by approximately 5%–15%, and HR$_{max}$ decreases by 6–10 beats/min each decade, starting at 25–30 years of age. However, the benefits of exercise include lowering the risk for cardiovascular morbidity and being associated with higher functional health and better cognitive function. Exercise or activity modifications for medical comorbidities and limitations are important. Aquatic (pool) therapy is particularly helpful for individuals with both peripheral joint and spinal facet arthropathies. Mind–body integrative approaches, such as yoga, Tai Chi, and Pilates, are safe and useful alternatives.

Diabetes Mellitus (eSlide 15.14)

The response to exercise in patients with type 1 diabetes mellitus depends on a variety of factors, including the adequacy of glucose control by exogenous insulin. Serum glucose concentrations in the general range of 200–400 mg/dL require medical supervision during exercise, and exercise is contraindicated for those with fasting glucose serum values greater than 400 mg/dL. Exercise-induced hypoglycemia is the most common problem during exercise, and it may last for up to 4–6 hours postexercise. Aerobic and resistance training guidelines for patients with type 1 diabetes mellitus are similar to those for the general population. However, additional precautionary measures include the following: frequent blood glucose monitoring, decreasing the insulin dose (e.g., by 1-2 units, as prescribed by the physician) or increasing carbohydrate intake (e.g., 10-15 g carbohydrate per 30 minutes of exercise) before an exercise session, avoiding exercise during times of peak insulin levels, eating carbohydrate snacks before or during prolonged exercise sessions, being able to detect the signs and symptoms of hypoglycemia and hyperglycemia, exercising with a partner, using proper footwear, avoiding exercise in excessively hot environments, avoiding jarring activities (if advanced retinopathy is present), and being aware of medications that can mask hypoglycemic or angina symptoms (e.g., beta-blockers).

Hypertension (eSlide 15.15)

Aerobic or endurance exercise training may be part of the initial nonpharmacologic treatment strategy, along with lifestyle modification, for individuals with mild-to-moderate essential hypertension. The recommended mode, frequency, duration, and intensity of exercise for patients with hypertension are generally similar to those for healthy individuals but with lower intensities (e.g., 40%-70% of $\dot{V}O_{2max}$). Resistance training may be incorporated but should not be the primary form of exercise. Exercise should be avoided if resting SBP is greater than 200 mm Hg and/or DBP is greater than 110 mm Hg. When exercising, the SBP should be maintained at less than 220 mm Hg and/or the DBP at less than 105 mm Hg.

Peripheral Vascular Disease (eSlide 15.15)

Patients with peripheral vascular disease (PVD) experience ischemic leg pain (claudication) during physical activity because of a mismatch between active muscle oxygen supply and demand. Pain is typically described as a burning, searing, aching, tightness, or cramping sensation in the calf, but it may originate from the buttock and radiate down the leg. The pain disappears with rest, but it may persist in severe cases. Treatment for severe PVD includes blood thinners, angioplasty, or bypass grafting. Weight-bearing exercise is preferred if tolerated, but non–weight-bearing exercise is a suitable alternative, with intensity limited by pain.

Myofascial Pain Syndrome and Fibromyalgia (eSlide 15.15)

Patients with myofascial pain syndrome or fibromyalgia will benefit from initial low-intensity aerobic exercise combined with stretching. On the basis of the physiologic response and maintenance of functional skills, the intensity of exercise is increased.

Organ Transplantation (eSlide 15.15)

Patients with an organ transplant are deconditioned and weak postoperatively, which can be partly attributed to their immunosuppressive medications. After heart transplantation, sinus node denervation is present, which makes the HR response an unreliable measure of exercise intensity. In these patients, the Borg Rate of Perceived Exertion Scale is preferred. Rehabilitation after solid organ transplantation appears highly beneficial. It also aids in psychological and physical recovery, thereby improving the quality of life.

Clinical Pearls

1. All energy-producing pathways are active during most exercises. However, different types of exercise place greater demands on different pathways.
2. The anaerobic threshold signifies the onset of metabolic acidosis and the peak work rate or oxygen consumption at which the energy demands exceed the circulatory ability to sustain aerobic metabolism.
3. Applying appropriate exercise prescriptions based on the physiologic response to exercises and the principle of specificity of training will ensure an appropriate training response and minimize the risk for injuries.
4. Although accepted teaching states that stretching is a preventive measure for athletic injuries, there is little conclusive epidemiologic evidence to support this idea.

BIBLIOGRAPHY
The complete bibliography is available on ExpertConsult.com.

Manipulation, Traction, and Massage

16

Reynaldo R. Rey-Matias

Understanding the basic principles behind manipulation, traction, and massage; their applications; and their potential for complications is highly important in physiatric practice.

• MANIPULATION

The International Federation of Manual Medicine defines *manipulation* as "the use of the hands in the patient management process using instructions and maneuvers to maintain maximal, painless movement of the musculoskeletal system in postural balance." These goals are accomplished by treatments that attempt to restore the mechanical function of a joint and normalize altered reflex patterns, as evidenced by the optimal range of movement, body symmetry, and tissue texture. Manual medicine can involve the manipulation of spinal and peripheral joints and myofascial tissues. Physiologic objectives behind the use of manipulation include decreasing nociceptive input, decreasing gamma gain of muscle spindles, enhancing lymphatic return, and improving circulation to tissues.

Overview of Various Types of Manual Medicine

Central to the application of manual medicine techniques is the barrier concept. This concept recognizes the limitation of motion of a normal joint in which asymmetric motion is present. Motion is relatively free in one direction, with loss of some motion in the other direction. Motion loss occurs within the normal range of movement for that joint (eSlide 16.1). The barrier concept implies that something is preventing the full range of movement of a joint. The term *pathologic barrier* was initially used to describe the point at which normal motion is limited. The term currently used is *restrictive barrier*, which means that no organic pathology can be seen under the microscope; these are functional restrictions. The new neutral position has shifted toward the direction of less restricted motion. This gives rise to positional asymmetry. Manipulation is designed to restore normal motion.

Manual medicine techniques can be classified in different ways. They may be classified as soft tissue, articulatory, or specific joint mobilization techniques. The terms *direct* and *indirect* are also used to classify the technique, with several types of technique in each category. Direct technique means that the practitioner moves the body part(s) in the direction of the restrictive barrier. Indirect technique means the practitioner moves the body part away from the restrictive barrier.

Direct techniques include the following:

1. *Thrust (impulse, high velocity, low amplitude):* The final activating force is operator force.
2. *Articulation:* Low velocity, high amplitude
3. *Muscle energy (direct isometric types):* The final activating force is a patient contraction.
4. *Direct myofascial release:* Load (stretch) tissues, hold, and wait for release.

Indirect techniques include the following:

1. Strain–counterstrain
2. Indirect balancing
3. Multiple names (functional, balanced ligamentous tension)
4. Indirect myofascial release
5. Craniosacral

Normal and Abnormal Coupled Spinal Motion

Flexion (forward bending) and extension (backward bending) are sagittal plane motions and are not coupled. However, rotation and side bending are coupled. The amount of pure rotation or pure side bending of spinal joints is limited and varies depending on the site within the spine. Rotation and side bending occur together in normal spinal joints. Fryette stated that when side bending is introduced in the absence of marked flexion or extension (termed *neutral*), a group of vertebrae rotate into the produced convexity, with maximum rotation at the apex. Rotation and side bending occur at opposite sides when compared with the original starting position. This is sometimes referred to as neutral mechanics or type 1 dysfunction. Nonneutral mechanics or type 2 dysfunctions involve a component of flexion or extension, with rotation and side bending to the same side. This is usually a single-segment motion, although several segments may be involved.

Somatic Dysfunction

Somatic dysfunction is a diagnostic term defined as impaired or altered function of related components of the somatic (body framework) system: skeletal, arthrodial, and myofascial structures and related vascular, lymphatic, and neural elements. Dysfunctions that can be palpated include changes in tissue texture, increased sensitivity to touch (hyperalgesia), altered ease or range of movement, and anatomic asymmetry or positional change. The *Glossary of Osteopathic Terminology* describes the following three ways of naming somatic dysfunction: *Type 1:* Where is it or what position is it in (e.g., right rotated)? *Type 2:* What will it do or what is the direction of free motion (e.g., right strain)? *Type 3:* What will it not do or what is the direction of restriction (e.g., restriction of left rotation)? A dysfunction should be named in three planes of motion, with the upper segment described in relation to the lower segment.

Physiologic Rationale for Manual Therapies

Increased gamma activity of muscle spindles results in increased alpha motor neuron activity of extrafusal fibers of skeletal muscles causing contraction. However, decreasing gamma gain activity is one mechanism that results in muscle relaxation. If the muscle spindle is stretched, increased activity of the gamma system stimulates muscle activity.

Examination

The mnemonic for a musculoskeletal examination is TART: *T*, tenderness or sensitivity; *A*, asymmetry (look); *R*, restriction of motion (move); and *T*, tissue texture abnormality (feel). The diagnosis of somatic dysfunction is based on a palpatory examination assessing TART. Terms to describe the "feel" might be *ease* and *bind* or *freedom* and *resistance* (eSlide 16.2). Segmental motion can also be tested using pressure applied through the hands, without relying on patient movement for diagnosis (eSlide 16.3).

Assessment of Fascia

Fascia is three dimensional and can form sleeves to compartmentalize, act as cables, or form diaphragms. Assessment of fascia starts with hand placement to perceive the combined vector force in the tissue. Assessment of an extremity would start with hand placement proximal and distal to the area. Examination of the fascia and myofascial structures may include looking for special "points" or "triggers." These include counterstrain tender points, myofascial trigger points of Simon and Travell, and acupuncture points.

Types of Manual Medicine Techniques

Manual medicine techniques can be classified in different ways, including soft tissue techniques, articulatory techniques, or specific joint mobilization. These are directly or indirectly applied. Combined techniques start with an indirect technique, and once the release has occurred, the practitioner may switch to a direct technique.

DIRECT TECHNIQUES

1. *Soft tissue techniques* are used to relax muscles and fascia. They usually involve applying a lateral force to stretch the muscle, direct longitudinal stretching, or careful kneading, similar to massage, but with a different treatment endpoint. The focus is on moving the tissue rather than on relaxing muscles.
2. *Articulatory treatment* moves a joint back and forth repeatedly to increase freedom of range of movement. It may be classified as a low-velocity, high-amplitude approach. Articulatory treatment is sometimes a form of soft tissue treatment in which the only way to access deep muscles is to move the origin and insertion (see eSlide 16.2). Articulatory treatment is very useful for stiff joints and older patients.
3. *Specific joint mobilization* may be accomplished in a number of ways:
   a. *Mobilization with impulse (thrust; high velocity, low amplitude)* is often considered synonymous with manipulation; it is used for restriction of motion in joints. An audible pop can occur with application of the technique. The thrust must be low amplitude, namely over a very short distance and of high velocity (eSlides 16.4, 16.5, and 16.6).
   b. *Muscle energy: direct isometric types* involve the patient to voluntarily move the body as specifically directed by the practitioner. This directed patient

action occurs from a precisely controlled position against a defined resistance applied by the practitioner. The initial classification of muscle energy techniques was based on whether the force was equal to (isometric), greater than (isotonic), or less than (isolytic) the patient force. These techniques have been used extensively by therapists and are often referred to as the contract–relax techniques. Muscle energy techniques require a specific diagnosis, incorporating all three planes of motion (Video 16.1). Most direct isometric muscle energy techniques involve the patient actively contracting the shortened muscle (sometimes referred to as the "sick" muscle). In muscle energy techniques, the final activating force is the patient's muscle contraction (eSlide 16.7).

c. *Direct myofascial release* is used to identify tissue restriction and to remove that restriction. The direct myofascial technique involves loading the myofascial tissues (stretch), holding the tissues in that position, and waiting for release. The term *creep* is applied to this phenomenon. When release occurs, there is additional lengthening of the tissues without an increase in the force being applied (eSlide 16.8). Direct myofascial release is a load-and-hold technique, which is essentially a zero-velocity technique.

INDIRECT TECHNIQUES

1. *Strain–counterstrain* is a type of manipulative treatment that uses spontaneous release by positioning and uses tender points to serve as a monitor to achieve the proper position. The neurophysiologic mechanism is based on the fact that shortening the muscle quiets the muscle and disrupts the inappropriate strain reflex. The use of counterstrain requires a structural evaluation and assessment of tender points. Tender points are tissue areas that are tender to palpation. They are sometimes described as "pea-like" areas of tension. Counterstrain is a very gentle technique with an extremely low risk for injury. However, patients can become very sore after counterstrain treatment. It is appropriate to caution patients that this might occur.

2. *Indirect balancing* positions the dysfunction in the direction of free motion, away from the restrictive barrier. The positioning involves achieving a balance of tension on all sides of the dysfunction. Indirect balancing techniques are indirect in that the operator moves the body part(s) away from the restrictive barrier until the tension on all sides of the joint is equal. Achieving the proper treatment position can be a challenge. However, when release occurs, it is very apparent to the treating clinician because there is a decrease in the overall tension surrounding the dysfunction.

Contraindications and Side Effects

Perhaps the most serious complication of cervical manipulation is a stroke associated with vertebrobasilar artery dissection. Most complications are associated with high-velocity thrusting techniques. eSlide 16.9 presents a list of conditions that are contraindications to the thrusting technique.

• TRACTION

Traction is a technique used to stretch soft tissues and separate joint surfaces or bone fragments using a pulling force. The force applied must be of sufficient magnitude and duration in the proper direction while resisting movement of the body with an equal and opposite force.

Types of Traction

Traction can be delivered by several different methods, including manual, mechanized, motorized, hydraulic, or inversion (which uses gravity) methods. Irrespective of the method, the surface resistance must be overcome. The resistance is approximately equal to half the weight of the body segment. The force can be continuous, sustained, or intermittent. Continuous traction uses a low force over a long period, such as 30–40 hours. Continuous traction is typically not well tolerated and is not commonly used. Sustained traction uses a larger force but for a shorter period (typically 30–60 minutes). Although sustained traction remains difficult to tolerate, it is commonly used in the lumbar spine with a split traction or autotraction table. Intermittent traction uses greater forces over shorter periods. The traction force can be increased or decreased during each treatment cycle and the duration of pull can be adjusted. The cycle is usually repeated for 15 to 25 minutes, with the traction phase ranging from 5 to 60 seconds, and the rest phase ranging from 5 to 15 seconds. The magnitude, duration, and direction of the pull can be varied.

Cervical traction is commonly performed using manual, mechanical, or motorized methods (with a head or chin sling) or with the use of a supine posterior distraction unit. The optimal angle of pull ranges between 20 and 30 degrees of flexion while 25 pounds of force are required to reverse the normal cervical lordosis and bring about the earliest distraction of vertebral segments. Mechanical cervical traction can be applied in the supine position, which reduces the weight of the head but increases frictional resistance. This position also allows for better control of the head by the patient and is typically more comfortable (eSlide 16.10).

Traction in the sitting position allows more accurate positioning for the correct angle of pull, but it usually affords less head control and is less comfortable.

Lumbar traction requires a significantly greater force to create distraction of the vertebral segments than cervical traction. Common traction systems include a thoracic or chest belt with a pelvic belt (eSlide 16.11), inversion, a split traction table, or an autotraction table. Split traction tables have a mobile half and a stationary half. Autotraction tables allow both segments of the table to move and are controlled by the patient. The patient assumes the most pain-free position and performs active traction by pulling on an overhead bar. The patient then uses his or her feet to activate a bar, which alternates compressive and distracting forces.

Physiologic Effects

Physiologic effects of traction have been extensively evaluated and reported. Traction can stretch muscles and ligaments, tighten the posterior longitudinal ligament to exert a centripetal force on the annulus fibrosis, enlarge the intervertebral space, enlarge the intervertebral foramina, and separate apophyseal joints.

Indications, Goals of Treatment, and Efficacy

There is no consensus on the definitive indications for traction, but the condition with the most support for its use is cervical radiculopathy. The use of traction for lumbar radiculopathy, neck pain, and low back pain is more controversial, with contradictions existing in the literature. In the absence of contraindications, traction can be used to treat any condition in which the physiologic effects of traction would be theoretically beneficial.

Contraindications

Absolute contraindications to traction include malignancy, infection (such as osteomyelitis or diskitis), osteoporosis, inflammatory arthritis, fracture, pregnancy, cord compression, uncontrolled hypertension or cardiovascular disease, and in the setting of a carotid or vertebral artery disease. Caution should also be exercised in the elderly, in the setting of midline disk herniations and in the lumbar region when abdominal problems are present. Inversion traction involves more risks because increases in blood pressure and decreases in heart rate are known to occur, leading to headaches and periorbital petechiae.

• MASSAGE

Massage is the term used to describe certain manipulations of the soft tissue of the body. Massage has been further defined as a group of procedures that are usually performed with hands and that include friction, kneading, rolling, and percussion of external tissues of the body.

Indications and Goals of Treatment

Massage has multiple effects on the body, including mechanical, reflexive, neurologic, and psychological effects. The goals of therapeutic massage are to produce relaxation, relieve muscle tension, reduce pain, increase mobility of soft tissues, and improve circulation.

Mechanical and Physiologic Effects

The mechanical pressure created by massage moves fluid from areas of relative stasis (low pressure) to higher pressure areas by creating a hydrostatic pressure gradient. Once fluids leave the cell or interstitial fluid, they can enter the lymphatic or vascular system. Valves within the lymphatic and venous system prevent return of the fluid to the tissue. Massage can also have an immediate effect on cutaneous blood flow, with hyperemia being noticed even with superficial techniques. Deep massage has an effect on the underlying fascia and deep connective tissues. Injuries to these deeper tissues can result in restrictions, adhesions, and scarring. These fascial constrictions can potentially cause restriction of fluid movement within the vasculature, as well as reduction in muscle activity. Deep massage can help release these restrictions, adhesions, and areas of microscarring.

Pain, inactivity, and debilitation result in insufficient muscle movement to mobilize fluids. This hypomobility can result in increased fluid stasis, producing a self-perpetuating positive feedback loop. This can result in the accumulation of not only fluids but also metabolic byproducts. These metabolic byproducts can create an osmotic influence on fluid shifts and result in stimulation of pain fibers. Massage increases the mobility of these metabolic byproducts and the dispersion of accumulated fluids.

Somatic afferent nerve fibers carry information from the somatic system to the spinal cord. Dysfunction within the somatic structures can result in increased afferent neural input. This increased input changes efferent activity at the same spinal cord level through interneurons, which can result in muscle hypertonicity and contraction.

Types of Massage

A vast array of techniques has been used to perform therapeutic massages. These techniques can be categorized by the geographic region of origin as either classic Western (European) or Eastern (Asian) forms of massage. The most common Western (European) techniques are those outlined by the Swedish system. The four basic massage strokes are effleurage, pétrissage, friction massage, and tapotement, as originally described by the French. Several treatment schemes combine massage with other techniques, such as structural reintegration, functional restoration, and movement therapies. Effleurage involves gliding the palms, fingertips, and/or thumbs over the skin in a rhythmic circular pattern with varying degrees of pressure. This stroke is performed by maintaining continuous contact with the skin and stroking from a distal to a proximal position on the extremities, torso, or spine (eSlide 16.12). This technique is often used as a prelude to more aggressive massage techniques or manipulation. Pétrissage is also known as "kneading massage." It involves both hands compressing the skin between the thumb and fingers. The tissue is grasped from the underlying skeletal structures, lifted, and massaged. Both hands rhythmically alternate in a rolling motion. Pétrissage (eSlide 16.13) is also considered as a compression massage, and several variations exist, including kneading or picking up, wringing, rolling, or shaking the tissue. Tapotement, or percussion massage (eSlide 16.14), uses rhythmic alternating contact of varying pressure between the hands and body's soft tissue. Various techniques are used to produce this type of massage, including hacking, clapping, beating, pounding, and vibration. Friction massage is a circular, longitudinal, or transverse pressure applied by the fingers, thumb, or hypothenar region of the hand to small areas. Cross-friction massage is perpendicular to the fibers. Very little motion occurs at the fingertips overlying the skin. The tissues are massaged by increasing the pressure applied from the superficial to deep tissues. The goal of friction massage is to break down adhesions in scar tissues, loosen ligaments, and disable trigger points. It is often uncomfortable and can even result in some bruising (eSlide 16.15). Other massage techniques include Tager psychological integration, Alexander and Feldenkrais techniques, "Rolfing" myofascial release, and manual lymphatic drainage. Shiatsu (*shi* ["finger"] and *atsu* ["pressure"]) is a Japanese type of body work based on acupuncture. Pressure is applied in particular meridians similar to acupuncture.

Evidence-Based Use of Massage

At least one large randomized controlled trial supports the use of massage in the treatment of anxiety and stress; arthralgias and various arthritides; fibromyalgia; lymphedema; musculoskeletal disorders, such as whiplash, low back pain, and sports-related injuries; and sleep disorders.

Contraindications

Massage should not be performed over areas of malignancy, cellulitis, or lymphangitis. Massaging these regions can cause mobilization of tumor cells into the vascular lymphatic supply or can cause the spread of infection. Areas of trauma or recent bleeding should not be treated with deep tissue massage. Mobilization of these areas can increase the propensity for rebleeding. Patients taking anticoagulants should be treated with gentler techniques and observed for bruising and ecchymosis. Deep tissue work should be used with extreme caution in people receiving anticoagulants or those who have a bleeding diathesis.

Massage should not be used over areas of known deep venous thrombosis or atherosclerotic plaques. This could dislodge vascular thrombi, resulting in embolic infarcts that affect the pulmonary, cerebral, or peripheral systems.

• CONCLUSION

Manipulation, traction, and massage have been an integral part of health care since ancient times. Research efforts, although in their infancy, have shown that a spectrum of beneficial physiologic and clinical changes can be associated with these modalities. Manipulation, traction, and massage are becoming increasingly recognized as valuable adjuncts to standard medical care. Many medical centers now have departments dedicated to the practice, education, and research of these areas.

Clinical Pearls

- The goals of manipulation or manual medicine are to help maintain optimal body mechanics and to improve motion in restricted areas. Enhancing maximal, pain-free movement in a balanced posture and optimizing function are major goals.
- Absolute contraindications to traction include malignancy, infection such as osteomyelitis or diskitis, osteoporosis, inflammatory arthritis, fracture, pregnancy, cord compression, uncontrolled hypertension or cardiovascular disease, and in the setting of carotid or vertebral artery disease
- Massage should not be performed over areas of malignancy, cellulitis, or lymphangitis. Areas of trauma or recent bleeding should not be treated with deep tissue massage. Mobilization of these areas can increase the propensity for rebleeding. Patients who are taking anticoagulants should be treated with gentler techniques and observed for bruising and ecchymoses. Massage should not be used over areas of known deep venous thrombosis or atherosclerotic plaques. Special care should be observed in patients with osteoarthritis or severe osteoporosis to avoid any excess range of motion or stretching that could alter articulating surfaces. Patients with low blood pressure might experience postural hypotension after treatment and should be observed carefully.

BIBLIOGRAPHY
The complete bibliography is available on ExpertConsult.com.

Physical Agent Modalities

17

Chueh-Hung Wu

The physiologic effects, indications, techniques, and precautions of various physical agent modalities, including cold, heat, ultrasound, electromagnetic waves, electricity, and mechanical force, are summarized in this chapter and eSlides.

• CRYOTHERAPY (eSlides 17.1 and 17.2)

Physiology

The major physiologic effects of cryotherapy (treatment involving lowering of local tissue temperature) include decreasing the nerve conduction velocity of pain fibers, reducing muscle spasm, and causing vasoconstriction, which may be followed by vasodilation.

Indications and Contraindications

Indications for cryotherapy include acute injury, acute swelling, hemorrhage and edema, acute contusion, acute muscle strain, acute ligament sprain, bursitis, tenosynovitis, tendinitis, muscle spasm or guarding, chronic pain, and myofascial trigger points. Contraindications include impaired circulation (e.g., Raynaud phenomenon, peripheral vascular disease), hypersensitivity to cold, skin anesthesia, open wounds or skin disorders (those that need cold whirlpools and contrast baths), and local infection.

Applications of Cryotherapy

Types of cryotherapy include ice packs, ice massage, cold whirlpools, chemical cold spray, and contrast baths. The primary action of cold spray is to stimulate Aβ nerve fibers to reduce the painful arc and muscle spasm. It can be used in the field to reduce pain and muscle spasm associated with an acute sports injury. Cold spray, in the technique of "spray-and-stretch," is also commonly used to relieve muscle spasms of myofascial pain syndrome. Contrast baths are used to treat subacute swelling. They produce alternating vasoconstriction and vasodilation, which reduce local edema.

• SUPERFICIAL HEAT (eSlides 17.3, 17.4, and 17.5)

Physiology

Thermotherapy, which can be divided into superficial heat and deep heat (diathermy), is used to increase tissue temperature. Superficial heating agents increase the temperature within the skin and subcutaneous fat. Deeper tissue heating is limited by vasodilation and the insulating properties of fat. Because of poor penetration (less than 1 cm), superficial heat generally only affects cutaneous blood flow and cutaneous nerve receptors. In addition to increasing local blood flow by applying heat, the higher cutaneous temperature also has an analgesic effect. Heat has the effect of relaxing skeletal muscle by simultaneously decreasing the stimulus threshold of muscle spindles and decreasing the gamma efferent firing rate.

Indications and Contraindications

Indications for thermal therapy include nonacute (longer than 6 weeks) inflammatory conditions, nonacute pain, subacute (6-12 weeks) muscle strain, subacute contusions, subacute ligament sprains, muscle guarding or spasm, decreased range of movement of a joint, and myofascial trigger points. Contraindications include acute musculoskeletal conditions, impaired circulation, peripheral vascular disease, skin anesthesia, open wounds, and infection.

Types of Devices and Techniques

HYDROCOLLATOR PACK

The most commonly used superficial heat method is the commercial hydrocollator pack.

PARAFFIN BATH

A paraffin bath (paraffin and mineral oil mixture) is a simple and efficient method for applying superficial heat, especially to small joints of the body such as the interphalangeal joints. It is most commonly used for rheumatoid arthritis and osteoarthritis. The combination of paraffin and mineral oil has a low specific heat, which enhances the patient's ability to tolerate heat from paraffin (compared with water at the same temperature) (Video 17.1).

INFRARED

Infrared is a superficial, dry heat modality, which tends to elevate superficial temperatures more than moist heat, but it may have a smaller depth of penetration. The advantage of an infrared lamp over other superficial heat modalities is that it can increase the temperature without touching the patient, making it the only superficial heating method appropriate for patients with skin defects.

HYDROTHERAPY

Hydrotherapy treats the patient through the medium of water. Water can provide warmth and coldness, moisten the soft tissues, and support the tissues. In addition to the thermal benefits of reducing pain, edema, and muscle spasm, a quick jet stream or stroking motion during whirlpool therapy has a local massage effect, which might cause further muscle relaxation and increase local circulation. When using a whirlpool, the patient can move the treated part easily in the whirlpool, which produces the additional benefit of exercise. A warm whirlpool is an excellent treatment for rheumatoid arthritis and osteoarthritis as it increases systemic blood flow and mobilization of the affected body part without exerting too much pressure on the joints.

• SPINAL TRACTION (eSlides 17.6 and 17.7)

Physiology

Spinal traction moves the spine overall and at each individual spinal segment. The amount of movement varies according to the position of spine, the amount of force, and the duration of traction. The major physiologic effects of spinal traction are derived from distraction of the spine, which may stretch ligaments, muscles, and facet joints; reduce disc pressure; facilitate return of the disc to its original position; decrease central pressure in the disc space and facilitate movement of the disc nucleus back to the central position; separate the joint surfaces, which releases the impingement of meniscal structures, synovial fringes, and osteochondral fragments between joint spaces; stretch specific paraspinal muscle groups, allowing better muscular blood flow; and activate muscle proprioceptors.

Indications and Contraindications

Spinal traction is indicated in patients with nerve impingement from disc herniation, spondylolisthesis, narrowed intervertebral foramen, spur formation, degenerative facet joints, joint hypomobility, discogenic pain, muscle spasm, and spinal ligament or connective tissue contractures. Contraindications include acute sprain or strain, acute inflammation, vertebral fracture or joint instability, pregnancy, tumors, bone disease, severe osteoporosis, and infection in bones or joints.

Techniques

When considering mechanical traction, several important parameters need to be set, including traction equipment, body position, force used, traction pattern (intermittent vs. sustained traction), and duration of traction. The effects of intermittent or sustained traction have been reported. In general, sustained traction is favored for treating intervertebral disc herniation because it produces a longer period of disc decompression, causing disc nuclear material to move centripetally and reducing the pressure of herniated disc on nearby nerve structures. However, intermittent traction is usually more comfortable than sustained traction with the same force, especially at higher forces.

• DEEP HEAT (Diathermy)

Ultrasound (eSlides 17.8, 17.9, and 17.10)
PHYSIOLOGY AND MECHANISM OF ACTION
The mechanism of heat transfer of ultrasound is conversion, which refers to the transformation of energy (e.g., sound or electromagnetic) into heat. Heat is produced when acoustic energy is absorbed, especially at or near the surfaces of structures with high attenuation coefficients, such as bone. The localized heating by ultrasound near bony surfaces (i.e., at soft tissue–bone interfaces) produces preferential hyperemia and increased extensibility of ligaments, tendons, and joint capsules. Ultrasound of higher frequency penetrates less into the tissues. Nonthermal effects of ultrasound include cavitation, media motion (acoustic streaming and microstreaming), and standing waves.

Sonophoresis

It has long been known that application of ultrasound to the skin increases its permeability and enables the delivery of various substances (most frequently, corticosteroid) into and through the skin via a process called sonophoresis or phonophoresis. Transdermal drug delivery offers several important advantages over traditional oral delivery or injections, including minimizing gastric irritation, first-pass effect, and injection pain.

CONTRAINDICATIONS AND PRECAUTIONS

Using the stroking technique for ultrasound allows a more even energy distribution over the site being treated. The stationary technique should be generally avoided because of the potential for standing waves and hot spots. Heat should be generally avoided in areas of impaired sensation or in patients with cognitive impairment. Heat can exacerbate acute inflammation, and thus ultrasound should be avoided in the management of acute tendinitis, arthritis, or ligament sprain. Applying ultrasound near structures that are vulnerable to thermal injury, such as nerves, the brain, eyes, reproductive organs, growing bone (with open epiphyses), and laminectomy sites, should be avoided. Heat may theoretically increase the rate of tumor growth or hematogenous spread; therefore ultrasound diathermy should be avoided in areas of known malignancy. Applying ultrasound near a pacemaker is generally contraindicated because ultrasound may cause it to malfunction. Ultrasound should be avoided near implants that contain plastic materials such as artificial hip joints with polyethylene liner or breast implants. In contrast to shortwave diathermy or microwave diathermy (MWD), ultrasound is believed to be the only type of diathermy that can be used in areas with surgical metallic implants.

• SHORTWAVE (eSlides 17.11 and 17.12)

PHYSICS

Shortwave diathermy (SWD) is a modality that produces heat by converting electromagnetic energy into thermal energy.

INDICATIONS AND EVIDENCE BASIS

Continuous SWD is the technique of choice when uniform elevation of temperature is required in deep tissues and inside joints. Subacute or chronic conditions respond well to continuous SWD, whereas acute lesions are better treated with pulsed SWD. Continuous SWD, when applied properly, is believed to have the ability to relieve pain and muscle spasm, resolve inflammation, reduce swelling, promote vasodilation, and increase soft tissue extensibility and joint range of movement.

CONTRAINDICATIONS AND PRECAUTIONS

In general, the common contraindications and precautions of SWD are similar to those for other methods of heating. Because of good bone penetration, SWD-induced heating of the epiphyseal plates in the long bones of children may affect growth; therefore injudicious application of SWD to a child may lead to long-term side effects. SWD is contraindicated in areas with metal implants and in patients with pacemakers or implanted deep brain stimulators.

Electromagnetic waves may selectively heat water; therefore, areas with excessive fluid accumulation, such as edematous tissue, moist skin, eyes, fluid-filled cavities, and a pregnant or menstruating uterus, should be avoided for both SWD and microwave treatment. Towels are usually necessary to be placed between the SWD applicator and treatment area to absorb moisture and avoid focal hot spots on body surfaces. A rule of "no water and no metal" is generally recommended when using both SWD and MWD.

Microwave

PHYSICS

Microwaves have a shorter wavelength than SWD. They generate heat by oscillating a high-frequency electrical field with a lesser extent of magnetic field to induce internal vibration of molecules with a high polarity.

INDICATIONS AND CONTRAINDICATIONS

Microwaves are absorbed to a large extent by water, so they are theoretically able to selectively heat muscle. Because of its limited penetration, microwaves are preferred for heating superficial muscles and shallow joints. It is typically used in patients with chronic neck pain, back pain, or arthritis.

MWD treatment should be avoided in areas close to epiphyses, reproductive organs, nervous system tissues, and fluid-filled cavities. MWD should not be used on or near a patient with a cardiac pacemaker or lead electrodes.

• EXTRACORPOREAL SHOCK WAVE THERAPY (eSlide 17.13)

PHYSICS

The shock waves used in medicine for extracorporeal shock wave therapy (ESWT) are high-intensity pulsed mechanical waves with a relatively low repetition frequency. Unlike therapeutic ultrasound, the temperature increase in the focal area is negligible for intensities used in therapeutic applications.

INDICATIONS AND MECHANISMS OF ACTION

The most widely accepted indications for ESWT are the treatment of plantar fasciitis, lateral epicondylitis, and rotator cuff calcified tendinopathy. The biological mechanisms are believed to involve the destruction of sensory unmyelinated nerve fibers and promotion of neovascularization. ESWT can stimulate bone remodeling; thus, it may be used as an alternative to surgical treatment for fractures, bony nonunion, and delayed union: settings in which it may yield better short-term clinical outcomes.

CONTRAINDICATIONS AND PRECAUTIONS

Contraindications to ESWT include bleeding disorders and pregnancy. Complications may include soft tissue swelling, ecchymosis or hematoma, skin redness or erosion, transient bone edema, nerve lesions, and increased pain.

• ELECTROTHERAPY

Physiology and Mechanism of Action

The mechanisms of action of electrotherapy devices in pain management can be broadly summarized as follows: (a) segmental inhibition of pain signals to the brain and the dorsal horn of the spinal cord (Melzack and Wall's gate control theory) and (b) activation of descending inhibitory pathways and stimulation of the release of endogenous opioids and other neurotransmitters, such as serotonin, gamma-aminobutyric acid, noradrenaline, and acetylcholine.

TRANSCUTANEOUS ELECTRICAL NERVE STIMULATION

Commonly used transcutaneous electrical nerve stimulation (TENS) units provide either conventional TENS (which produces a tingling sensation) or low-frequency TENS (which produces a burning, needling sensation). In painful diabetic peripheral polyneuropathy and myofascial trigger points, TENS units have been found to be effective for up to 3 months.

INTERFERENTIAL CURRENT (eSlide 17.14)

Interferential current therapy (IFC) employs alternating medium-frequency electrical current signals of slightly different frequencies, which penetrate tissues more easily and are less prone to neuronal adaptation than TENS. IFC therapy has been successfully used in a variety of musculoskeletal and neurologic conditions, as well as in the management of urinary incontinence for up to 3 months.

IONTOPHORESIS

Iontophoresis is the technique of using the charges of ions and particles to drive them across tissues and membranes under the influence of an imposed electrical field. It can be useful for local or systemic drug delivery because it avoids first-pass hepatic metabolism and drawbacks associated with oral or intravenous routes, such as gastric irritation and variability of serum concentrations.

Precautions and Complications

Electrotherapy devices should not be used near implanted or temporary stimulators because of the potential for interference with the function of these devices. Abnormal vascular responses may develop when electrotherapy is used near sympathetic ganglia or the carotid sinus. IFC should not be used near open incisions or abrasions because of the potential for concentration of the electrical current at these sites. Electrotherapy devices should not be used near the gravid uterus because of potential adverse effects on fetal development or the possibility for stimulating uterine contractions. A deep venous thrombosis may be dislodged and propagated (resulting in an embolus) if electrotherapy induces stimulation of vascular smooth muscle in the area. Other precautions include insensate skin and patients with cognitive impairment.

• LOW-LEVEL LASER THERAPY (eSlide 17.15)

Physics and Bioeffects

Low-level laser therapy (LLLT) involves the use of relatively low light energy (less than 100-200 mW). The potential physiologic benefits of LLLT appear to be nonthermal; it can have a stimulating effect on target tissues. LLLT is used to decrease pain and inflammation, stimulate collagen metabolism and wound healing, and promote fracture healing.

Indications and Evidence Basis

LLLT may have a role in wound care, especially for diabetic foot ulcers. Following LLLT, pain is immediately reduced in patients with acute neck pain and over a period of 1–5 months in those with chronic neck pain. LLLT also reduces pain in the wrists, fingers, knees, and temporomandibular joints, as well as the pain associated with lateral epicondylitis.

Contraindications and Precautions

Precautions should be taken to ensure that the LLLT beam does not hit the eye directly or after reflection off a shiny surface. LLLT should not be used in areas with cancerous tissue.

• SUMMARY

Physical agent modalities are commonly used in the daily practice of physiatrists to relieve patient discomfort. Future research may focus on defining the best parameters of modality settings such as treatment dosage, duration, and frequency. Exploring the mechanism of treatment effects on tissues may also broaden our knowledge and aid in selecting the most appropriate modalities for various pathologies.

Clinical Pearls

1. Cryotherapy is generally used to treat acute injury, whereas thermotherapy is primarily used for subacute and chronic conditions. Heating produces modest increases in nerve conduction velocity, whereas cooling produces dramatic decreases in conduction velocity.
2. Depth of penetration is arbitrarily divided into deep and superficial. Superficial heat therapy includes hot packs, paraffin baths, infrared therapy, and hydrotherapy. Deep therapy includes ultrasound diathermy, shortwave diathermy, and microwave diathermy.
3. In Hubbard tanks, when only a portion of the body is immersed, more extreme temperatures can be used. For whole body immersion, neutral temperatures (34°C-36°C or 93°F-97°F) should be used to prevent core temperature fluctuations.
4. Ultrasound diathermy should be avoided near nerves, brain, eyes, reproductive organs, and growing bones (with open epiphyses), but it may be the only diathermy that can be used in areas with surgical metallic implants.
5. "No water and no metal" is recommended when considering the use of shortwave diathermy or microwave diathermy.
6. The lower frequencies used in shortwave diathermy and microwave diathermy have the advantage of increased depth of penetration but the disadvantages of greater beam dispersion and the need for larger applicators.
7. The potential physiologic effects of low-level laser therapy appear to be nonthermal.

BIBLIOGRAPHY
The complete bibliography is available on ExpertConsult.com.

18 | Integrative Medicine in Rehabilitation

Tian-Shin Yeh

Integrative medicine, emphasizing communication and education, is a patient-driven approach to lifestyle changes and overall improvement of well-being. An integrative approach to pain management and rehabilitation across neurologic and musculoskeletal disorders may drive enhanced outcomes.

• INTEGRATIVE MEDICINE (eSlide 18.1)

Complementary and integrative medicine (CIM) is a holistic, interdisciplinary approach to health, designed to treat the person and not just the disease. CIM combines conventional medicine with complementary and alternative medicine (CAM) when there is strong evidence of safety and effectiveness of the CAM. It encompasses Eastern and Western philosophies, as well as the individual and family. The goal is to concurrently treat the mind, body, and spirit.

• COMPLEMENTARY AND ALTERNATIVE MEDICINE (eSlide 18.2)

The National Center for Complementary and Alternative Medicine (NCCAM) uses the term "complementary health approaches" and defines two specific sub-groups of CAM: natural products (i.e., herbs and supplements, such as vitamins) and mind–body practices (including acupuncture, massage, meditation, mindfulness, movement therapies, relaxation techniques, spinal manipulation, yoga, and traditional Chinese medicine such as tai chi and qigong). Complementary medicine involves nonmainstream treatments that are often used in conjunction with conventional medicine. Alternative medicine, in contrast, involves the use of CAM instead of conventional medicine. According to the 2007 National Health Interview Survey, back pain (17.1%), neck pain (5.9%), and joint pain (5.2%) were the most common conditions that prompted CAM use.

Complementary and Alternative Medicine Practices (eSlide 18.3)

WHOLE MEDICAL SYSTEMS

Traditional Chinese medicine uses specific diagnostic evaluations, such as pulse and tongue assessment, and treatments such as herbal prescriptions and acupuncture.

Ayurveda from India is based on the theory of the three doshas (Tridoshas; the elements of life force or energy), which must be at equilibrium for good health. Yoga and herbal medicines are also components of Ayurvedic medicine.

Homeopathy focuses on two theories: "like cures like" (i.e., the disease can be treated or cured by a substance that produces similar symptoms in healthy people) and "law of minimum dose" (i.e., the principle of dilution: the effect is greater at the lowest dose of the medication).

MIND–BODY MEDICINE

Research has identified interactions between the brain and immune system, suggesting the existence of a mind–body connection. Yoga, tai chi, qigong, mindfulness-based (MB) cognitive therapy, and MB stress reduction programs are a few common MB interventions. These approaches are being used in psychotherapy and for the management of pain.

MANIPULATIVE AND BODY-BASED PRACTICES

Osteopathy. Osteopathic medicine, including manual manipulation of the spine, appears to play a role in the management of various types of pain, such as low back pain.

Massage. Massage is a general term for pressing, rubbing, and manipulating the skin, muscles, tendons, and ligaments to aid in relaxation and recovery from injury.

Movement Therapies. Common forms of movement therapy include tai chi, qigong, and yoga.

Acupuncture (eSlide 18.4). Acupuncture is a form of energy medicine. The traditional Chinese explanation is that life energy (Qi) flows through the body and over its surface to nourish the tissues through channels called meridians. Pain and illness are considered to occur when the flow of Qi becomes blocked or unbalanced. Acupuncture can unblock the obstructions and reestablish the flow of Qi through needle placement at points along the meridians, thus allowing the return of homeostasis. The modern scientific explanation is that acupuncture stimulates the nervous system to release chemicals in the muscles, spinal cord, and brain. These chemicals will either change the experience of pain or trigger the release of other chemicals and hormones, influencing the body's internal regulating systems. Acupuncture has been clinically demonstrated to be effective for low back pain, lateral epicondylitis, headaches, nausea, and vomiting.

Supplements (eSlide 18.5). S-Adenosylmethionine (SAM-E), a substance produced and used in the liver, has been shown to be as effective as nabumetone and celecoxib in the treatment of knee osteoarthritis (OA). The efficacy of glucosamine and chondroitin sulfate for treating arthritis has been controversial. Other supplements include vitamin D, N-acetylcysteine (NAC), methylsulfonylmethane (MSM), alpha-lipoic acid (ALA), magnesium, strontium, and fish oil.

QIGONG (eSlide 18.6)

Qigong is a "moving" mindfulness practice that uses slow graceful movements with coordinated breathing to promote the circulation of Qi within the body, thereby enhancing overall health, relaxation, and mental focus. A literature review concluded that evidence of health benefits from tai chi or qigong is strongest for bone health, cardiopulmonary fitness, balance, and factors associated with preventing falls and improving the quality of life and self-efficacy. Qigong may also reduce pain and improve sleep and mood status in patients with fibromyalgia or cancer.

TAI CHI (eSlide 18.7)

Tai chi, often referred to as "meditation in motion," involves performing a series of movements in a slow and graceful manner. It can enhance cardiovascular fitness, muscular strength, balance, physical function, quality of life, and performance of activities of daily living and reduce stress, anxiety, and depression. Tai chi can be safely recommended for patients with OA, rheumatoid arthritis, fibromyalgia, and Parkinson disease.

Yoga (eSlide 18.8). Many styles of yoga exist. Yoga has been shown to significantly improve standing balance and performance on the sit-to-stand and 4-m walk tests, as well as reduce sympathetic activity and/or increase vagal modulation. Studies support the use of yoga as a feasible intervention for patients who have had a stroke or traumatic brain injury.

Meditation/Mindfulness (eSlide 18.9). There are numerous types of meditation, such as guided imagery, mindfulness meditation, and prayer. By focusing attention, meditation has long been used for relaxation and stress reduction. Studies have also shown that it can help reduce pain and improve mood.

• ECONOMICS OF COMPLEMENTARY AND INTEGRATIVE MEDICINE (eSlide 18.10)

Research supports the use of CIM as a cost-effective option. CIM practices that include chiropractic manipulation, acupuncture, massage, reflexology (foot massage), music therapy, relaxation response stress reduction, and guided imagery may reduce pain, decrease medication use, and lower health care expenditures.

• CONCLUSION

Integrative medicine includes all health and wellness practices that best serve each individual. Future research may continue to explore the mechanisms of these approaches and the effectiveness of their application for diverse conditions (eSlide 18.11).

Clinical Pearls

1. Spinal manipulation, most often provided by chiropractors, is beneficial for low back pain. Its contraindications include severe osteoporosis, spinal epidural infection, and spinal metastasis. The most common side effect is local discomfort. The risk of death or permanent neurologic sequelae from stroke after cervical spine manipulation is 1 in 1,000,000 (eSlide 18.12).
2. Reiki involves the manipulation of energy fields using specific hand positions. It can be performed at a distance and does not require focused attention by the patient.
3. The Dietary Supplement Health and Education Act of 1994 exempts manufacturers from having to prove the safety or efficacy of their herbal products.
4. Studies have suggested the following indications for complementary and alternative medicine in integrative rehabilitation:
   1) Pain management: osteopathy, acupuncture (needle shock typically occurs during the first treatment), massage, qigong, tai chi, yoga, meditation, reflexology (based on the principle of microsystem), vitamin D, NAC, and fish oil
   2) Arthritis: acupuncture, tai chi, SAM-E, glucosamine and chondroitin (full effects can take up to 2 to 4 months), MSM, strontium ranelate, fish oil, cat's claw, devil's claw
   3) Cardiorespiratory fitness enhancement, balance improvement, and fall prevention: movement therapies
   4) Relaxation or stress reduction: massage, meditation, qigong, tai chi, yoga

BIBLIOGRAPHY
The complete bibliography is available on ExpertConsult.com.

Computer Assistive Devices and Environmental Controls

19

Shih-Ching Chen

Assistive technology (AT) devices allow people with disabilities to participate in activities of daily living. The AT evaluation team should determine goals and suggest appropriate AT devices and services to promote the use of AT by patients and their caregivers. Clinical assessments and physician responsibilities are summarized in this chapter.

• DEFINING ASSISTIVE TECHNOLOGY (eSlide 19.1)

The term *assistive technology* describes tools used to enable people with disabilities to walk, eat, see, and otherwise conduct and participate in activities of daily living. Public law defines AT as "any item, piece of equipment or product system whether acquired commercially off the shelf, modified, or customized that is used to increase or improve functional capabilities of individuals with disabilities." This definition also includes a second component, defining AT services as "any service that directly assists an individual with a disability in the selection, acquisition, or use, of an assistive technology device."

• OVERVIEW OF ASSISTIVE TECHNOLOGY DEVICES (eSlides 19.2 and 19.3)

AT devices are designed to facilitate functional abilities and to meet the needs of humans. Considering one's own interaction with technology gives insight into issues involved in the concept of the human-technology interface (HTI). Interaction commonly occurs through dials, switches, keyboards, handlebars, joysticks, or handgrips. Typical interfaces for direct selection, such as a computer keyboard or television remote control, are used by individuals with abilities to accurately choose an intended item because all possible options are presented at once and will be directly selected by individuals. Scanning switches that come in many styles (e.g., tongue touch, sipping and puffing, eye blink), the eye gaze switch, and the head mouse are examples of indirect selection methods used by severely disabled individuals to interact with their environment. HTI is also applicable for completing the feedback loop from devices back to the user. Good assessment skills and a focus on patients and their goals and needs are essential for HTI success and preventing abandonment of AT devices.

• ASSISTIVE TECHNOLOGY FOR COMMUNICATION DISORDERS (eSlides 19.4 and 19.5)

AT devices that meet the needs of people with many types of speech and language impairments are commonly called augmentative and alternative communication (AAC) devices. The use of AAC devices should be encouraged along with all other available communication modalities, such as gestures, vocalizations, sign language, and eye gaze. Nonelectronic AAC systems can be created with digital photographs, pictures from books or catalogs, or a marker to draw letters, words, phrases, or pictures. Digital voice output devices allow recording and storing of simple phrases in the memory of the device. When the user wants to speak, he or she simply presses a button and the device speaks the prerecorded message. However, these devices are not appropriate for individuals who need or want to communicate complex thoughts or feelings.

Synthesized speech is created by the software that uses rules of phonics and pronunciation to translate alphanumeric text into spoken output through the speech synthesizer hardware. Because numerous AAC applications (apps) are currently available, the use of touchscreen tablets, such as the iPad, has become highly popular and mainstream. Advantages of these systems are that they allow users to speak on any topic and use any word they wish. Among the latest developments for people who are completely locked-in are speech-generating devices that can be activated by a simple eye blink or by visually gazing on the desired area of the screen. The speech enhancer processes speech sounds for people with dysarthria, enabling improved speech recognition by others. The user wears a headset with a microphone attached to a portable device, and after processing, the clarified voice is projected via speakers.

• ASSISTIVE TECHNOLOGY FOR MOBILITY IMPAIRMENTS (eSlides 19.6 and 19.7)

Motor impairments greatly affect the ability of individuals to interact with their environment. Early intervention and supportive caregivers and family members who are available to create modifications and incorporate AT devices into activities of daily living can help people compensate for impaired motor skills. Individuals can fully participate in life because many tasks can be accomplished through computers. Computers can perform education-related and work-related tasks and can monitor and control an unlimited array of devices and appliances at home, work, and school. Many AT devices have been developed to help individuals with upper body mobility impairment in using computers. Alternative computer keyboards come in many shapes, sizes, and layouts; onscreen keyboards are visible on the computer monitor. Voice recognition (VR) software has become essential for computer access for many individuals with motor impairment. AT solutions can include crutches, a rolling walker, a powered scooter, or a manual or powered wheelchair for individuals with lower body mobility impairments. Simple environmental modifications or adaptations can be indispensable facilitators for these individuals and might be all that is needed to increase participation.

• ASSISTIVE TECHNOLOGY FOR ERGONOMICS AND PREVENTION OF SECONDARY INJURIES (eSlides 19.8 and 19.9)

A rapidly growing area of concern for AT practitioners is the development of repetitive strain injuries (RSIs). Over the past few years, an entire industry of

AT has been developed to deal with repetitive motion disorders. Electronic aids to daily living (EADL) provide alternative control of electrical devices within the environment and increase independence in activities of daily living. This technology is also referred to as environmental control units (ECUs). EADLs can be controlled directly by pressing a button with a finger or pointer or by voice command or controlled indirectly by scanning and switch activation. EADLs are primarily used at the home but can also be used at work or school.

• ASSISTIVE TECHNOLOGY FOR HEARING IMPAIRMENTS (eSlide 19.10)

Hearing impairment and deafness affect the feedback loop in the human–environment interaction. AT devices, such as hearing aids and FM (frequency modulation) or radio wave systems, can be used to facilitate both auditory input and speech output. Other types of AT devices provide a visual representation, such as flashing lights of the auditory signal. Cochlear implants are inserted surgically with an electrode array placed within or around the cochlear structure when the hearing system is impaired at the level of the middle ear or cochlea. This system requires a battery pack worn on the body or behind the ear. It also requires an experienced audiologist to teach the individual to use acoustic cues produced by the cochlear implant as a substitute for natural hearing. Another recent adaptation for people with significant hearing impairments is computer-assisted real-time translation. This AT solution involves a specially trained typist or stenographer who records what is being spoken on a computer. The text is then projected onto a display, resulting in close to "real-time" translation. For individuals who wear hearing aids, the environmental adaptations frequently support individuals who are deaf or hard of hearing. Lip movements and gestures can also be helpful.

• ASSISTIVE TECHNOLOGY FOR VISUAL IMPAIRMENTS (eSlide 19.11)

The term *visual impairment* technically encompasses all types of permanent vision loss or low vision. AT solutions conventionally involve the use of simple handheld magnifiers, large-print reading materials, or mobility devices (e.g., a white cane) for safe and efficient travel. High-contrast tapes or markers can also be used to indicate hazards in the environments. Braille text is still the first choice of many individuals for reading. Computers fitted with a speech synthesizer and specialized software allow navigation of the desktop, operating system, applications, documents, and the entire Internet. Any digital text can be heard aloud by the individual using this software. For individuals with some visual ability, screen magnification software enables the user to choose the amount (2–20 times) and type of magnification preferred for optimal computer access. Many magnification applications combine enlargement with speech synthesis or text-to-speech. People with visual impairment usually keep the setup of their home and work environments constant because this helps in locating items. To supplement these less technical aids, some individuals use electronic travel aids that have the capability of detecting obstacles missed by a cane. This technology uses ultrasound or information embedded in the environment, expressly for users who have limited vision.

• ASSISTIVE TECHNOLOGY FOR COGNITIVE OR LEARNING DISABILITIES (eSlides 19.12)

AT systems are being used to assist people with cognitive disabilities to learn new jobs/tasks and/or to prompt people through the various steps of a given task. Another system enables developers to use context-aware sensors in a multitude of environments and technologies to facilitate the safety, capacity, and well-being of people with cognitive disabilities using batteryless micropower sensors. There are a number of both low-technology and high-technology solutions available to assist literacy development, such as audiobooks or text-to-speech software that provides anticipation or multisensory feedback on the computer. VR can sometimes be helpful for people with learning disabilities. Some AT software systems provide auditory or visual prompts for individuals with cognitive disabilities. These system can be set up to prompt an individual through each step of a task.

• SELECTING APPROPRIATE ASSISTIVE TECHNOLOGIES (eSlide 19.13)

Abandonment

Depending on the type of technology, nonuse or abandonment can be as low as 8% or as high as 75%. On an average, one-third of more optional ATs are abandoned, most within the first 3 months. To prevent abandonment, the AT team should include the individual with a disability and consider his or her opinions and preferences during the evaluation process.

• PRINCIPLES OF CLINICAL ASSESSMENT

The goal of an AT evaluation is to determine whether AT devices and services have the potential to help an individual meet his or her activity or participation goals at home, school, work, or play. Other goals include (1) providing a safe and supportive environment, (2) identifying the need for AT services, (3) modifying or customizing ATs as needed, and (4) developing a potential list of recommended devices. Professionals from various disciplines should be chosen as members of the AT evaluation team based on the identified needs of an individual with the disability. It is not appropriate for an AT vendor to be called in to perform an AT evaluation, but the vendor can demonstrate its products and assist in setting up the equipment for evaluation when requested by the team. However, other team members, including the end user and his or her family, should perform the evaluation and make the final recommendations.

Phase 1 Assistive Technology Assessment

Phase 1 of the assessment process begins when a referral is received. Standard demographic and impairment-related information and clinical assessments are collected. The team leader takes responsibility for ensuring that the individual, his or her family, and any other significant individuals are invited for the evaluation. The team identifies the life roles, the specific activities engaged in, and any problems the individual has in fulfilling these life roles. The team prioritizes the order in which to address barriers to participation, and a specific plan of action is developed. As time goes on, further assessments should be performed and needs should be noted. The assessment team includes the individual and his or her caregivers as primary members.

Phase 2 Assistive Technology Assessment

Once the team has agreed on a specific plan of action and those things that "must" occur, phase 2 of the assessment process begins. AT devices are tested along with various adaptations, modifications, and placements to ensure appropriate matching of the technology to the individual. Because many devices require extensive training and follow-up, it is essential that realistic information about training and learning time be provided and appropriate resources within the local community be identified. With very few exceptions, the wise course of action involves borrowing or renting the AT device before making a final purchase decision. Consumers and their families should always be informed so that they can make the final decision regarding when and where the equipment will be delivered. AT professionals, in consultation with the physician, should also anticipate future needs, and final decisions should consider both the expected performance and durability of the device.

Writing the Assistive Technology Assessment Report

The evaluation report documents the AT assessment process and must include several components. First and foremost, it is helpful to use layman's terms to help case managers, educators, and others unfamiliar with ATs understand the process. The report should focus on the funding requested to purchase the technology. It is also extremely important that all components of the AT device be included in the list of recommended equipment because devices are often recommended for purchase as a "system." Besides purchasing AT devices, paying for the AT services is important to avoid low use or abandonment. Finally, it is also important to include the vendors' contact information.

• PHYSICIAN RESPONSIBILITIES (eSlides 19.14 and 19.15)

Prescribing the Technologies

The following items should be considered when prescribing AT devices and certifying medical necessity. The physician must provide evidence of individual medical necessity for the specific AT, and health insurance companies require an "appropriate" prescription that includes mention of the comprehensive assessment process, individual's motivation, availability of training, and potential functional outcome(s) for the patient.

Documentation in the Health Care Record

In addition to prescribing and certifying medical necessity on various forms, physicians must maintain a system that tracks device performance and maintain complete patient health care records that include details such as the diagnosis, patient's condition, prognosis, functional limitations, interventions and results, and a list of all assistive devices. This comprehensive health care record supplies the background information needed to substantiate the need for AT devices and services, regardless of the funding source.

Funding Letters of Medical Necessity

Physicians are frequently asked to write "letters of medical necessity" to help ensure that the AT needs of patients are met. These letters should include the diagnosis and functional limitations of the patient. In addition, there should be a statement about the patient's inability to perform specific tasks, such as activities of daily living, work activities, or functional walking.

The letter should also include a paragraph stating why the equipment is necessary and a rationale for choosing this specific equipment. It also requires a description of the specific equipment features and listing of all the required components.

• FUNDING ASSISTIVE TECHNOLOGY

Funding sources for AT devices and services are private or government medical or health insurance and the coverage is based on existing laws and regulations.

The five steps in developing a funding strategy are as follows: (1) surveying the funding resources available to the individual, (2) identifying various funding sources for various steps in the AT intervention, (3) preparing a funding plan with the patient and family members or advocates, (4) assigning responsibilities to specific individuals for the funding of each step of the AT intervention, and (5) preparing the necessary written documentation for the funding source so that there is a record in the event an appeal is needed.

• CONCLUSION

The growing culture of inclusion is changing traditional concepts about disability and impairment. Future research regarding AT should include opinions of individuals with disabilities and their families and use mainstream technologies to provide more opportunities for participating in activities of daily living.

Clinical Pearls

1. Assistive technology (AT) devices are designed to facilitate functional abilities and to meet the needs of humans throughout their varied life stages and roles.
2. In addition to professionals from various disciplines chosen as AT evaluation team members, the AT team should also include individuals with disabilities and their families.
3. AT device use and requirements will change with time as individuals mature and take on different life roles.
4. Physicians should prescribe AT devices, maintain well-documented health care records, write the AT assessment report, and assist patients in finding a funding source.

BIBLIOGRAPHY
The complete bibliography is available on ExpertConsult.com.

COMMON CLINICAL PROBLEMS

Bladder Dysfunction 20

Shih-Chung Chang

Urinary tract neurophysiology, types of bladder dysfunction, and management strategies for bladder dysfunction are summarized in this chapter.

• NEUROANATOMY AND PHYSIOLOGY

Detrusor and Sphincter Muscle Characteristics

Detrusor contraction is initiated by an increase in intracellular calcium, and detrusor relaxation is associated with influx of potassium into detrusor smooth muscle cells. Collagen forms nearly 50% of the bladder wall in healthy individuals. The majority of distal sphincters are slow-twitch striated fibers, and pelvic floor muscles are a mixture of fast-twitch and slow-twitch striated fibers.

Lower Urinary Tract Pharmacology: Receptors and Neurotransmitters (eSlide 20.1)

Cholinergic muscarinic (M_2 and M_3) receptors are distributed in the body of the bladder, trigone, bladder neck, and urethra. The M_2 cholinergic muscarinic receptors structurally predominate in normal bladders, but the M_3 receptors may be functionally more important for bladder contraction. Cholinergic nicotinic receptors are primarily located in the striated sphincter. Adrenergic receptors (predominantly α_1) are concentrated in the trigone, bladder neck, and urethra. Norepinephrine-containing nerve cells are distributed in the paravesical and intramural ganglia, which maintain continence by producing contraction of the bladder neck and urethral smooth muscle. β_2-Adrenergic and β_3-adrenergic receptors produce relaxation at the bladder neck on initiation of voiding and relax the bladder body to enhance storage. The main effector transmitter for urethra contraction is norepinephrine (via the α_1 receptors), and the relaxation of the urethra is caused by the release of nitric oxide in the urethral wall, which is mediated by acetylcholine in the pelvic ganglia.

Lower Urinary Tract Innervation (eSlides 20.2 and 20.3)

Peripheral innervations include pelvic (parasympathetic), hypogastric (sympathetic), and pudendal (somatic) nerves. Bladder filling sensory information is transferred back to the central nervous system via afferent Aδ fibers in the pelvic nerve. In pathologic and inflammatory states, the capsaicin-sensitive vanilloid receptors and C-afferent fibers play a major role in detrusor overactivity.

MICTURITION REFLEX

The pontine micturition center (PMC) coordinates the activity of the bladder and sphincter during micturition. Disruption of pathways between the PMC and sacral outflow to the bladder lead to detrusor sphincter dyssynergia. Afferent axons form bladder synapses with the Onuf nucleus (pudendal nerve nucleus at the lateral border of the ventral horn of S_2, S_3, and S_4), which allows inhibition of pelvic floor activity during voiding. Voluntary control of the pelvic floor is achieved through afferents that ascend to the sensory cortex and the synapse of descending fibers from the motor cortex with the pudendal nucleus.

Lower Urinary Tract Function

Neonates and infants have involuntary reflex voiding, but approximately 90% of children have volitional control of voiding by 5 years of age. For healthy adults, there is only a minimal increase in intravesical pressure but with increasing activity of the pelvic floor and voluntary sphincter during the bladder filling phase. Voiding is initiated by voluntary relaxation of the pelvic floor with subsequent release of inhibition of the detrusor reflex at the pontine level. Urinary frequency, urgency, and incontinence with incomplete emptying are common in older adults. This may result from detrusor underactivity, benign prostate hyperplasia, impaired sphincter activity, loss of cerebral inhibition due to minor strokes, collagen deposition in the bladder wall, secondary polyuria from inadequate antidiuretic hormone secretion at night, reduced renal concentrating ability, and mobilization of lower extremity edema during sleep.

• CLASSIFICATION OF NEUROGENIC BLADDER DYSFUNCTION (eSlide 20.4)

Neurogenic bladder dysfunction can be classified as anatomic (supraspinal, infrasacral, peripheral autonomic, and muscular lesions) or functional (storage ability and activity and coordination of the detrusor and sphincter).

Evaluation of Neurogenic Bladder Dysfunction

Careful history and physical examinations, including volume of fluid intake and output, frequency of urinary tract infections (UTIs), presence of neurologic disorders, and assessment of pelvic floor muscle and rectal tone and reflexes (bulbocavernosus, cremasteric, and anal reflexes), are important basic evaluations.

Diagnostic Testing for Neurogenic Bladder Dysfunction (eSlides 20.5 and 20.6)

Indications for upper tract evaluation include symptoms suggestive of pyelonephritis, history of renal disease, spinal cord lesions, and myelodysplasia. A simple baseline screening test, such as an ultrasound, is sufficient for patients with a stroke, Parkinson disease, and multiple sclerosis because the involvement of the upper tract is infrequent in these patients.

Upper Tract Tests

Ultrasonography (US) is adequate for imaging chronic obstruction and dilation, scarring, renal masses (both cystic and solid), renal stones, bladder wall thickness, bladder irregularity, presence of bladder stones, and measurement of postvoid residual (PVR) urine, but not for evaluating acute ureteral obstruction. A kidney, ureter, and bladder x-ray (KUB) is often combined with US to identify possible ureter or bladder stones. Computed tomography (CT) or CT urogram can detect small bladder stones in patients with an indwelling catheter and a collapsed bladder and is useful in the evaluation of possible acute upper tract obstruction by stones.

Isotope studies, such as a technetium-99m dimercaptosuccinic acid (DMSA) scan or technetium-99m mertiatide (MAG-3) renogram, can be used to evaluate differential function, functional area of the renal cortex, and urinary tract drainage. Iothalamate is used in excretory urography and in measuring the glomerular filtration rate.

Lower Tract Tests

Urinalysis and culture and sensitivity testing should be performed for all patients with a neurogenic bladder disorder or new lower urinary tract symptoms, as well as before invasive procedures. The PVR is clinically useful when compared with previous recordings and in conjunction with the bladder pressure, clinical symptoms, and appearance of the bladder wall. Cystography is used to detect ureteral reflux and to evaluate the outline and shape of the bladder.

Urodynamic and videourodynamic studies (eSlides 20.7 and 20.8) can be used to evaluate the filling and voiding phases of the lower urinary tract. Indications for videourodynamic studies include the following: patients with incomplete spinal cord lesions with incontinence but with incomplete emptying; those with mechanical obstruction with neuropathy; assessment of detrusor contraction, bladder neck obstruction, and striated sphincter dyssynergia (eSlide 20.9); before sphincterotomy; patients in whom pharmacotherapy has failed; before bladder augmentation, continent diversion, or placement of an artificial sphincter or a suprapubic catheter; and for assessment of deterioration of the upper urinary tract and frequent relapses of symptomatic bacteriuria. Normal bladder compliance should be greater than 30 mL/cm H_2O, and less than 10 mL/cm H_2O is considered to be poor compliance. Sphincter electromyography (EMG) can be combined with cystometrogram (CMG) or videourodynamic studies. Normal sphincter EMG increases gradually as bladder capacity is reached during the filling phase and becomes silent just before voiding. With detrusor sphincter dyssynergia, sphincter EMG activity increases when a reflex detrusor contraction occurs. The only routine indication for cystoscopy is long-term indwelling catheter (suprapubic or urethral) use. Cystoscopy is also indicated after CT urogram in patients who have gross or microscopic hematuria that cannot be attributed to UTI, stones, or trauma.

Nonpharmacologic Treatment of Neurogenic Bladder Dysfunction (eSlides 20.10 and 20.11)

A timed voiding program helps patients with detrusor overactivity urinate before actual detrusor contraction occurs. Suprapubic tapping or jabbing over the bladder causes a mechanical stretch reflex of the bladder wall and subsequent contraction; it may be effective for patients with paraplegia. Patients with areflexia and infrasacral lesions may be able to void using a Valsalva or Credé maneuver. Patients with paraplegia and a spastic pelvic floor can achieve effective voiding by stretching the anal sphincter and then emptying the bladder by the Valsalva maneuver.

Urine collection devices include external catheters, indwelling catheters (urethral or suprapubic), clean intermittent catheterization, and protective garments. The clean intermittent catheterization program requires a low-pressure bladder of adequate capacity (greater than 300 mL) and enough outflow resistance to maintain continence. People with a spinal cord injury (SCI) at C6 and below can often manage self-catheterization.

Surgical Treatment of Neurogenic Bladder Dysfunction

To increase bladder capacity (eSlide 20.12), options include bladder augmentation (with or without continent catheterizable stoma) and an ileal conduit. Bladder augmentation is used for patients with detrusor hyperactivity, reduced compliance, and decreased functional storage capacity that do not respond to medical therapy. An ileal conduit used as a urinary diversion strategy is recommended for conditions in which the bladder cannot be preserved. To increase bladder contractility, electrical stimulation with electrodes implanted on the bladder wall, pelvic nerves, sacral roots, and conus is used to elicit detrusor contraction. To increase bladder outlet resistance, options include injection therapy into the bladder neck and urethra to increase tissue bulk under and around the bladder neck, a fascial sling, or an artificial sphincter. To decrease bladder outlet resistance, sphincterotomy is usually indicated in patients with SCI who are unable or unwilling to perform self-catheterization, with bladder neck obstruction resulting from primary hyperactivity or bladder wall hypertrophy that occurs because of chronic striated sphincter dyssynergia. After the procedure, obstruction from recurrence of the stricture or dyssynergia may occur. A urethral stent is used after failed sphincterotomy or as a substitute for sphincterotomy.

Pharmacologic Treatment of Neurogenic Bladder Dysfunction (eSlide 20.13)

Antimuscarinic agents (such as propantheline bromide, hyoscyamine, and oxybutynin) and muscarinic receptor antagonists (such as darifenacin, solifenacin, and trospium) are used for the suppression of detrusor activity. Cholinergic agonists (bethanechol) can be used to increase detrusor activity. Adrenergic antagonists (such as terazosin, doxazosin, tamsulosin, and silodosin) are used to reduce symptoms that result from benign prostate hypertrophy and to increase bladder emptying. Tamsulosin can also decrease symptoms of autonomic dysreflexia in suprasacral SCI. Mirabegron (which acts on β_3-adrenergic receptors) showed efficacy for overactive bladder symptoms. Cystoscopic injection of botulinum toxin type A can be used in patients with neurogenic detrusor overactivity that is refractory to medications.

Differential Diagnosis of Neurogenic Bladder Dysfunction

Patients with stroke, dementia, brain tumors, or trauma typically have frequency and urge incontinence but coordinated voiding and complete emptying. Patients with Parkinson disease commonly have urinary frequency, urgency, and urge incontinence, and 50% of these individuals complain of difficulty voiding. In patients with multiple sclerosis (brain and spinal cord lesions), 90% develop bladder hyperactivity and incomplete emptying. Bladder areflexia is present in multiple sclerosis with predominant conal lesions.

The detrusor reflex of patients with spinal cord lesions usually returns within the first 6 months after a period of spinal shock. Because of loss of inhibitory and coordination control from higher centers, incomplete sustained detrusor contraction and impaired voluntary control of the pelvic floor may occur. Patients with an incomplete lesion may have urgency and adequate emptying, but patients with a complete lesion may have reflex incontinence and incomplete emptying because of detrusor sphincter dyssynergia. Excessive sympathetic activity can also lead to detrusor bladder neck dyssynergia in patients with high complete tetraplegia.

Conus, cauda equina, and peripheral nerve lesions may lead to an areflexic or noncontractile and insensate bladder. Autonomic neuropathy, secondary to diabetes or multiple system atrophy, may result in a noncontractile and insensate bladder. Myelodysplasia frequently produces a mixed pattern of lower urinary tract dysfunction, but the most common is a hyperactive or noncompliant bladder with dyssynergia or a nonrelaxing sphincter.

Complications of Neurogenic Voiding Dysfunction (eSlides 20.14 and 20.15)

BACTERIURIA

UTIs are common in patients with a neurogenic bladder. *Escherichia coli, Proteus, Klebsiella, Pseudomonas, Serratia, Providencia*, enterococci, and staphylococci are common organisms in patients with catheter-associated UTI. Patients with mild to moderate illness can be treated with oral fluoroquinolone (ciprofloxacin, levofloxacin, or gatifloxacin) or trimethoprim-sulfamethoxazole, but trimethoprim-sulfamethoxazole does not provide coverage against *Pseudomonas aeruginosa*. In more seriously ill and hospitalized patients, piperacillin plus tazobactam, ampicillin plus gentamicin, or imipenem plus cilastatin provide coverage against most expected pathogens.

AUTONOMIC DYSREFLEXIA

In patients with SCI, autonomic dysreflexia symptoms (sudden hypertension, sweating, piloerection, headache, and reflex bradycardia) can be elicited from nociceptive sources (such as a distended bladder), especially if the injury is above T6. Prevention of nociceptive stimuli is the best strategy. Nitroglycerin ointment, prazosin, or captopril can be used if symptoms persist even after the elimination of the stimulus. Phenoxybenzamine (an adrenergic antagonist) has been used to prevent autonomic dysreflexia.

HYPERCALCIURIA AND STONES

Hypercalciuria occurs in patients with SCI because of the loss of calcium from bones as a result of immobility and may lead to renal and bladder stone formation. Bladder stones are effectively treated with cystoscopy and laser lithotripsy. Small stones and particles can be dissolved by bladder irrigations with 30 mL of hemiacidrin (Renacidin) solution. Growing calculi or renal pelvis stones should be treated by extracorporeal shock wave lithotripsy before ureter obstruction occurs. Percutaneous approach is the preferred method for larger stones (greater than 3 cm diameter).

LOWER AND UPPER URINARY TRACT CHANGES

Bladder trabeculation occurs in most SCI patients. Sacculation and diverticula occur when obstruction and high pressure are severe, which may lead to ureteral reflux. Ureteral reflux or high bladder pressure without reflux can cause upper tract dilation. If reflux or ureteral dilation occur, intermittent catheterization, antimuscarinic medication, or botulinum toxin injections can be used to lower the bladder pressure. If the bladder pressure improves but reflux persists, surgical repair of the reflux should be considered. If bladder pressure does not respond, urinary diversion is indicated.

Clinical Pearls

1. Patient failures with pharmacologic treatment of neurogenic bladder dysfunction are frequently due to intolerable side effects (e.g., dry mouth, drowsiness, hypotension). Careful medicine selection and close monitoring of side effects during pharmacologic treatment are important.
2. Autonomic dysreflexia is a dangerous syndrome found in patients with a spinal cord injury (SCI), which should be immediately treated. All patients with SCI and their caregivers should be aware of this problem.
3. Ultimate goals of bladder management are to prevent upper tract deterioration, reduce morbidity, and improve the patient's quality of life. A careful history and physical examination, appropriate diagnostic testing, and classification of bladder dysfunction are important for individualized management to achieve these goals in each patient.

BIBLIOGRAPHY
The complete bibliography is available on ExpertConsult.com.

Neurogenic Bowel: Dysfunction and Rehabilitation

21

Yu-Hui Huang

The epidemiology, neuroanatomy, physiology, pathophysiology, evaluation, and management of neurogenic bowel are summarized in this chapter.

• EPIDEMIOLOGY AND IMPACT

Neurogenic bowel dysfunction results from autonomic and somatic denervation and produces fecal incontinence, constipation, and difficulty with evacuation (DWE), as well as upper gastrointestinal symptoms. The prevalence of DWE ranges from 10% to 50% among the hospitalized or institutionalized older population. Bowel continence is one of the greatest predictors of return to home for survivors of a stroke. More than one-third of surveyed people with spinal cord injury (SCI) rated bowel and bladder dysfunction as having the most significant effect on their lives. Almost one-third of people with SCI report worsening of bowel function 5 years after their injury, with 33% developing megacolon. These problems significantly affect nutrition and health and can create considerable psychological, social, and emotional trauma. When restoring normal defecation is not possible, social continence (predictable and adequate defecation without incontinence) becomes the goal.

• NEUROANATOMY AND PHYSIOLOGY OF THE GASTROINTESTINAL TRACT

Neural control of the gastrointestinal tract involves the central nervous system (CNS; brain and spinal cord), autonomic nervous system (sympathetic and parasympathetic), and enteric nervous system (ENS) (eSlides 21.1 and 21.2).

Enteric Nervous System (eSlide 21.3)

The ENS is a distinct system with its own set of neurons that coordinate sensory and motor functions. It includes sensory neurons, interneurons, and motor neurons, which are organized and situated in two layers: the submucosal (Meissner) plexus and the intramuscular myenteric (Auerbach) plexus. The ENS has automatic feedback control with reflex circuits that coordinate motor patterns [migrating motor complex, digestive activity, and giant migratory contractions (GMCs)]. It is the key to proper functioning of the entire gastrointestinal tract and the coordination of the segment-to-segment function.

Enteric Nervous System Relationship to the Spinal Cord and Brain

Sensory information from vagal afferents in the ENS is relayed to two main areas: (1) the nodose ganglia (caudal ganglion of the vagus) and consequently to the nucleus tractus solitarius and area postrema in the medullary area of the brainstem, which send signals to the rostral centers in the brain (this pathway does not reach the level of consciousness) and (2) the dorsal motor nucleus of the vagus (DVN) and the nucleus ambiguus, which share the information with the forebrain and brainstem, creating the dorsal vagal complex. Brain influences (conscious and nonconscious) are translated to the dorsal vagal complex, where the DVN and nucleus ambiguus represent the efferent arm of the reflex pathway. Spinal afferents (splanchnic and pelvic) send sensory impulses to the dorsal root ganglia (or prevertebral sympathetic ganglia), which are conducted to the dorsal column nuclei. This pathway plays a greater role in nociceptive transmission than the spinothalamic or spinoreticular tracts. The somatosensory cortex regulates the awareness and recognition of pain, and the paralimbic and limbic areas contribute to the cognitive and affective aspects of pain.

Gastrointestinal Neuromotor System

The gut wall is composed of "self-excitable" smooth muscles that contract in an all-in-one manner. They spontaneously respond to stretch and can function independently of neural or endocrine control. The interstitial cells of Cajal act like a pacemaker and allow the propagation of electrical slow waves into the circular muscle layer, which generates spontaneous muscle contraction. The aboral direction of propulsive activity throughout the digestive tract is achieved by segmental inactivation of inhibitory motor neurons distally. Sympathetic nervous system stimulation tends to promote the bowel's storage function by enhancing anal tone and inhibiting colonic contractions, whereas parasympathetic activity enhances colonic motility.

Gastrointestinal Tract Motility and Physiology (eSlide 21.4)

The gastric fundus acts as a reservoir, which accommodates incoming food, and the antrum is a mixer that generates propulsive waves. Intestinal motility has two patterns: (1) the interdigestive migrating motor complex pattern, which occurs during fasting and is influenced by the hormone motilin, and (2) the postprandial segmentation pattern of motility, which is induced by vagal efferents and gradually develops into giant migrating contractions (GMCs) sustained through long portions along the small and large bowel. The colon functions to serve as a reservoir for food waste, reabsorbs fluids and gases, provides an environment for the growth of bacteria, and absorbs certain bacterial breakdown products. The "gastrocolonic response" or "gastrocolic reflex" refers to the increased colonic activity (GMCs and mass movements) that occurs in the first 30–60 minutes after a meal. It is modulated both by hormonal and neural (spinal cord–mediated vesicovesical reflexes) effects and is often therapeutically used to enhance bowel evacuation. The rectum is usually empty until just before defecation. Continence is maintained by the anal sphincter mechanism, which consists of the internal anal sphincter (IAS), external anal sphincter (EAS), and puborectalis muscle. The resting anal canal pressure is largely determined by the angulation at the anorectal junction by the puborectalis sling and internal sphincter tone; only 20% of the pressure is attributable to the EAS (although it is physically larger than the IAS). The EAS (innervated by the S2-S4 nerve roots via the pudendal nerve) and puborectalis muscle (innervated by direct branches from the S1 to S5 roots) are the only striated skeletal muscles whose normal resting state is tonic contraction.

Normal defecation begins with rectosigmoid distention by approximately 200 mL of feces. Two reflexes emerge after rectosigmoid distention: the rectorectal reflex, in which the bowel proximal to the bolus contracts and the bowel distal to it relaxes, and the rectoanal inhibitory reflex, characterized by reflex relaxation of the IAS and stretching of the puborectalis muscle, correlated with the urge known as "the call to stool." One can then volitionally contract the levator ani to open the proximal anal canal and relax the EAS and puborectalis muscles to produce defecation, which may be aided by a Valsalva maneuver. However, one can elect to defer defecation by volitionally contracting the puborectalis muscle and EAS. The reflexive IAS relaxation subsequently fades, usually within 15 seconds. The EAS generally tenses in response to a small rectal distention via a spinal reflex, although reflexive relaxation of the EAS occurs in the presence of greater distention. These spinal cord reflexes are centered in the conus medullaris and are augmented and modulated by higher cortical influences. When cortical control is disrupted (in patients with SCI), the EAS reflexes usually persist and allow spontaneous defecation.

• PATHOPHYSIOLOGY OF GASTROINTESTINAL DYSFUNCTION

The pathophysiology of common symptoms generated from neurogenic bowel dysfunction is presented in eSlide 21.5.

Upper Motor Neurogenic Bowel (eSlides 21.6, 21.7, and 21.8)

Any destructive CNS process above the conus can lead to upper motor neurogenic bowel (UMNB) pattern of dysfunction. Spinal cortical sensory pathway deficits lead to decreased sensation of defecation, but some patients with SCI have some residual sensation, possibly mediated by an autonomic nervous system pathway. Colonic compliance was previously reported to be impaired, but recent studies have indicated that it is normal. The presence of rectal sphincter dyssynergia (passive filling of the rectum leads to increased sphincter tone) might be known as impaired colonic compliance, and it often results in DWE. Colorectal transit times were reported to be significantly prolonged in supraconal SCI patients, especially during the acute phase, with the total gastrointestinal transit time reported to be 3.93 days (control group, 1.76 days). The transit time of the rectosigmoid portion tended to be less severely prolonged than that of the colon because of sparing of the sacral reflex arc. Patients with UMNB also have a normal or increased anal sphincter tone, a palpable puborectalis muscle sling, a normal anal verge appearance, and intact sacral reflexes, including the anocutaneous (or anal wink), vesicorectal (increased EAS pressure in response to increased intraabdominal pressure), and bulbocavernosus reflexes.

Lower Motor Neurogenic Bowel

Polyneuropathy, conus medullaris or cauda equina lesions, pelvic surgery, vaginal delivery, or even chronic straining during defecation can impair the autonomic and somatic innervation of the rectosigmoid and anus. Lower motor neurogenic bowel (LMNB) dysfunction might produce fecal incontinence (pudendal denervation), distal colonic sluggishness (parasympathetic denervation), and prolonged transit time. The addition of constipation and DWE to fecal incontinence compounds difficulties, and a large bolus impaction can contribute to paradoxical liquid incontinence by a ball-valve effect. The physical examination shows a decreased anal tone, an impalpable puborectalis muscle ridge, and a shortened anal canal (normal, 2.5-4.5 cm in length) on digital examination, a flattened and "scalloped" contour during anal-to-buttock inspection, and absent or decreased sacral reflexes (anocutaneous and bulbocavernosus reflexes).

Diagnostic Testing
Diagnostic tests and their purposes are listed in eSlide 21.9.

• MANAGEMENT

Management of Nausea, Vomiting, Bloating, and Early Satiety
Management of acute episodes includes resting the bowel, supplementing nutrition, maintaining fluid and electrolyte balance, and minimizing drugs that affect mobility. For chronic subocclusive states, strategies include enteral nutrition, enterostomies, and total parenteral nutrition.

Management of Diarrhea
Impaction can result in diarrhea and incontinence and can be evaluated by history, physical examination, and abdominal x-rays. Diarrhea associated with *Clostridium difficile* colitis due to repeated use of antibiotics should be treated with metronidazole (for mild to moderate colitis) and oral vancomycin (for severe or complicated disease).

Management of Defecation Dysfunction: Constipation and Fecal Incontinence
GOALS OF THE BOWEL PROGRAM
The goals of the bowel program are as follows: (1) regular passage of stool on a daily or every-other-day basis, (2) bowel evacuation at a consistent time of the day (morning or evening), (3) complete emptying of the rectal vault with every bowel care session, (4) stools that are soft, formed, and bulky, and (5) completion of bowel care within half an hour (at most, within an hour). In 95% of individuals, defecation frequency is between three times per day and three times per week (eSlide 21.10).

DIETARY CONSIDERATIONS
The main goal of dietary choices is to achieve soft but well-formed, bulky stools. Fiber increases stool bulk and plasticity. A diet that daily contains fiber, at least 38 g for men and 25 g for women, is recommended (15 g initially and gradually increased as tolerated).

MEDICATIONS
Currently available and emerging medications for constipation are listed in eSlides 21.11, 21.12, and 21.13.

Management of Upper Motor Neuron Defecatory Dysfunction
Digital stimulations, rectal stimulant medications, enemas, or electrical stimulations can cause reflex relaxation of the IAS and EAS. Anorectal colonic reflexes would subsequently increase motility of the left colon, causing defecation. The presentation of stool to the rectum can be associated with GMCs and mass

movements, and this can be habituated. Digital rectal stimulation should be performed for 20 seconds and repeated every 5–10 minutes until bowel care is completed. Rectal stimulant suppositories and mini-enemas with bisacodyl or glycerin are applied approximately 30 minutes before the intended bowel care, followed by digital rectal stimulation. When digital rectal stimulation and rectal medications are not sufficient to achieve the goals of the bowel program, oral colon stimulants, stool softeners, or both are commonly used. Oral laxative abuse can cause dysfunction of the ENS.

Management of Lower Motor Neuron Defecatory Dysfunction

In LMNB, the bowel is areflexic, and the most effective way to completely empty the rectum is through manual disimpaction or the use of cleansing enemas (water, soapsuds, mineral oil, or milk and molasses) one to two times per day. To avoid incontinence, it is imperative to keep the stools well-formed and bulky and to empty the rectal vault more regularly. Use of oral medications as outlined for the UMNB might likewise be warranted if stool is not efficiently reaching the rectum in a timely manner. Biofeedback and behavior training could be effective in subjects with incomplete neurogenic deficit and children with myelomeningocele.

Progressive Steps in a Bowel Habituation Program

See eSlides 21.14 and 21.15 for the protocol of this program.

Physical Interventions

BOWEL IRRIGATION

Transanal irrigation with a unique enema system, including a pump and a rectal balloon catheter (Peristeen, Coloplast), or with only water irrigation was found to be helpful.

ABDOMINAL MASSAGE

Abdominal massage from the cecum, throughout the colon, to the rectum for 5 minutes can promote better bowel movements in people with SCI.

FUNCTIONAL ELECTRICAL STIMULATION OR FUNCTIONAL MAGNETIC STIMULATION

An abdominal belt with electrodes for electrical stimulation of abdominal muscles in people with tetraplegia was shown to improve colonic transit time.

Surgical Options

GASTRIC ELECTRICAL STIMULATION

Surgically implanted electrical pacemakers for patients with gastroparesis showed improved gastric emptying, but the device remains impractical for clinical use.

GASTROSTOMIES AND ENTEROSTOMIES

Gastronomies and enterostomies provide nutrition and are beneficial for patients with gastroparesis or with intestinal or colonic pseudoobstruction.

SURGERY FOR CHRONIC INTESTINAL OR COLONIC PSEUDOOBSTRUCTION

Subtotal colectomy with ileorectostomy has been found to be the most effective treatment for chronic colonic pseudoobstruction.

PELVIC FLOOR SLING
Transposition of innervated muscle graft can replace puborectalis function and restore the acute anorectal junction angle for subjects with sacral nerve deficits.

ELECTROPROSTHESIS
A transplanted sacral anterior root stimulator, used in patients with SCI to manage neurogenic bladder, was also found to be beneficial for managing neurogenic bowel.

ANTEGRADE CONTINENCE ENEMA
Antegrade enemas are delivered via a catheterizable appendicocecostomy stoma. They should be considered in clinical scenarios of prolonged bowel care time, recurrent fecal impactions, or poor or intermittent response to rectal medications.

COLOSTOMY
Colostomy is indicated in four general scenarios: (1) when conservative treatments have failed, (2) when repetitive bowel impactions occur, (3) when pressure ulcers or other skin lesions occur that cannot be effectively healed because of frequent soiling, or (4) when intrinsic bowel deficits exist.

• COMPLICATIONS
For people with gastroparesis or intestinal pseudoobstruction, primary complications are chronic malnutrition, dehydration, and electrolyte imbalance. Persistent impaction can result in progressive distention and cecal ischemia, causing perforation or even resulting in death. Other gastrointestinal complications reported by patients with SCI include gastroesophageal reflux, premature diverticulosis, rectal bleeding caused by hemorrhoids, and autonomic dysreflexia.

• TREATMENT OUTCOMES
Bowel habituation training in children with myelomeningocele by means of suppositories, digital stimulation, or both resulted in 83% of compliant patients having less than one incontinent stool per month. Although all patients with complete SCI have episodic fecal incontinence, this is a chronic problem in only 2%. DWE appears to be a progressive problem that develops 5 years or more after SCI.

• CONCLUSION
The management of neurogenic bowel dysfunction should be based on the type of neurologic disease (upper motor neuron or lower motor neuron) and careful evaluation of patients, including a thorough past history and physical examination. Management is a stepwise approach, and each strategy needs an observation period of 10–14 days. New medicines are emerging, and we hope that new treatment strategies (such as botulinum toxin injection) or surgeries can offer some benefit for these patients.

Clinical Pearls

1. Neural control of the gastrointestinal tract involves the central nervous system, autonomic nervous system, and enteric nervous system (ENS). The ENS is a distinct system with its own set of neurons that coordinate sensory and motor functions.
2. The "gastrocolonic response," occurring 30–60 minutes after a meal, is often therapeutically used to enhance bowel evacuation.
3. The resting anal canal pressure is largely determined by the puborectalis sling and internal sphincter tone; only 20% of the pressure is attributable to the external anal sphincter (EAS).
4. Defecation is accomplished by the rectorectal reflex, rectoanal inhibitory reflex, contraction of the levator ani, and relaxation of the external sphincter and puborectalis muscles.
5. Patients with upper motor neurogenic bowel (UMNB) have a prolonged colorectal transit time (less severe over the rectosigmoid portion), a normal or increased anal sphincter tone, a palpable puborectalis muscle sling, a normal anal verge appearance, and an intact sacral reflex.
6. Patients with lower motor neurogenic bowel (LMNB) have a significantly prolonged colorectal transit time (especially over the left colon), a decreased anal tone, an impalpable puborectalis muscle ridge observed during digital examination, a shortened anal canal, a flattened contour observed during anal-to-buttock inspection, and absent or decreased sacral reflexes.
7. Goals of a bowel program should include regular passage of stool on a daily or every-other-day basis, evacuation at a consistent time of the day, and completion of bowel care within half an hour (at most, within an hour).
8. For patients with UMNB, digital rectal stimulation and rectal medications can be used to induce sacral reflexes to help defecation.
9. For patients with LMNB, the most effective way of completely emptying the rectum is through manual disimpaction or use of cleansing enemas.
10. Bowel training should follow a stepwise approach, as shown in eSlides 21.14 and 21.15; each step is added only after a 10- to 14-day consistent trial of the previous step has been ineffective.

BIBLIOGRAPHY
The complete bibliography is available on ExpertConsult.com.

22 Sexual Dysfunction and Disability

Tunku Nor Taayah Tunku Zubir

Sexuality, a complex aspect of human life, has physiologic and psychosocial influences. Disability often has a dramatic negative impact on sexual functioning, without changing the inherent human yearning that sexuality affords. This chapter, an overview of sexual function and dysfunction, emphasizes the sexual challenges of people with disabilities.

• SEXUAL RESPONSE AND BEHAVIOR

Human Sexual Response

The classic model of human sexual response by Masters and Johnson depicted women and men as having similar sexual responses, namely the four phases: excitement, plateau, orgasm, and resolution.

However, they noted differences between the sexes. For example, men tend to pass through each phase faster and have one orgasm per cycle, whereas women can achieve multiple orgasms within the same cycle. They also noted that women could be "stalled" at the plateau phase, thereby passing straight to resolution without an orgasm. A newer sexual response model describes three phases: desire, excitement, and orgasm. Desire is the "specific sensation motivating individuals to initiate or respond to sexual stimulation," which always precedes arousal. A new model for the female sexual response, addressing differences between sexes (eSlide 22.1), emphasizes that sexual response in women is much more complex than that in men.

Sexual Behavior and Aging

The frequency of sexual activity is well documented to decline with age, which is an important contributor to the quality of life throughout the life span. Factors that influence this decline include sexual dysfunction caused by medical illness, increasing frailty, medication side effects, vulvovaginal atrophy, vaginal dryness, decreased testosterone, and psychosocial barriers such as decreased partner availability and cognitive decline.

• TYPES OF SEXUAL DYSFUNCTION

According to the *Diagnostic and Statistical Manual of Mental Disorders*, fifth edition (DSM-5) (eSlide 22.2), sexual dysfunction is most frequently classified as causing "significant distress" for a minimum of 6 months, with symptoms present 75%–100% of the time (with the exception of medication-induced sexual dysfunction disorder). Details of the types of male and female sexual dysfunction are summarized in eSlides 22.3 and 22.4.

• SEXUAL DYSFUNCTION IN DISABILITY AND CHRONIC DISEASE

Factors that can cause sexual dysfunction in people with a disability or chronic disease are primary physical changes, secondary physical limitations, psychosocial contributions, effect of comorbid conditions, and medication-related factors.

Spinal Cord Injury

The frequency of sexual activity and the level of sexual satisfaction decreases in both men and women after spinal cord injury (SCI). The type of sexual dysfunction that a patient will experience depends on the spinal cord level and the degree of completeness of the injury. Upper motor neuron (UMN) SCI allows for reflexogenic erection in men because of an intact parasympathetic sacral reflex arc. Psychogenic erection, however, is not usually possible unless the injury is incomplete. Ejaculation is difficult for these patients as it is sympathetically mediated from T11-L2. Lower motor neuron (LMN) SCI is associated with preserved integrity of the thoracolumbar sympathetic outflow tract, and thus psychogenic erections and ejaculation are theoretically more likely to be intact, but reflexogenic erections are not. The prevalences of erectile and orgasmic dysfunction in men with SCI are summarized in eSlides 22.5 and 22.6.

Orgasmic ability is preserved in 38%–50% of men with complete UMN SCI, 78%–84% of men with incomplete UMN injury, and 0% of men with complete LMN injury. Women with SCI have been shown to have similar sexual responses as men, with arousal and vaginal lubrication being the female correlates to penile erection. Fertility in men with SCI is impaired because of decreased ability to ejaculate and also poor semen quality. Fertility in women with SCI is preserved once menstruation resumes.

Stroke, Traumatic Brain Injury, Multiple Sclerosis, and Other Neurologic Disorders

The most common findings in men who have had a stroke are erectile and ejaculatory dysfunction (40%–50%) and decreased sexual drive. Women tend to experience decreased sexual drive, decreased vaginal lubrication (approximately 50%), decreased orgasm (approximately 20%–30%), and decreased overall sexual satisfaction. The prevalence of sexual dysfunction after a traumatic brain injury has been reported to be 4%–71%. The types of sexual dysfunction include reduced sexual desire and frequency of sexual activity in both sexes; erectile dysfunction (ED) and ejaculatory dysfunction in men; and dyspareunia, anorgasmia, and reduced lubrication in women. Hypersexual behavior and hyperorality can particularly occur in people with injuries to the limbic system, prefrontal regions, or bilateral temporal poles. Depression after brain injury is the most sensitive indicator of sexual dysfunction. In multiple sclerosis (MS), sexual dysfunction is present in 40%–80% of women and 50%–90% of men. Parkinson disease is often associated with low testosterone levels and therefore decreased sexual drive, ED, and premature or delayed ejaculation. In women, decreased lubrication and involuntary urination can occur during intercourse.

Chronic Pain and Rheumatologic Disease

In patients with chronic pain, sexual dysfunction is often related to physiologic, pharmacologic, and psychological factors. In patients with rheumatologic diseases, sexual function can be primarily affected by joint pain, stiffness, and fatigue. The hip joint is most often implicated in leading to sexual difficulties.

Diabetes Mellitus and Cardiovascular Disease

ED is three times more common in people with diabetes mellitus than in those without the disease, with prevalence estimates ranging from 35% to 75%. Other types of sexual dysfunction include premature ejaculation and hypoactive sexual desire disorder. Hypertension, coronary artery disease, and congestive heart failure have all been associated with an increased prevalence of sexual dysfunction. ED has been noted in 40%–95% of men with hypertension and is correlated with the duration of the disease.

• SEXUAL DYSFUNCTION RELATED TO MEDICATION USE IN INDIVIDUALS WITH DISABILITY

Sexual dysfunction is a common side effect of many medications routinely used by patients with disabilities. Table 22.1 presents an overview of sexual dysfunction associated with various commonly encountered classes of medications.

• EVALUATION OF SEXUAL DYSFUNCTION

Sexual History Taking

A thorough inquiry regarding sexual dysfunction should include obtaining information about the medical, sexual, and psychosocial history of the patient. There are multiple validated tools for assessing sexual dysfunction. The ALLOW, PLISSIT, and BETTER models are three different approaches (eSlide 22.7).

The Brief Sexual Symptoms Checklist is a self-report tool that can be a useful adjunct to the physician's comprehensive sexual history (Fig. 22.1).

Physical Examination

A complete and comprehensive examination should include neurologic examination, paying particular attention to reflexes such as the anal wink and bulbocavernosus reflexes. These reflexes evaluate the integrity of the pudendal nerve and should be performed in both men and women.

TABLE 22.1   Medications and Sexual Dysfunction[a]

Drug Category	Drug Class[b]	Impact on Sexual Function[c]
Cardiac	Diuretics (**thiazides, spironolactone,** loop diuretics, chlorthalidone)	ED, decreased sexual desire, impaired ejaculation, retrograde ejaculation
	Centrally acting sympatholytics (clonidine, α-methyldopa)	ED, decreased sexual desire
	β-Blockers	ED, decreased sexual desire (men and women)
	α-Blockers (prazosin, terazosin)	ED, priapism (rare), retrograde ejaculation
	Vasodilators (hydralazine)	Priapism (rare)
	Antiarrhythmics (**digoxin,** disopyramide)	ED, decreased sexual desire
	Anticholesterolemics (statins, fibrates, niacin)	ED, decreased sexual desire

TABLE 22.1	Medications and Sexual Dysfunction[a]—cont'd	
Drug Category	Drug Class[b]	Impact on Sexual Function[c]
Psychiatric	**Selective serotonin reuptake inhibitors (SSRIs)**	Ejaculatory dysfunction, anorgasmia (men and women), decreased sexual desire (men and women), ED
	Serotonin–norepinephrine reuptake inhibitors (SNRIs)	ED, decreased sexual desire
	Tricyclic antidepressants (TCAs)	Decreased sexual desire, ED
	Trazodone	Priapism
	Antipsychotics	Decreased sexual drive (men and women), ejaculatory or orgasmic dysfunction, ED, priapism
	Benzodiazepines	Orgasmic dysfunction (women), delayed ejaculation, decreased sexual desire
	Neurostimulants (methylphenidate, amantadine)	Hypersexual behavior
Gastrointestinal	**H$_2$-Blockers** (especially **cimetidine**)	ED, decreased sexual desire, painful erections, gynecomastia
	Proton pump inhibitors	ED, gynecomastia
	Metoclopramide	Decreased sexual drive, ED
Other	Baclofen (especially **intrathecal baclofen**)	Ejaculatory dysfunction, ED, decreased orgasmic function (men and women)
	Gabapentin, pregabalin, other anticonvulsants (**phenytoin**)	Ejaculatory dysfunction, anorgasmia (men and women), decreased sexual desire (men and women)
	Opioids	Decreased sexual desire, anorgasmia, ED, hypogonadism
	Tramadol	Delayed ejaculation
	NSAIDs	ED
	Corticosteroids	Decreased sexual desire
	Methotrexate	ED, decreased sexual desire, gynecomastia

[a]From references 24, 29, 53, 59, 88, 134, 139, 176, 187, 200, 204, 207, 212.
[b]The medications that most commonly cause sexual side effects are listed in boldface.
[c]The most common effects are listed first.
ED, erectile dysfunction; *NSAIDs,* nonsteroidal antiinflammatory drugs.

Diagnostic Evaluation

Recommended laboratory tests for all men and women with sexual dysfunction include complete blood cell count, chemistry panel, fasting glucose test, and fasting lipid profile. Other laboratory tests that are warranted on the basis of history and physical examination findings include thyroid function studies and serum free testosterone, prolactin, and prostate specific antigen levels. Measurements of other sex hormones, such as estrogen, follicle-stimulating hormone, luteinizing hormone, or total testosterone, have been shown to have a far less utility in a majority of individuals.

Brief sexual symptom checklist: men's version

Please answer the following questions about your overall sexual function in the past **3 months** or more.

1. Are you satisfied with your sexual function?
     ☐ Yes   ☐ No
   If no, please continue.
2. How long have you been dissatisfied with your sexual function?

3a. The problem(s) with your sexual function is: (mark one or more)
     ☐ 1 Problems with little or no interest in sex
     ☐ 2 Problems with erection
     ☐ 3 Problems with ejaculating too early during sexual activity
     ☐ 4 Problems taking too long, or not being able to ejaculate or have orgasm
     ☐ 5 Problems with pain during sex
     ☐ 6 Problems with penile curvature during erection
     ☐ 7 Other:
3b. Which problem is most bothersome (circle) 1 2 3 4 5 6 7
4. Would you like to talk about it with your doctor?
     ☐ Yes   ☐ No

Brief sexual symptom checklist: women's version

Please answer the following questions about your overall sexual function in the past **3 months** or more.

1. Are you satisfied with your sexual function?
     ☐ Yes   ☐ No
   If no, please continue.
2. How long have you been dissatisfied with your sexual function?

3a. The problem(s) with your sexual function is: (mark one or more)
     ☐ 1 Problems with little or no interest in sex
     ☐ 2 Problems with decreased genital sensation (feeling)
     ☐ 3 Problems with decreased vaginal lubrication (dryness)
     ☐ 4 Problems reaching orgasm
     ☐ 5 Problems with pain during sex
     ☐ 6 Other:
3b. Which problem is most bothersome (circle) 1 2 3 4 5 6
4. Would you like to talk about it with your doctor?
     ☐ Yes   ☐ No

FIG. 22.1 The Brief Sexual Symptom Checklist for men and women. (Redrawn from Hatzichristou D, Rosen RC, Broderick G, et al: Clinical evaluation and management strategy for sexual dysfunction in men and women, *J Sex Med* 1:49–57, 2004.)

• TREATMENT OF SEXUAL DYSFUNCTION

Male Hypoactive Sexual Desire Disorder

The primary causes of hypoactive sexual desire include hypogonadism and low testosterone levels and are also due to psychosocial factors such as variant arousal patterns or conflicts about sexual orientation. Secondary hyposexual disorder in men is considered to develop most frequently in response to other types of sexual dysfunction, such as ED or premature ejaculation, or as a result of medications. Treating primary sexual dysfunction and changing the type or dosage of medication will often improve a patient's sexual desire.

Erectile Dysfunction

ED is known to be associated with advanced age, cardiovascular disease, diabetes, dyslipidemia, smoking, obesity, and depression. The treatment of ED was revolutionized with the approval of sildenafil, the first of the now ubiquitous phosphodiesterase 5 (PDE5) inhibitors. PDE5 inhibitors have been studied and proven effective for ED in patients with cardiovascular disease, hypertension, diabetes, SCI, MS, and depression. These medications have been reported to significantly improve erectile function, as evidenced by successful vaginal penetration in as many as 79%–87% of patients. The medications are strictly contraindicated in patients taking nitrates for chest pain.

Second-line treatments after the failure of PDE5 inhibitor treatment include intracavernosal injection therapy, intraurethral alprostadil [medicated urethral system for erection (MUSE)] therapy, topical alprostadil, and vacuum constriction devices. Intracavernosal penile injections have been used for decades, with treatment satisfaction rates of 87%–93.5%, a relatively low rate of adverse effects, and a rapid onset of action (eSlide 22.8).

High discontinuation rates have been noted. Discontinuation can occur because of penile pain and complications such as priapism and Peyronie disease. Intraurethral alprostadil therapy with the MUSE system can be an alternative for patients who cannot take PDE5 inhibitors and who do not want to try more intracavernosal injection therapy (eSlide 22.9). Vacuum constriction devices (eSlide 22.10) have efficacy rates as high as 90%, but satisfaction rates tend to be lower because of the unnatural appearance of the erection, penile pain, and trapped ejaculate. Constriction devices are contraindicated in patients with a history of severe bleeding disorder, priapism, or severe penile curvature.

Third-line treatments for ED include surgical options such as penile prostheses (eSlide 22.11).

Premature Ejaculation

Premature ejaculation is often caused by a combination of organic, psychogenic, and relationship-related factors. Neurobiological and genetic variations have been recently proposed as contributing factors. The mainstay of treatment for premature ejaculation until recently was cognitive-behavioral therapy and psychological counseling. Selective serotonin reuptake inhibitors (SSRIs) are the most commonly used medication for premature ejaculation, with paroxetine being the most effective, followed by fluoxetine and sertraline. In addition to dapoxetine, which is a new short-acting SSRI, tramadol has been shown to be an excellent on-demand treatment for premature ejaculation.

Delayed Ejaculation, Anejaculation, and Anorgasmia in Men

Assisted ejaculation methods that have been shown effective for fertility treatment in men with SCI, MS, and other disabilities include penile vibratory stimulation (PVS) and rectal probe electroejaculation (EEJ) (eSlides 22.12 and 22.13).

PVS is the most commonly used technique because it is able to produce superior sperm quality, is more comfortable and preferable to patients, and can be used in a home setting. PVS only produces ejaculation in 60%–80% of men, whereas EEJ is successful in 80%–100% of men. Chemically assisted ejaculation is also a possibility, particularly with the combination use of midodrine and PVS to improve ejaculation success rates. Pharmacologic treatment for ejaculatory and orgasmic dysfunction in men remains largely unproven, although some medications have shown modest benefit.

Female Sexual Interest/Arousal Disorder

Despite limited research, psychotherapy remains the mainstay for the treatment of female sexual interest/arousal disorder. Sexual behavioral techniques, sex therapy, and couples counselling have been shown to be beneficial by helping reduce anxiety and exaggerated sexual expectations. Pharmacologic treatments for female hypoactive sexual desire include testosterone therapy, tibolone, melanocortins, flibanserin, and a combination of testosterone and PDE5 inhibitors or buspirone.

Female Orgasmic Dysfunction

Beneficial treatments include cognitive-behavioral therapy (which focuses on decreasing anxiety and promoting changes in attitudes and sexual thoughts), sensate focus therapy, and direct masturbation. These behavioral treatments have been shown to be effective in 60% of women.

Genitopelvic Pain/Penetration Disorder

This disorder encompasses both dyspareunia and vaginismus. Prevalence rate of vaginismus has been reported to be 1%–6%, and recent research disputes the classic definition of vaginismus because muscle spasm and even pain are not always present. Dyspareunia and vaginismus have a variety of organic and psychogenic causes, and proper treatment depends on etiology.

• CONCLUSION

A thorough understanding of the diagnosis and treatment of sexual dysfunction within the context of disability, as well as a willingness to openly discuss sexuality with patients, will enable the physician to have a significant impact on a patient's quality of life and provide comfort and hope to those who need it most (eSlide 22.14).

Clinical Pearls

Low-flow (or ischemic) priapism is a medical emergency, and all patients with an erection that lasts for more than 4 hours should visit the nearest hospital. High-flow and stuttering priapism are usually benign and self-limiting in duration.

BIBLIOGRAPHY
The complete bibliography is available on ExpertConsult.com.

Spasticity

23

Gerard E. Francisco

• SPASTICITY AND THE UPPER MOTOR NEURON SYNDROME

Spasticity is a significant complication of many neurologic conditions. In itself, spasticity predisposes to other complications, such as joint contractures and joint deformities, and as a comorbidity, spasticity amplifies the effects of weakness and other motor disorders and contributes to limitations in activity and participation. Although it has become common practice to label any condition presenting as muscle tightness as "spasticity," it is important to point out that spasticity is only one of myriad consequences of the upper motor neuron (UMN) syndrome (eSlide 23.1).

• EPIDEMIOLOGY

Because of the lack of a strict definition and standardized methods for clinically measuring spasticity, estimates of the incidence and prevalence of spasticity vary.

• PATHOPHYSIOLOGY

The exact pathophysiology of spasticity has not yet been determined. Various pathomechanisms have been suggested to explain the evolution of spasticity following an insult to the central nervous system (eSlide 23.2).

Abnormal Regulation of the Stretch Reflex

Excitability of the spinal stretch reflex arc is maintained by descending regulation from the inhibitory dorsal reticulospinal tract and the facilitatory medial reticulospinal and vestibular spinal tracts, as well as by intraspinal processing of the stretch reflex. Recent reports suggest that abnormalities in the supraspinal pathways predominate, whereas intraspinal mechanisms likely represent plastic rearrangement secondary to an imbalance of excitatory and inhibitory descending inputs to the intraspinal network. Abnormal intraspinal processing could result from the following: (1) increased afferent input to the spinal motoneurons; (2) altered interneuronal reflex circuits producing enhanced motoneuronal excitability, including reduced presynaptic inhibition of Ia afferents, group Ib facilitation (instead of inhibition), group II facilitation, and reduced reciprocal inhibition; and (3) changes in the intrinsic properties of spinal motor neurons. Disruption of descending inputs could cause spinal motoneurons to activate voltage-dependent persistent inward currents. These persistent inward currents can lead to the development of plateau potentials in motoneurons and self-sustained firing in response to a transient input. These changes in reflex circuits and intrinsic properties of spinal motoneurons can lead to a decreased reflex threshold, which has been considered as the primary change in patients with spasticity.

DOES SPASTICITY RESULT FROM MALADAPTIVE PLASTICITY?

Motor recovery commences almost immediately after the onset of a central nervous system lesion, when reversible changes begin to resolve. For instance, regardless of the type (hemorrhagic or not) or location (cortical or subcortical) of a stroke, a relatively predictable pattern of recovery sets in after the event. Brunnstrom empirically described the stereotypical stages of motor recovery from flaccidity to full recovery of motor function, which are summarized in eSlide 23.3. As a stroke survivor improves, progression from one recovery stage to the next occurs in an orderly manner toward recovery of normal movement, but evolution may be arrested at any stage.

Interestingly, as motor recovery after a stroke progresses, spasticity decreases. However, the same pattern of motor recovery and emergence and disappearance of spasticity may not be seen in patients with UMN syndrome caused by other etiologies. A period of "shock" after the initial injury (traumatic or other acquired injury) is commonly observed, which is followed by a gradual return of reflexes and not by a sudden progression to hyperreflexia. This implies that there must be some sort of neuronal plastic change after the initial injury. This process occurs at any time, but it is usually seen between 1 and 6 weeks after the initial injury. Plastic rearrangement occurs within the brain and spinal cord and is regarded as an attempt to restore function through the emergence of novel neuronal circuitry. This process often results in muscle overactivity and hyperreflexia, and thus spasticity. The emergence and disappearance of spasticity in the course of complete motor recovery collectively imply that the presence of spasticity reflects a phenomenon of abnormal plasticity. Spasticity may be maintained after its emergence by arresting further plastic rearrangement and recovery. Spasticity is a manifestation of maladaptive plasticity is further supported by recent studies demonstrating that abnormal cortical reorganization can be modulated by interventions directed at decreasing spasticity.

Peripheral Contribution

Spasticity can be differentiated from hypertonia arising from other mechanisms by its dependence on the speed of the muscle stretch. However, spasticity may be explained not only by hyperreflexia but also by changes in mechanical properties of muscles. The increased mechanical resistance may be caused by alterations in tendon compliance and physiologic changes in muscle fibers. These muscle property changes may be adaptive and secondary to paresis. When a paralyzed muscle is held in a shortened position, it loses sarcomeres to "adjust" its length so that it can produce optimal force at the shortened muscle length. As a result, muscle fibers are almost twice as stiff as in nonspastic muscles. These changes in the mechanical properties of muscles occur gradually and may also lead to contracture and increased muscle stiffness and are not easily detected during usual clinical examination. The effect of blood flow restriction on Ia afferent activity has also been implicated. Animal studies have shown that a decrease in blood flow can increase Ia afferent firing by fusimotor activation of group III and IV afferents that respond to the accumulation of metabolites within the muscle.

CLINICAL PRESENTATION, GOAL-SETTING, AND ASSESSMENT

Problem Identification

Obtaining a thorough, yet focused, history is of paramount importance in guiding the examination and formulation of mutually agreed upon treatment goals and plans. When a patient presents with tight muscles and limb deformities and complains of an inability to perform certain tasks, it is often tempting to attribute all the problems to spasticity. The clinician should keep in mind that spasticity is one of the multitude of problems resulting from UMN disease. Weakness is often the primary cause of limitations rather than spasticity. Thus although spasticity is present, it may not be the immediate cause of a particular problem; instead, the problem may be a consequence of different, but related, UMN pathologies (eSlide 23.4).

POSTURAL ABNORMALITIES

Although the clinical presentation varies widely in individuals within and across patient populations, certain postural patterns are commonly observed (eSlides 23.5, 23.6, and 23.7). These patterns are manifestations of an imbalance between agonist and antagonist strength and hypertonia. Thus, a flexed elbow posture is not necessarily due to solely flexor muscle group hypertonia, but it may be caused by a combination of hypertonic flexors and weak extensors. Alternatively, the flexor and extensor muscle groups may both be hypertonic, but the former predominates.

IMPAIRED MOVEMENTS

Just as with abnormal postures, impaired movements usually result from interactions between spasticity, weakness, and other features of the UMN syndrome, such as loss of coordination and dexterity, dystonia, or sustained muscle contraction.

FUNCTIONAL LIMITATIONS

Activity limitations are even more complex as the causes of impaired movement are not only further aggravated by abnormalities other than the UMN disorder but also are a direct result of the underlying disease. Tactile and proprioceptive sensory loss, visual field cut, hemineglect, and cognitive difficulties (such as learning a novel task and procedural sequencing) can magnify the motor challenges imposed by spasticity and weakness. Thus a rehabilitation effort that will be effective in enhancing activity participation should address not just spasticity and deficits in strength and coordination but also concurrently tackle any related impairments.

Goal-Setting

An important component of assessment and management decision-making is to set treatment goals that are mutually agreed upon by the patient (or caregiver) and clinician. Identifying goals a priori provides a context for identifying pertinent problems and their solutions and helps manage utilization of resources. It is not uncommon for patients to desire goals of regaining normal form and function, but because this is not always achievable, a discussion regarding goal-setting prior to initiating treatment can help manage expectations regarding treatment outcomes. Goal-setting can also help identify the best treatment strategy at a particular time in the course of a person's rehabilitation and recovery.

Clinical Assessment

Spasticity assessment typically consists of a combination of quantitative and qualitative measures. eSlide 23.8 presents a practical clinical examination sequence. Although it is true that quantitative measures are desirable because of their inherent objectivity and reliability, they may not be practical and may discourage clinicians from assessing and managing spasticity. Ideal measures include biomechanical and electrophysiologic tests, but many of the devices needed to carry out these tests are not available to a typical clinician, and the time needed to perform them properly may impose excessive demands in a busy practice. Thus a combination of clinical measures, some of which appear to correlate with biomechanical and electrophysiologic assessments, is a practical approach.

• BIOMECHANICAL ASSESSMENT: SPASTICITY OR CONTRACTURE?

Resistance to passive stretch is composed of three components: passive muscle stiffness, active muscle stiffness, and neurally mediated reflex stiffness. Experimentally, total joint stiffness is first measured in response to a controlled angular perturbation (eSlide 23.9).

Electrophysiologic Measurements

Reflex stiffness from torque-angle relations can be obtained quantitatively, as described previously. However, certain precautions should be taken when interpreting this reflex stiffness. Mechanical properties of the muscle, such as viscosity and change, are influenced by stretching velocities. Analysis of the neuromuscular response via electromyography (EMG) can provide electrophysiologic insight into measurement of spasticity. In spastic muscles, a normal passive stretch can elicit an exaggerated stretch reflex response. The angle at which an EMG response is first detected when the limb is displaced at one or more velocities is defined as the threshold of the stretch reflex. The threshold indicates the onset of motoneuronal recruitment in response to an external stretch.

• MANAGEMENT

Nonpharmacologic

Although spasticity is a neurologic condition, its obvious manifestations are physical; thus physical modalities are considered a mainstay of first-line treatment for spasticity because they are widely available and relatively innocuous compared to drugs. Passive stretching has been shown to be effective in reducing tone and increasing range of movement in patients with brain injury. Splinting and casting are often used in the acute cases of sustained stretching. Casting alone seems sufficient to prevent contracture and reduce spasticity if the intervention is initiated early after a severe brain injury. A systematic review of the use of upper extremity casting found a high variability in casting protocols, which indicates that there is no consensus regarding the technique. In the clinical setting, individualized stretching has shown promise in reducing wrist and finger spasticity and improving passive range of movement.

Electrical stimulation may be temporarily used to reduce spasticity. A novel technique involving electrical stimulation triggered by voluntary breathing demonstrated reduction in spasticity. However, the efficacy of electrical stimulation in reducing spasticity has not been observed in more recent studies.

Pharmacologic

There is more than one way to approach the pharmacologic management of spasticity. eSlide 23.10 presents a treatment decision algorithm. Historically, a step-ladder paradigm was followed, which began with the least invasive treatment and culminated with surgical procedures when nonoperative options failed. More recently, this sequential approach has been abandoned in favor of concurrent use of both "noninvasive" and "invasive" strategies, such as using injection therapy concurrently with therapeutic exercises or using injection therapy for residual focal spasticity in people with generalized spasticity managed simultaneously with intrathecal drugs. The current approach reflects a better appreciation of the magnitude of the problem: that spasticity alone does not account for the presenting problem, that other features of UMN syndrome contribute significantly, and that different treatments may be required to increase the chances of a successful outcome.

ORAL SPASMOLYTICS

Various medications with different mechanisms of action have been used to treat spasticity. eSlide 23.11 summarizes common medications used for spasticity and their mechanisms of action.

Baclofen is an analog of gamma-aminobutyric acid (GABA), the most potent inhibitory neurotransmitter. It binds to $GABA_B$ receptors that are widespread in Ia sensory afferent neurons and alpha motor neurons. Adverse effects of baclofen include drowsiness and weakness, which are shared by other oral spasmolytics. Abrupt discontinuation of baclofen may result in a withdrawal syndrome, characterized by rebound spasticity, hallucinations, and seizures.

Tizanidine is believed to exert its effects by inhibiting the facilitatory ceruleospinal tracts and the release of excitatory amino acid from spinal interneurons. In addition to the typical side effects of oral spasmolytics, hepatotoxicity may also occur with tizanidine. Being a central alpha-2 adrenergic receptor agonist, tizanidine should be used with caution in patients with hypotension or those who are concomitantly taking other alpha-agonists, such as clonidine. Likewise, caution should be used when coadministering tizanidine with fluoroquinolone antibiotics, which may increase serum concentrations of tizanidine. Tizanidine is a peculiar spasmolytic in that it has a dose-dependent antinociceptive effect, which is presumably due to reduced release of substance P and decreased activity of excitatory amino acids at the spinal level.

The use of benzodiazepines as first-line treatment for spasticity has been limited because of concerns regarding their side effects (mainly drowsiness, sedation, reduced attention, and memory impairment) and the potential for physiologic dependence. They appear to be used more often when spasticity is accompanied by other conditions that are also amenable to benzodiazepine therapy, such as seizures, anxiety, insomnia, and muscle spasms or other movement disorders. Similar to baclofen, benzodiazepines exert their effects through modulation of GABAergic transmission, but unlike baclofen, which binds to $GABA_B$ receptors, benzodiazepines bind to $GABA_A$ receptors.

Another GABAergic agent, gabapentin, is commonly used for the treatment of seizures and neuropathic pain, but it also decreases muscle hypertonia through selective inhibition of voltage-gated calcium channels containing the $\alpha2\delta$-1 subunit.

Unlike baclofen and tizanidine, which act on the central nervous system, dantrolene sodium is a spasmolytic that acts directly on skeletal muscle. It appears that direct or indirect inhibition of the ryanodine receptor, which is the major calcium release channel of skeletal muscle sarcoplasmic reticulum, is fundamental in the molecular action of dantrolene. Inhibition of the receptor leads to a decrease in the intracellular calcium concentration. Because of the potential for hepatotoxicity, regular monitoring of liver function is recommended during dantrolene treatment.

Other agents have also been observed to exert a spasmolytic effect in various patient populations with UMN disease. One of these agents is the alpha-adrenergic agonist clonidine, which has more affinity for alpha-2 adrenergic receptors than alpha-1 adrenergic receptors. The potassium-channel blocker 4-aminopyridine, which is thought to enhance neural transmission by improving axonal conduction and synaptic neurotransmitter release, has been shown to reduce spasticity in patients with spinal cord injuries (SCIs). Cyproheptadine, a serotonergic antagonist, has likewise been demonstrated to decrease spasticity in people with SCIs. Cannabis and its active ingredient delta-9-tetrahydrocannabinol are believed to decrease spasticity, especially in individuals with pain. However, its use is limited because of concerns about potential cognitive impairment and a possible increased risk of psychosis associated with cannabis.

FOCAL TREATMENT: BOTULINUM TOXINS

Chemodenervation using botulinum toxins has become a widely used spasticity treatment. It is preferred for the management of focal spasticity or when the treatment plan targets a particular muscle. Botulinum toxins exert their effects through inhibition of acetylcholine release at the neuromuscular junction. Their clinical effects do not become manifest until several days after an injection, largely because of the complex process involved. The process requires three main steps: (1) internalization of the toxin, (2) reduction and translocation of the disulfide bonds holding the toxin's light and heavy polypeptide chains together, and (3) inhibition of acetylcholine release.

Consensus and review papers support the use of botulinum toxins for the management of spastic conditions in pediatric and adult populations. There are now several botulinum toxins commercially available. Their properties are compared in eSlide 23.12.

FOCAL PHARMACOLOGIC TREATMENT: NERVE BLOCKS (NEUROLYSIS)

Prior to the introduction of botulinum toxins, nerve blocks using either alcohol or phenol were the only option for focal spasticity management. They were used in the 1950s to chemically ablate nerve to manage cancer-related pain and were subsequently applied to relieve spasticity. Over time, percutaneous nerve blocks using phenol or alcohol proved to be effective in controlling focal spasticity across different populations, including spasticity occurring secondary to cerebral palsy, traumatic brain injury, and stroke. Phenol 5%–7% and alcohol 35%–60% denature proteins in neural tissues, leading to blockade of nerve transmission. In addition, phenol appears to produce degeneration of muscle spindles and damage both afferent and efferent nerve fibers. This chemical denervation is thought to be irreversible and leads to permanent control of spasticity; however, this is not commonly observed clinically, as spasticity tends to return several months after a percutaneous neurolytic block. This may be explained by partial nerve regrowth and sprouting.

Percutaneous injections can be performed at either the nerve or motor branch level, guided by electrical stimulation or ultrasound. Because phenol is also an anesthetic, especially at concentrations less than 3%, the muscle relaxation commonly observed immediately after an injection is due to its anesthetic effect. The neurolytic effect may not set in until a few hours later, as it takes some time for the effects on neural tissues to develop. Care must be exercised when injecting nerves with a significant sensory component to mitigate the risk of developing postinjection dysesthesia. Other side effects include localized swelling and excessive weakness. Inadvertent intravascular injection or systemic absorption may result in cardiovascular effects, such as hypotension, or central nervous system effects, including tremors or convulsions. eSlide 23.13 presents comparisons between botulinum toxins and phenol.

INTRATHECAL THERAPIES

As early as the 1950s, intrathecal phenol was used to reduce pain and spasticity. Its popularity has waned because of its many potential complications (such as sensory, respiratory, bladder, bowel, and sexual dysfunction) and the introduction of baclofen, which appears to have a better adverse effect profile. The use of intrathecal phenol is now limited to specific situations in which severe spasticity cannot be managed through any of the other currently available techniques.

The physiologic effects of intrathecal baclofen (ITB) include a decrease in monosynaptic and polysynaptic reflex responses and a reduction in resistance to passive stretch. At the cellular level, ITB's mechanism of action is similar to that of oral baclofen; however, the intrathecal route provides more direct access to GABA$_B$ receptors in the spinal cord because the blood-brain barrier does not have to be traversed. Thus intrathecal administration produces greater hypertonia reduction and reflex inhibition at doses lower than those required for the oral formulation, which decreases the risk of adverse events.

ITB is usually considered only when less invasive management options are ineffective in controlling spasticity. However, ITB may be warranted within the first few months of disease onset when spasticity of the lower limbs is so severe that waiting for other less invasive options to take effect is likely to produce more complications. A situation in which very early use has been shown to be beneficial is in a person with severe dysautonomia following a traumatic brain injury.

The most common drug-related side effect of ITB is hypotonia. Other side effects include somnolence, headache, convulsion, dizziness, and urinary retention. Pump-related adverse events include pump stalling, but catheter-related problems, such as dislodgement, fracture, and kinking, are more common. Finally, clinician-related complications, such as dosing and programming errors that can lead to either underdosing or overdosing, may occur. Early recognition of withdrawal due to pump or catheter malfunction is important to allow expedient intervention and avoid potentially serious (and rarely fatal) outcomes. eSlide 23.14 presents an algorithm for the assessment of suspected ITB withdrawal syndrome.

SURGICAL INTERVENTION
Surgical management of spasticity is a well-accepted treatment option for contractures, as it primarily addresses joint deformities rather than the spasticity itself. eSlide 23.15 presents more information regarding specific surgical options.

Clinical Pearls

- Although spasticity is a common complication of many neurologic conditions, it does not exclusively account for functional deficits, which may arise from the other features of the upper motor neuron syndrome (UMNS).
- Abnormal regulation of the stretch reflex due to an imbalance between excitatory afferent and descending inhibitory inputs is widely acknowledged as pathomechanism of spasticity.
- Spasticity and the other features of UMNS result in postural abnormalities, impaired movements, and functional limitations.
- Systematic clinical examination starts with observation of the patient's active movements, followed by passive stretching of the limbs and concurrently performing scales such as Ashworth (or its modified version) and Tardieu method. A functional assessment, when appropriate, should be performed as well.
- The patient and clinician must have mutually agreed on treatment goals, which are based not only on the severity, but also the significance (i.e., functional impact) of spasticity.
- Nonpharmacologic management, such as sustained stretching, is as important as pharmacologic management because it addresses the peripheral component of spasticity.
- Drug therapies are delivered focally (e.g., neurolysis, chemodenervation), intrathecally, or systemically (e.g., oral spasmolytics), depending on several factors, such as the anatomic extent of spasticity and tolerance of drug adverse effects.

BIBLIOGRAPHY
The complete bibliography is available on ExpertConsult.com.

24 Chronic Wounds

Julia Patrick Engkasan

This chapter summarizes the pathophysiology, treatment, and prevention of common chronic wounds, including pressure, neuropathic, ischemic, and venous ulcers.

• DEFINITIONS OF CHRONIC WOUNDS

Pressure Ulcers

A pressure ulcer is defined as a localized injury to the skin and/or underlying tissue (usually over a bony prominence) that results from pressure or pressure combined with a shear force, friction, or both. Obesity, congestive heart failure, chronic obstructive pulmonary disease, cerebrovascular disease, diabetes mellitus, spinal cord injury, and the use of corticosteroids during hospitalization are significant risk factors for pressure ulcers.

Diabetic, Ischemic, and Neuropathic Ulcers

The combination of neuropathy, arteriosclerosis, and microvascular disease creates a high-risk situation for the development of ischemic or neuropathic diabetic foot ulcers in individuals with diabetes. Neuropathic ulcers result from repetitive trauma to hyposensate distal extremities, usually on weight-bearing bony prominences. Ischemic ulcers occur on extremities with impaired arterial inflow caused by arteriosclerotic and microvascular diseases.

Chronic Venous Leg Ulcers

Chronic venous or edematous ulcers of the leg typically arise on the lower third of the leg. They are associated with impaired venous return, incompetence of venous perforators, or loss of integrity of leg fascia (e.g., from trauma) in patients with normal arterial inflow. Chronic venous leg ulcers begin as aberrancies in the peripheral venous system, which manifest as varicose veins, and end as discrete chronic ulcers.

• HEALING AND PATHOPHYSIOLOGY OF CHRONIC WOUNDS (eSlide 24.1)

Process of Normal Healing

Surgically induced skin wounds heal by primary intention, whereas wounds with large tissue defects heal by secondary intention. The major phases of wound healing are inflammation, proliferation or provisional matrix formation, repair, and remodeling. Remodeling of the preexisting tissue, scaffolding, and cleanup of extracellular and pathogen debris characterize the inflammatory phase of wound healing. In the proliferation phase, the extracellular matrix (ECM) components attach to "integrins."

This evolving framework is reinforced by type I collagen, which is secreted in sections (fibrils) and self-assembles extracellularly. Over this framework, a "ceiling"

TABLE 24.1	Comorbidities Associated With Chronic Wounds
Condition	Pathophysiologic Effect Related to Wound Healing
Spinal cord injury	Vasomotor instability (>T6 level), insensitivity, denervation atrophy, spasticity, contractures, bowel or bladder alterations
Older adult	Reduced skin elasticity and altered skin microcirculation, comorbidities, reduced healing rate noted clinically and in animal models
Diabetes	Insensitivity, microangiopathy, altered inflammatory response, foot deformities (intrinsic minus, Charcot), blunted reactive hyperemia, reduced incision-breaking strength and wound contraction in diabetic models
Malnutrition	Negative nitrogen balance, cachexia, immunosuppression
Anemia	Local hypoxia
Arteriosclerosis	Local hypoxia
End-stage renal disease	Transient dialysis-related hypoperfusion, arteriosclerosis, microangiopathy
Steroid medications	Reduced healing rate in animal models, immunosuppression
Transplant recipients	Immunosuppression
Smoking	Hypoxia, vasoconstriction, increased blood viscosity
Parkinson disease	Immobility
Osteoporosis	Bony prominences
Upper motor neuron disease	Immobility, contractures, bowel or bladder alterations
Dementia	Immobility, malnutrition, contractures, bowel or bladder alterations
Acutely ill (intensive care unit-related)	Hypotension, immobility, bowel or bladder alterations, malnutrition, increased metabolic demands
Noncompliance, abuse, and neglect	Multifactorial

of epidermal cells advances over the defect to provide a durable cover, accompanied by collateral neovascularization that supplies oxygen and nutrients. Remodeling of the dermal matrix occurs after closure. During remodeling, collagen fibers are preferentially retained along lines of stress, forming a functional cicatrix.

Pathophysiology of Chronic Wounds (Table 24.1)

PATHOMECHANICS

Pathomechanics refers to the noxious application of pressure on and shear stress tangential to the skin surface. Prolonged pressure leads to ulcers if it exceeds the tissue capillary pressure of 32 mm Hg. Deep muscle layers that cover bony prominences are often exposed to higher stresses than the overlying skin. This makes the muscle even more prone to ischemia and infarction. By lowering the ulceration threshold, shear stresses exacerbate the tendency for ulceration caused by pressure.

CHRONIC HYPOXIA

Chronic hypoxia results from poor inflow of blood, typically caused by arteriosclerotic narrowing proximal to the hypoxic skin. Chronic ischemia blunts several processes, including granulation tissue deposition, proliferation of fibroblasts, mononuclear cell infiltration, delayed epithelialization, and the probability of wound closure.

REPERFUSION INJURY

Ischemia-reperfusion injury involves reactive oxygen species that overwhelm endogenous antioxidants, resulting in a cascade of events, including mast cell degranulation, recruitment of neutrophils to the endothelial wall, arteriolar constriction that limits tissue perfusion, and increased vascular permeability leading to inflammation and edema.

EDEMA, IMPAIRED OXYGEN, AND NUTRIENT EXCHANGE

Edema is one of the major factors associated with the pathogenesis and maintenance of chronic wounds. Venous ulcers extravasate fibrinogen and fluid across the microvasculature endothelium because of venous congestion and backpressure, leading to excess protein-rich interstitial fluid.

GROWTH FACTOR ABNORMALITIES

Growth factor abnormalities also impair wound healing. They may include reduced factor synthesis, increased protein or matrix sequestration, increased breakdown of factors, or insensitivity of the target cells.

CHRONIC INFLAMMATION

Bacterial colonization and local infection impede healing. Wounds that have greater than 10^5 organisms per gram of tissue tend to not heal and are "stuck" in the inflammatory stage.

• CLINICAL WOUND ASSESSMENT

Wound Area and Volume Assessment (eSlide 24.2)

The perpendicular wound length (maximum length measured in the direction of head to toe) and width (maximum width measured from side to side) is the most straightforward method of documenting linear wound dimensions. Manual tracing, a useful and inexpensive technique, involves drawing the wound outline on a piece of clear plastic.

Perfusion Assessment (eSlide 24.3)

The ankle-brachial index (ABI) is the ratio of the systolic blood pressure of the ankle to that of the arm (brachium). The normal ABI is 0.8–1.3. ABI is measured using a portable Doppler instrument and a blood pressure cuff. A series of cuffs can be used to obtain a pulse volume recording, which involves the continuous monitoring of pressure within cuffs applied to the thigh, calf, and ankle. These segmental pressure traces are checked for bilateral symmetry and waveform shape.

A direct and absolute measure of microcirculation is transcutaneous oxygen partial pressure ($TcPO_2$). The normal $TcPO_2$ is greater than 50–60 mm Hg. Wound healing is considered to be impaired at pressures less than 40 mm Hg, and a $TcPO_2$ of 20 mm Hg is associated with rest pain and ischemic ulcers. The most complete picture of lower extremity perfusion comes from combining $TcPO_2$ and segmental pressure measurements.

• GENERAL PRINCIPLES OF TREATMENT

Wound Bed Preparation

Chronic wounds tend to be heavily colonized by bacteria. As wounds heal and bacterial virulence decreases, wound appearance transforms from black to yellow, then to dull red and finally to bright red. The therapeutic processes for "coaxing" a chronic wound to granulate have been referred to as "wound bed preparation."

Once the wound bed is prepared, the goal is to maintain a moist environment so that the epithelium advances and attaches to the underlying tissues.

Débridement

Wound débridement methods include surgical, sharp, mechanical, enzymatic, and autolytic débridements. Surgical débridement is indicated for abscesses or wounds that traverse tissue planes and have a moderate-to-high risk of significant bleeding. Sharp débridement is commonly performed in the outpatient setting as part of routine wound care; it is accompanied by minimum blood loss.

Mechanical débridement is accomplished by whirlpool treatments, forceful irrigations, or use of wet-to-dry dressings. Enzymatic debriding agents are used to treat well-perfused, partially necrotic pressure ulcers. They are applied with daily change of dressings until the wounds are free of slough or eschar. Enzymatic débridement may increase pain and drainage, requiring adjustments of dressing change schedules. Autolytic débridement involves the use of natural proteases and collagenases in wound fluids to digest nonviable material. Pain associated with débridement can be managed with topical analgesia. A local anesthetic, such as lidocaine 5% or EMLA cream (a eutectic mixture of lidocaine 2.5% and prilocaine 2.5%), can be applied up to 15 minutes before débridement. Premedication with a fast-acting oral nonopioid analgesic, oral opioid analgesic, or both can also be helpful.

Dressings (eSlide 24.4)

The primary dressing is contiguous with the wound surface, and the secondary dressing is applied external to the primary dressing. The secondary dressing is used for absorption, protection, or fixation.

Hyperbaric Oxygen Therapy

Hyperbaric oxygen therapy (HBOT) involves the therapeutic delivery of oxygen at a partial pressure at least 10-fold greater than the oxygen partial pressure of ambient air. HBOT enhances the natural mechanism of phagocytosis, reduces inflammation and reperfusion injury, releases endothelial progenitor stem cells from bone marrow, and enhances cross-linking of collagen in the ECM.

Gene Therapy and Exogenous Application of Growth Factors

Gene therapy refers to the insertion of a desired gene into recipient cells. Exogenous application of growth factors has been proposed as a means of promoting wound healing because these factors are often deficient in chronic wound environments.

Stem Cell Therapy

Adult stem cells can undergo "differentiation" into other cells, as they are adipogenic, osteogenic, and neurogenic. Bone marrow–derived stem cells, mesenchymal cells, and adipose tissue–derived stem cells can be used.

Platelet-Rich Plasma (eSlide 24.5)

Platelet-rich plasma (PRP) is an autologous concentration of platelets suspended in plasma. It is derived from whole blood that has undergone centrifugation to separate the PRP from the red blood cells. The platelets degranulate and release a variety of growth factors involved in wound healing, including platelet-derived growth factor, vascular endothelial growth factor, and transforming growth factor.

Therapeutic Ultrasound

Ultrasound applied to wounds results in two types of therapeutic effects: thermal and nonthermal. Thermal effects include increased blood flow and collagen extensibility; they manifest as increased tissue temperature. Nonthermal effects are largely attributable to acoustic streaming and cavitation.

Electrical Stimulation and Electromagnetic Therapy

Application of electrical stimulation facilitates the migration of epithelial cells and promotes wound healing.

Negative Pressure Wound Therapy

Topical negative pressure (TNP) treatment involves negative pressure (–125 mm Hg) applied on the wound surface to promote wound healing. TNP increases local blood flow, reduces edema and wound exudates, decreases bacterial colonization, stimulates cell proliferation, induces granulation tissue, and provides a moist wound environment.

• DIAGNOSIS AND TREATMENT OF SPECIFIC ULCER TYPES

Pressure Ulcers (eSlides 24.6, 24.7, 24.8, and 24.9)

PRESENTATION

The National Pressure Ulcer Advisory Panel classifies pressure ulcers in stages based on the extent of the lesion, as revealed on clinical observation (Stages I-IV). Recently added to the staging system is suspected deep tissue injury, in which the skin is intact but discolored.

TREATMENT

The mainstay of pressure ulcer treatment is evidence-based medical and nursing care, including continence care. Areas with a pressure ulcer should be relieved of any source of pressure. The wound area, depth, undermining, and appearance should be assessed at least weekly, and treatment should be modified accordingly. Periodic débridement and drainage management are essential to promote healing.

PREVENTION

Education, inspection, and optimization of continued pressure and shear stress are the keys to preventing the first or recurrent ulcerations. Pressure-relieving surfaces are required for patients who have impaired sensation. However, some pressure ulcers are unavoidable, notably at the end of life. The Norton and Braden scales are reliable and valid risk assessment tools.

Uncomplicated Chronic Venous Ulcers (eslide 24.10)

PRESENTATION

Patients with chronic venous ulcers usually have a history of a previous venous ulcer, dependent edema, previous deep venous thrombosis, pelvic surgery, vein stripping, or vein harvest for coronary artery bypass graft. Peripheral pulses are typically intact.

An ABI is required before starting treatment. If the ABI is normal, standard care (including compression) works well for most stasis ulcers. If arterial disease is suspected, segmental studies are useful to ensure that therapeutic compression is safe. Measurement of $TcPO_2$ is considered when the ABI is less than 0.8.

TREATMENT
Compression is the mainstay of treatment for chronic venous ulcers. Two major types of compression are used: elastic and nonelastic. Elastic compression provides compression of 30–40 mm Hg continuously, depending on the elastic compression brand. Nonelastic, nonstretch compression (classically the Unna paste boot) serves as a "fascial envelope" against which calf muscles can increase pressure during ambulation and reestablish a venous ankle pump.

PREVENTION
Compression of 20–30 mm Hg must be a lifelong practice. The patient remains at risk for recurrence because the underlying venous or fascial anatomic defect remains.

Uncomplicated Neuropathic Ulcers (eSlide 24.11)
PRESENTATION
Neuropathic or "insensate" foot ulcers can occur as a result of an acquired or a congenital sensory neuropathy. Diabetic foot insensitivity most often affects the plantar forefoot first; thus neuropathic ulcers commonly affect the plantar surface of the toes, halluces, or metatarsal heads. Neurotrophic osteoarthropathy (Charcot foot) frequently causes midfoot collapse and plantar-grade subluxation of the navicular or cuboid bone. The physical examination of an uncomplicated foot ulcer typically shows intact peripheral pulses, but sensation is diminished or absent in the vicinity of the ulcer.

TREATMENT
Treatment strategies involve "off-weighting" the ulcer, which promotes healing by reducing mechanical irritation, inflammation, and edema. This is achieved through prescribing orthoses, assistive devices, weight-relief shoes, physical therapies, and limited weight bearing. A total contact cast (TCC) is considered the "gold standard" of care. It is lightweight and mainly designed for protection, immobilization, and uniform pressure application. TCC is contraindicated when the $TcPO_2$ is less than 35 mm Hg or the ABI is less than 0.45 in the affected leg.

Other simpler off-loading techniques including a healing shoe, forefoot relief shoe (i.e., "half shoe"), removable cast walker, and DH walker. The DH walker is a well-padded knee-high "boot" with removable hexagonal insole pieces. It is effective for wounds involving the toes or metatarsal heads. The insoles of healing shoes have prominences proximal to or surrounding the plantar ulcers to relieve excessive pressures at the ulcer site; they can be effective in healing digital plantar ulcers. The half shoe reduces pressure on forefoot ulcers because the forefoot is "hanging in space."

PREVENTION
The most cost-effective predictor of the risk of neuropathic ulceration is an abnormal result identified during testing with the 5.07 Semmes–Weinstein monofilament. People who are found to be at risk may be prescribed orthopedic Oxford shoes with a high toe box, removable PPT-Plastazote insoles, and a modified rocker bottom.

Ischemic Ulcers (eSlide 24.12)

PRESENTATION

Patients with ischemic ulcers typically have peripheral arterial disease, with calcification, stenosis, or blockage of arteries anywhere from the aortic bifurcation to the plantar and digital arteries. In addition to arteriosclerosis, patients with ischemic wounds have a microvascular disease or a microcirculation abnormality, which contributes to chronic local hypoxia. Ischemic leg and foot ulcers may be one of multiple subtypes: pure, postsurgical, venous, pressure, or neuroischemic.

Neuroischemic ulcers (i.e., neuropathy is present) typically occur at areas of trauma or repeated pressure. They are generally located on the foot margins, such as the lateral heel, lateral fifth metatarsal head, and medial hallux. Pressure-related ischemic wounds also occur at the foot margins. A postsurgical ischemic wound can occur as a result of dehiscence of a residual limb incision within an ischemic region. Venous ischemic wounds can occur anywhere on the leg and foot and are associated with edema or venous insufficiency. Pure ischemic ulcers occur in the setting of acute proximal arterial blockage, distal emboli, or macroangiopathy or microangiopathy not otherwise classified. Ischemic ulcers tend to be exceedingly painful for sensate patients, exacerbated by leg elevation, and relieved by placing the leg in a dependent position. In addition to wound pain, the skin over the affected area is hairless and appears fragile and friable.

DIAGNOSTIC TESTS

Pulse volume recordings might show an asymmetrically low value, although an ABI of less than 0.4 is not uncommon and tends to carry a poor prognosis. A useful definition of ischemia is a periwound $TcPO_2$ less than 20 mm Hg.

TREATMENT

If the wound is truly ischemic, a vascular surgical referral is needed to determine whether proximal flow can be reestablished by angioplasty or a bypass procedure. Conservative, nonsurgical, standard wound care must be optimized, including liberal use of padding and weight-relief strategies. Many experts have advocated keeping ischemic wounds dry in an effort to avoid "wet gangrene." Techniques that address pathomechanics are crucial and involve optimizing gait mechanics, with limited weight-bearing on or near the ischemic wound. Overly aggressive rehabilitation of a patient with an ischemic wound can be detrimental.

PREVENTION

Frequent skin checks and vigilance are required. In the posthealing phase of venous ischemic wounds, careful attention should be paid to the compression pressure to avoid necrosis (e.g., use of 5-10 mm Hg antiembolism stockings or 10-20 mm Hg compression hose rather than 20-30 mm Hg stockings). Cigarette smoking lowers $TcPO_2$, which complicates healing of chronic wounds and makes recurrence more likely.

• WOUND INFECTIONS (eSlide 24.13)

Presentation

The signs and symptoms of local infection are increased pain, friable granulation tissue, wound breakdown (i.e., small openings in newly formed epithelial tissue not caused by reinjury or trauma), and a foul odor. Outpatient management of infections requires treatment with broad-spectrum oral antibiotics that are effective against gram-positive and gram-negative bacteria and anaerobes. Patients with systemic infection benefit from hospitalization, close monitoring, and intravenous antibiotics.

Osteomyelitis

Approximately 25% of all nonhealing ulcers are accompanied by a bone infection. The diagnosis of osteomyelitis should be considered and either confirmed or excluded at the time of the initial presentation. Osteomyelitis is most easily diagnosed by imaging studies. Plain films are positive for osteomyelitis if they show reactive bone formation and periosteal elevation. Plain films are the least expensive imaging study, but have limited sensitivity and specificity. Conventional three-phase bone scan is more sensitive for osteomyelitis than plain films, but it has limited specificity. Adding indium leukocyte scanning improves sensitivity, and when combined with a three-phase bone scan, the sensitivity of indium leukocyte scanning is 100% and the specificity is 81%. Magnetic resonance imaging reveals anatomic details and is extremely sensitive for showing the presence of marrow edema on T2-weighted images. It also has a high specificity.

Surgical Management of Infection

Frank tissue invasion, abscess, frank purulence, fistulae, or acute osteomyelitis require débridement in the operating room because the infection will not resolve with antibiotics alone. Musculocutaneous flaps can help heal osteomyelitis and limit further damage caused by shearing, friction, or pressure. Split-thickness skin grafts can also be used to repair recalcitrant venous ulcers and neuropathic ulcers. Reconstruction, osteotomies, or tendon recessions could be performed to relieve the source of pathomechanical risk factors.

Revascularization has become the standard care for limbs at risk of requiring an amputation. Angioplasty and arterial bypass produce similar results, although angioplasty produces lower periprocedural morbidity for high-risk wound patients. Limb amputation should only be performed as a last resort. It should be reserved for these situations: the limb is unsalvageable, revascularization surgery is too risky, life expectancy is very low, or limb salvage is not expected to produce any functional gains.

Nutrition

Major signs of poor nutrition include a body weight less than 90% of ideal body weight, a serum albumin less than 3.5 g/mL, or a serum prealbumin less than 15 mg/mL. Nutritional therapy for patients with stage III or stage IV pressure ulcers includes a total energy intake of 30–35 kcal/kg/day; protein intake of 1.2–1.5 g/kg/day, by means of oral, enteral, or parenteral routes; and fluid intake of 1 mL/kcal.

• CONCLUSION

Chronic wound care encompasses managing local wound, optimizing the musculoskeletal function of patients, prescribing orthoses and modalities, understanding gait biomechanics, and ensuring protected weight-bearing. Although there is a proliferation of new treatment options, the foundations of chronic wound management remain good dressing practices and aggressive preventive measures.

1. The hospitalization rate for dysvascular lower extremity amputation has not been reduced despite the introduction of preventive strategies. People with diabetes are 13 times more likely to be admitted for lower extremity amputation than the general population.
2. A low ankle-brachial index (ABI) with a good transcutaneous oxygen ($TcPO_2$) indicates good collateral arteries with adequate blood circulation.
3. Wound bed preparation aims to reduce the bacterial count, remove dead tissue, and reduce drainage to stimulate the epithelialization process.
4. The strategy of "off-weighting" the ulcer is a fundamental approach for pressure, neuropathic, and ischemic ulcers. This is achieved by using orthoses, special shoes, and limited weight bearing.
5. Check the ABI and possibly the $TcPO_2$ (if the ABI is <0.8) before application of compression therapy for stasis ulcers.
6. Long-acting opioids (e.g., oxycodone slow release, morphine sulfate slow release, and fentanyl transdermal patches) are indicated for treatment of intractable wound pain. Short-acting opioids (e.g., codeine, oxycodone, morphine sulfate, and hydromorphone) may be used simultaneously to manage breakthrough pain.

BIBLIOGRAPHY
The complete bibliography is available on ExpertConsult.com.

Vascular Diseases

25

Blessen C. Eapen

There is a broad differential diagnosis for lower extremity vascular disease. It is thereby important to understand the pathophysiology, clinical evaluation, and diagnostic testing modalities of these conditions to facilitate optimization of management by selecting the appropriate diagnosis and treatment.

• ARTERIAL DISEASES

Peripheral arterial disease (PAD) is a disease of aging, which commonly presents with intermittent claudication or symptoms of critical limb ischemia. The symptoms usually occur distal to the level of stenosis. If the patient is active, intermittent claudication is the typical presenting complaint, and if the patient is inactive, PAD may present with rest pain, ulceration, dependent rubor, or gangrene (eSlide 25.1). The clinical presentation of acute arterial occlusion is described as the "6 Ps": pain, pallor, paresthesia, paralysis, pulselessness, and polar (cold sensation). Some or all of these symptoms may be present (eSlide 25.2). The presence of intermittent claudication indicates that there is an inadequate supply of arterial blood to contracting muscles. It is brought on by walking and relieved by rest (without a change of position), and it is described as leg numbness, weakness, buckling, aching, cramping, or pain. When claudication abruptly increases, one must consider thrombosis in situ or an embolic event.

Vasculitic Syndrome

Polyarteritis nodosa is an acute necrotizing vasculitis that primarily affects small and medium-sized arteries. It is a systemic disorder that may involve the kidneys, joints, skin, nerves, and various other tissues.

   Thromboangiitis obliterans (Buerger disease) is a nonatherosclerotic segmental vasculitis that affects small and medium-sized arteries and veins of the extremities. It is strongly associated with tobacco exposure. The first manifestation of Buerger disease may be superficial phlebitis, and if smoking is discontinued, the process is frequently arrested.

• ARTERIAL EVALUATION (eSlide 25.3)

Noninvasive Arterial Studies

The *ankle-brachial index (ABI)* provides objective data about arterial perfusion of the lower limbs. The ABI refers to the ankle to arm systolic blood pressure ratio; a normal ABI is 1.0–1.4. ABI values above 1.4 indicate noncompressible arteries. ABI values from 0.91–0.99 are considered "borderline," are mildly diminished when they are ≤0.90 and ≥0.80, are moderately diminished between 0.50 and 0.80, and are severely decreased when <0.50.

   Segmental pressure measures the arterial closing and opening pressures at a specific anatomic location. It is often used to determine the location of arterial stenosis. Gradients of 10–15 mm Hg between adjacent sites may represent physiologically important obstruction.

Continuous wave Doppler (Video 25.1): A change from triphasic to monophasic waveforms provides reasonable accurate information about the location and extent of specific lower extremity lesions. Doppler waveform analyses are reliable even in highly calcified vessels that are not amenable to pressure determinations (eSlide 25.4).

Transcutaneous oximetry ($TcPO_2$) values provide a very sensitive means of assessing skin perfusion and the potential for cutaneous healing at a specific site. $TcPO_2$ values below 20–30 mm Hg suggest inadequate perfusion for healing (eSlide 25.5).

Imaging Techniques

Computed tomography angiography has become a standard noninvasive imaging modality for vascular anatomy and pathology (eSlide 25.6). Magnetic resonance angiography can be used to determine the morphology of blood vessels and assess the blood flow velocity. Contrast angiography is the "gold standard" for lower extremity arterial evaluation (eSlide 25.7).

• MANAGEMENT (eSlide 25.8)

Risk Factor Management

Risk factors for PAD should be rigorously assessed. PAD should be treated aggressively with a combination of 3-hydroxy-3-methylglutaryl-coenzyme A (HMG-CoA) reductase inhibitors (statins) (to achieve a low density lipoprotein goal of <70 mg/dL in patients with atherosclerotic disease), angiotensin converting enzyme inhibitors, antiplatelet agents, and beta-blockers (if there is a history of coronary disease). Cigarette smoking has been identified as an independent predictor of vascular disease and the reason why vascular procedures and interventions fail.

Rehabilitation

Patients should wear protective footwear at all times and monitor their extremities carefully for redness or skin breakdown. Lower extremity exercise in the form of a structured or a supervised walking program is critical for patients with PAD. Ambulation can help develop collateral blood flow and may lead to resolution or improvement of intermittent claudication.

Revascularization

Revascularization was once considered for patients with rest pain, impending tissue loss, significant limitations of lifestyle, or who failed medical treatment, but endovascular intervention, coupled with aggressive proactive medical management, is replacing this conventional paradigm.

Intermittent Pneumatic Compression

Intermittent pneumatic compression has been shown to improve walking distance. The extent of improvement is comparable to that seen with supervised exercise. External compression briefly raises the tissue pressure, which empties the underlying veins and transiently reduces the venous pressure, but it does not occlude arterial blood flow.

• VENOUS DISEASE

Chronic venous disease is a spectrum of diseases and disorders of the limbs, with spider veins and varicosities on one end of the spectrum and edema, skin changes (e.g., stasis dermatitis, hyperpigmentation), and ulceration at the other end (eSlide 25.9).

Venous Thromboembolism

Predisposing risk factors for deep vein thrombosis (DVT) include prolonged immobilization, estrogen use, previous DVT, a family history of thrombosis, and hypercoagulable state. Thrombosis may occur anywhere, but it most commonly involves the deep veins of the leg. Once a thrombosis forms, several events may occur: (1) it may propagate, (2) it may embolize, (3) it may be removed by fibrinolytic activity, or (4) it may undergo organization, including recanalization and retraction. Patients with risk factors should receive appropriate prophylaxis. Phlegmasia cerulea dolens is a rare complication of DVT.

Chronic Venous Insufficiency

Venous insufficiency can be the result of various factors, including heredity, local trauma, thrombosis, and intrinsic defects in the veins or valves themselves.

• VENOUS EVALUATION (eSlide 25.10)

Continuous wave Doppler can be used as a screening tool to test the integrity of the venous system. It identifies the presence of venous obstruction or incompetence, quantifies the severity of the venous disease, and localizes abnormalities to a particular segment of the limb.

Duplex ultrasound has become the method of choice for testing veins of the superficial, deep, and perforating systems.

Contrast venography of the lower extremities remains a powerful, but decreasingly used, tool in the evaluation of both acute and chronic DVT (eSlide 25.11).

D-Dimer levels have a high sensitivity for patients with acute venous thrombosis but low specificity for acute thrombosis. They can also be elevated in other clinical conditions.

• MANAGEMENT (eSlide 25.12)

Compression Therapy

The mainstay of treatment for chronic venous insufficiency is compression therapy. Knee-length graduated compression stockings (with a pressure of 30-40 mm Hg at the ankles) are prescribed. Graduated compression that provides decreasing pressure from distal to proximal surface has been the standard of care for both thromboprophylaxis and management of venous and lymphatic disorders. To prevent postthrombotic syndrome, compression stockings should be used routinely after a proximal DVT for a minimum of 1 year.

Elevation

When elevation is used for edema control, the extremity is typically elevated above the level of the heart. The leg should be elevated whenever possible, and long periods of standing or sitting with the dependent legs should be avoided.

Intermittent Pneumatic Compression

Lower extremity volume can be stabilized with an intermittent pneumatic compression pump (at 40–50 mm Hg). Compression wraps should be used between pumping sessions. Intermittent pneumatic compression is contraindicated in patients with congestive heart failure and venous obstruction.

Exercise

The value of exercise in the management of chronic venous insufficiency has not been conclusively demonstrated. Exercises involving the leg musculature, such as walking, bicycling, or swimming, promote muscle tone in the calf and enhance venous return.

• LYMPHATIC DISEASE (eSlide 25.13)

Lymphedema is the most frequent form of obstructive lymphatic disease because of lymph drainage failure. Lymphedema may be characterized as either high-lymph or low-lymph output failure.

Classification of Lymphedema

Secondary lymphedema occurs much more commonly than primary lymphedema. It is because of disrupted lymphatic flow resulting from infection, trauma, tumor, obstruction, surgery, or radiation. The most common cause of secondary lymphedema worldwide is filariasis, and the most common cause in the United States is breast cancer.

• EVALUATION

The differential diagnosis for a new-onset unilateral limb lymphedema is broad. In addition to systemic reasons for edema accumulation, the presence of acute DVT postphlebitic syndrome, chronic venous insufficiency, tumor obstruction, chronic infection, and lipidemia should all be considered.

Imaging Techniques

Lymphoscintigraphy is the standard evaluation tool to establish lymphatic flow patterns.

• TREATMENT OF LYMPHEDEMA (eSlide 25.14)

Complex decongestive therapy for lymphedema includes the following: (1) skin care management and treatment of infection, (2) specialized massage techniques to promote the movement of lymph, (3) compression of the lymphedematous region, and (4) elevation and exercises to reduce swelling and supplement the massage therapy.

Compression

Lymphedematous regions may be compressed with bandages (elastic or low-stretch) or graduated compression garments. Graduated compression garments are necessary to prevent fluid reaccumulation once a reduced and stable limb volume is achieved.

Elevation

Elevation of a lymphedematous limb can decrease the hydrostatic pressure gradient from the vasculature to the tissues and reduce the amount of fluid and protein moving out of the capillaries.

Exercise

Exercise improves mobility and muscular activity and leads to internal compression of lymph vessels. Lymph drainage is stimulated by intermittent pressure changes between muscles and external compressive bandages or garments. Resistance exercises seem to increase strength, decrease exacerbations of lymphedema, and decrease symptoms of lymphedema.

Vasopneumatic Compression Therapy

Vasopneumatic compression therapy pumps increase the total tissue pressure in edematous limbs and push tissue fluid back into blood capillaries. Total tissue pressures of 40–50 mm Hg are sufficient to remove fluid and lessen the risk for tissue damage.

• CONCLUSION

Arterial, venous, or lymphatic dysfunction may be the primary issue or comorbidity in patients who undergo rehabilitation. A detailed vascular history, thorough examination, and selected diagnostic tests should be inherent in the rehabilitation evaluation. When identified early, interventions such as exercise, appropriate compression, positioning, protection, and proper footwear may ameliorate the need for more aggressive medical and surgical treatments in patients with vascular disease.

Clinical Pearls

- Clinical presentation of acute arterial occlusion is described as the "6 Ps": pain, pallor, paresthesia, paralysis, pulselessness, and polar (cold sensation). Critical limb ischemia is clinically evident by the presence of rest pain, ischemic ulcers, or gangrene.
- Thromboangiitis obliterans (Buerger disease): Skip lesions are a classic finding on arteriogram and patients have a high risk of requiring an amputation.
- An ankle-brachial index (ABI) below 0.5 represents severe peripheral arterial disease (PAD) and has a poor prognosis for functional impairment, amputation, myocardial infarction, stroke, and death. An ABI value above 1.3 indicates the presence of vessel wall calcification and is uninterpretable.
- The best initial treatment for mild PAD involves modification of risk factors, cessation of tobacco use, and participation in a regular exercise program. Arteriography is the study of choice while preparing for vascular reconstructive surgery.
- Venous insufficiency is commonly associated with a history of previous venous thrombosis. The risk of venous ulcer formation is greatest with venous ambulatory pressures exceeding 80 mm Hg.
- Focal occlusive disease is most likely to benefit from transluminal percutaneous angioplasty, and focal diffuse disease would most likely benefit from a bypass procedure.
- Prosthetic vascular grafts are reserved for situations in which autogenous venous grafts are not feasible. Prosthetic grafts are associated with a higher risk of infection.
- Chronic severe lymphedema can lead to lymphangiosarcoma, which should be considered in patients with worsening of chronic skin changes. Surgery involving excisional debulking is indicated when the limb size markedly impairs function.

BIBLIOGRAPHY

The complete bibliography is available on ExpertConsult.com.

26 Burns

Amaramalar Selvi Naicker

Significant advances in management have resulted in an increase in survival after burn injury. As a consequence, burn survivors, who are often young adults, have long-term sequelae that impact schooling, return to work, and community reintegration. The future of burn care will be challenged by the expense and complexity of treatment, as well as an aging population.

• EPIDEMIOLOGY OF BURN INJURIES (eSlide 26.1)

In North America, up to 1 million burns require treatment annually and over 10 times as many burns occur worldwide. Among individuals with burns, the mortality rates are higher in low-income and middle-income countries. Predictors of burn mortality include increasing age, a higher total body surface area (TBSA) affected, and the presence of an inhalation injury.

• ACUTE PHYSIATRIC ASSESSMENT OF THE BURNED INDIVIDUAL (eSlides 26.2, 26.3, 26.4, and 26.5)

In the inpatient setting, the burn physiatrist may manage different medical aspects of burn care as part of a larger team. In the outpatient setting, the physiatrist should be competent in managing small, nonoperative burns, yet also be able to recognize individuals who may benefit from hospital admission, acute excision, and reconstruction of their wounds or scars.

Size, location, and depth of the burn injury are important predictors of complications and mortality. TBSA may be calculated using the Lund and Browder chart or by following the "rule of nines" (Fig. 26.1). Thermal burns are classified as superficial, partial-thickness, or full-thickness injuries. Superficial wounds (e.g., sunburns) are red and painful, with little exudate. They usually heal within 7 days and have a low risk of scarring. Partial-thickness burns are further classified as superficial and deep. Superficial partial-thickness burns are painful and have mild to moderate wound exudate and serous-filled blisters. They usually heal within 7–14 days and have a low risk of scarring, but may produce skin pigmentation. Deep partial-thickness burns have fewer blisters and moderate to extensive wound exudate. These burns are painful and often heal within 14–28 days, but the prolonged inflammatory phase increases the risk of scarring. Full-thickness burn injuries damage all of the epidermis and dermis and extend to the deeper structures. The burned skin may have reduced somatic sensation, but pain arises from underlying necrotic tissue, surrounding burns, or damage to nearby structures. These wounds typically appear pale with minimal exudate and have significant scarring, which arises from either the full-thickness injuries themselves or from treatment with skin grafts. Acute intervention to excise necrotic tissue and reconstruct the wound is indicated.

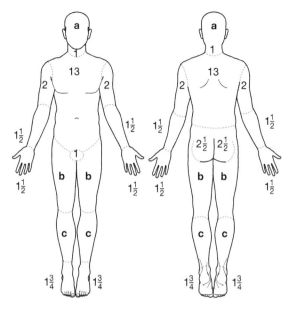

FIG. 26.1 The Lund and Browder method for calculation of burn size is reliable for children with different body proportions. (From Artz CP, Moncrief JA, Pruitt BA: *Burns: a team approach,* Philadelphia, 1979, Saunders, with permission.)

Electrical injuries differ from thermal injuries. High-voltage (>1000 V) injuries are usually work-related, whereas most low-voltage (<1000 V) injuries occur at home. The extent of soft tissue damage may be greater than expected, as electrical current will affect the tissues with the least electrical resistance, resulting in peripheral and central nervous system damage. Myocardial necrosis and arrhythmias may occur; however, individuals who do not have an arrhythmia in the first 24 hours are at a lower risk of developing later arrhythmias. High-voltage electrical injuries account for a large number of burn-related amputations and neuropathies. Ocular complications, such as cataracts or macular holes, may occur late after the injury.

Other types of acute burn injury, such as frostbite, may occur from environmental or industrial exposure to cold. Burns may also occur in association with the medical use of ionizing radiation. Various other conditions, such as Stevens-Johnson syndrome, toxic epidermal necrolysis (TEN), necrotizing fasciitis, and Fournier gangrene (which will require excision and subsequent split-thickness skin grafting), are complex to care for and rehabilitate.

• ACUTE WOUND CARE (eSlide 26.6)

Removal of necrotic material and the establishment of a clean, moist wound tissue bed are the primary goals of acute wound management. Among the large number of commercially available products, silver sulfadiazine remains a mainstay in burn care. Other dressings include biosynthetic, silver-based, or hydrogel dressings. Tense blisters can be drained, allowing the separated epithelium to act as a temporary biological dressing. Immersion hydrotherapy is no longer practiced, as the tanks may lower core body temperature or sodium levels, may be a source of gram-negative bacteria such as *Pseudomonas*, and may cause cross-contamination of wounds. Acute burn pain is magnified by procedural pain associated with dressing changes, mobility, stretching, and surgery. Opioids remain the mainstay of pain care, whereas adjuncts, including distraction, hypnosis, or anxiolytics, may be particularly useful in pediatric individuals.

• ACUTE SURGICAL PROCEDURES FOR BURN INJURIES (eSlide 26.7)

Wound edema and the fluids required for resuscitation after a burn injury may increase the risk of developing compartment syndrome. Escharotomies in the limbs and trunk can be performed to relieve pressure. After an escharotomy, the limb should be elevated and splinted in a neutral position for 24 hours before initiating passive range of movement. Early excision of necrotic tissue and eschar, combined with autologous, split-thickness skin grafting, has greatly improved survival after burn injury. Donor skin is removed with the use of a powered dermatome and placed on the surgically prepared wound bed, where it is held in place by staples, sutures, or dermal glues. A compressive postoperative dressing is then applied to the skin graft area. The donor site heals spontaneously in 2 weeks. To improve adherence of the skin graft, the grafted site is typically immobilized in the immediate postoperative phase; however, rehabilitation therapies can be initiated a few days later to improve function and reduce the length of hospital stay.

• CLINICAL PROBLEMS FOLLOWING BURN INJURIES (eSlide 26.8)

Presence of Inhalation Injury

Inhalation injury is a significant risk factor for morbidity following burns. Poor oxygenation and toxic smoke components put the burned individual at risk of developing hypoxic brain injury. Inhalation injuries also increase the risk of developing pneumonia, adult respiratory distress syndrome, and multisystem organ failure.

• CATABOLISM AND METABOLIC ABNORMALITIES

In all individuals with burn injuries greater than 30% TBSA, significant metabolic abnormalities occur, which result in the loss of bone mineral density, reduced lean body mass, and increased insulin resistance. Progressive loss of lean body mass is associated with increasing loss of function and an increased risk of pneumonia and poor wound healing. Management of this hypermetabolic state has been improved with the use of anabolic agents and beta-blockers, as well as exercise (including passive therapies to improve respiration), splinting, and positioning to minimize the risk of contracture. Dysphagia can also develop from exposure to inhaled irritants, mechanical complications of tube placement, or neurologic injury; it can be a barrier to achieving adequate nutrition. Thus, the increased caloric and nutritional needs of patients with burn injuries should be addressed with early enteral feeding and nutritional supplementation.

• PERIPHERAL NEUROPATHY

Approximately 10% of burned individuals will develop peripheral neuropathy from direct thermal injury, electrical current, compression, or metabolic derangements. Deeper and larger TBSA burns are more likely to be associated with axonal neuropathies. Mononeuropathy and polyneuropathy patterns are often seen. Electrodiagnostic studies can help define the extent of nerve injuries.

• HETEROTOPIC OSSIFICATION (eSlide 26.9)

There is an increased risk of developing heterotopic ossification (HO) after burn injuries. The most common site is the elbow. Treatment and prevention of HO remain controversial, but emphasis is placed on early and frequent mobilization and appropriate positioning. Surgical resection is only considered when the bone is mature. The role of bisphosphonates is not well defined.

• HYPERTROPHIC SCARRING (eSlide 26.10)

Hypertrophic scarring is the most common complication after burn injury. It involves raised, red, painful, pruritic, and contracted scarring within the margins of the original injury. A few months after the injury, scars will increase in volume and erythema, but regress several months later. Keloid scars invade surrounding tissues. Younger individuals, patients with darker skin pigmentation, injuries with a prolonged inflammatory healing phase, and wounds that have been open longer than 3 weeks tend to be associated with a higher incidence of hypertrophic scarring.

The best treatment is to prevent scarring through adequate wound care. Deficiencies of sweat and sebaceous glands cause pruritus. Oral diphenhydramine, doxepin, hydroxyzine, and gabapentin have all shown some efficacy in relieving pruritus in large regions of scarring caused by burns. Treatment includes regular use of a moisturizing cream, avoidance of mechanical insults, minimization of direct heat and sun exposure, use of pressure garments, application of silicone gel sheeting, and intralesional injection of corticosteroids. Therapies based on little evidence, such as massage, pulsed dye laser, and interferon-α, are also being tried.

• CONTRACTURES (eSlide 26.11)

Contractures commonly occur in the shoulder, elbow, and knee joints. Treatment entails splinting, positioning, and range of movement exercises. The appropriate positioning for burned individuals has been described in an attempt to minimize burn scar contracture development. Evidence supports early splinting and therapy for deep burns of the axilla to prevent contracture formation. The shoulder can likely be safely positioned in 90 degrees of flexion with 10 degrees or less of horizontal adduction to take any potential stress off the brachial plexus.

Risk Factors for the Development of Depression in   BOX **26.1**
Burn Survivors

Preburn affective disorders (mood disorders)
Coping styles (adult individuals who engage in both avoidance and approach strategies of
    coping report greater symptoms of depression compared with those who use only one
    of these or other alternative strategies)
Demographic characteristics, such as female sex
Burn injury characteristics, such as individuals with head or neck burns
Disposition variables, such as a longer hospital stay

• PSYCHOSOCIAL ADJUSTMENT (eSlides 26.12 and 26.13)

Comprehensive, interdisciplinary rehabilitation treatment should focus on both physical and psychological complications, such as depression and anxiety disorders, which can have a negative impact on recovery. Several risk factors predispose to the development of depression in burn survivors (Box 26.1). Post-traumatic stress disorder is not uncommon. Predictors of a poorer body image include burn characteristics, social and emotional variables, and the individual's coping style. An individual's expression of sexuality remains inseparable from body image and self-esteem.

• COMMUNITY REINTEGRATION (eSlide 26.14)

Community reintegration is an important aspect of every burn rehabilitation program because the ultimate goal is to return the individual as close as possible to his or her preinjury life, including work, school, home, recreational, and community activities. Early identification of those at risk for prolonged unemployment and subsequent referral to comprehensive rehabilitative services that include work hardening, vocational training programs, and workplace assessment are important steps in facilitating a quick and successful return to work.

Clinical Pearls (eSlide 26.15)

- Burn care requires a multidisciplinary approach.
- Specialized rehabilitation units in the acute care setting have been shown to reduce the length of hospital stay and improve function.
- Knowledge of the common sequelae of complications following burns is important in preventing and treating these complications (including reflex sympathetic dystrophy [RSD], which, although rare, is difficult to treat).
- Awareness of household items that can cause burns, such as barbeque pits, hot irons, and electric blankets, is important for prevention.

BIBLIOGRAPHY
The complete bibliography is available on ExpertConsult.com.

Acute Medical Conditions

27

Norhayati Hussein

Medical rehabilitation encompasses the needs of patients with cardiopulmonary disorders, renal dysfunction, and debility. These conditions may present as primary or secondary reasons for rehabilitation in addition to other primary disabilities. A degree of frailty is a common feature of these underlying conditions.

• ASSESSMENT OF CARDIOPULMONARY FUNCTION AND EXERCISE CAPACITY

Cardiopulmonary rehabilitation begins with taking a thorough history and performing a thorough physical examination. It is important to understand the basic terminology of exercise and the effects of physiologic conditions on cardiopulmonary exercise capacity.

• BASIC TERMINOLOGIES OF EXERCISE

Aerobic capacity is a measure of the work capacity of an individual; it is expressed as the maximal oxygen uptake (Vo_{2max}). Oxygen consumption (Vo_2) increases linearly with workload, up to the Vo_{2max}. Maximal exercise capacity assessment can assist in rating disability and planning exercise and recovery programs.

Maximum *heart rate (HR)* decreases with age and is best determined by exercise testing. It can also be estimated using either the Karvonen equation or this equation: [maximum HR = 220 − age (in years)]. Physical conditioning can alter the slope of the relationship between the HR and Vo_2, with improved conditioning lowering the slope so there is less increase in HR for a given Vo_2. HR is a useful exercise indicator because of the linear relationship with Vo_2, except when certain medications that can alter the HR response are used.

Stroke volume (SV) is the volume of blood ejected during left ventricular contraction. Maximal SV increases with exercise. The greatest increase in SV occurs during the early exercise phase. The SV increase is sensitive to postural changes, with the smallest increase occurring in the supine position. SV increases in a curvilinear manner, achieving a maximum at approximately 40% of Vo_{2max}.

Cardiac output (CO) is a product of the HR and SV. It has a linear relationship with work and is the primary determinant of Vo_{2max}. CO is higher in the upright position.

Myocardial oxygen consumption (Mvo_2) is the oxygen consumption of the heart muscle. It increases in proportion to the workload of the myocardium. When the Mvo_2 exceeds the maximum coronary artery oxygen delivery, myocardial ischemia and angina can occur. The *rate pressure product* (*RPP*; [HR × systolic blood pressure (SBP)]/100) is directly related to the Mvo_2. Compared with erect exercises, supine exercises have a higher Mvo_2 at low intensity and a lower Mvo_2 at high intensity.

• AEROBIC TRAINING

Aerobic training involves physical exercises that increase the cardiopulmonary capacity (i.e., the VO_{2max}). The benefits of aerobic training are reduced cardiac risk and improved cardiac conditioning. Aerobic training prescriptions must include four components: intensity, duration, frequency, and specificity.

Components of Aerobic Training

The *intensity* of exercise is defined as how difficult an exercise is. It can be prescribed in terms of a target HR, a metabolic equivalent of task (MET) level, or an intensity level measured in watts. The usual intensity target for cardiac primary prevention is an HR that is 80%–85% of the predicted maximum HR or the peak HR determined during an exercise tolerance test. For secondary prevention, exercise should be at a safe level of 60% or more of the maximum HR to achieve a training effect.

The *duration* of exercise for cardiac conditioning usually requires 20- to 30-minute sessions, in addition to 5- to 10-minute warm-up and cool-down periods.

The *frequency* is the number of exercise sessions performed over a fixed time period. The recommended frequency of aerobic training is 5 times per week for moderate-intensity exercise.

The *specificity* of exercise refers to the type of activities performed. Training benefits specifically relate to the type of activity.

Effects of Aerobic Training

Aerobic capacity: Maximum aerobic capacity increases with aerobic training. The resting VO_2 is stable, as is the VO_2 at a given workload. The changes are specific to the trained muscles.

Cardiac output: Maximum CO increases, whereas resting CO is stable. Resting SV increases, with a corresponding decrease in the resting HR.

Heart rate: Resting HR decreases with aerobic training and is lower at any given workload. The maximum HR is unchanged.

Stroke volume: SV increases at rest and is maintained at a lower HR, resulting in a lower RPP for a given level of exertion.

Myocardial oxygen capacity: Maximum MVO_2 usually does not change, but at a given workload, MVO_2 decreases with training. This reduces episodes of angina.

Peripheral vascular resistance (PVR): Aerobic training reduces arterial and arteriolar tone, thereby decreasing cardiac "afterload" and PVR. The reduction in PVR results in a lower RPP and a lower MVO_2 at a given workload and at rest.

• CARDIAC REHABILITATION

Cardiac Rehabilitation Programs

Cardiac rehabilitation programs typically consist of primary and secondary prevention strategies. *Primary prevention* strategies are initiated prior to a cardiac event and focus on modification of cardiac risk factors. *Secondary prevention* strategies are used after manifestation of cardiac disease. They focus on reducing the risk of subsequent cardiac events and associated complications. Secondary prevention includes all features of primary prevention. Cardiac rehabilitation is indicated after myocardial infarction, angina, congestive heart failure, revascularization procedures, and heart transplantation. Various cardiac conditions impose specific physiologic abnormalities and effects on exercise capacity (eSlide 27.1).

Cardiac Rehabilitation After Myocardial Infarction

The phases of cardiac rehabilitation are as follows:

Acute Phase (Phase 1) and Inpatient Rehabilitation Phase (Phase 1B): These start at the acute phase following a cardiac event and end at discharge from the hospital. The acute phase is characterized by early mobilization (eSlides 27.2, 27.3, and 27.4).

Training Phase (Phase 2): This is an outpatient training phase, which encompasses secondary prevention strategies, intense education, and aerobic conditioning.

Maintenance Phase (Phase 3): This phase is necessary to maintain the benefits of phases 1 and 2. Patients seek to continue aerobic exercises and maintain lifestyle modifications.

Cardiac risk factor modification is performed during all phases. For patients who were not hospitalized at the time of cardiac diagnosis, the goals are essentially phase 2 and phase 3 cardiac rehabilitations.

Cardiac Rehabilitation Programs for Specific Conditions

ANGINA PECTORIS

The goal of cardiac rehabilitation in individuals with angina is to lower the HR. This will reduce the RPP and Mvo_2, thus reducing episodes of angina.

Cardiac Rehabilitation After Revascularization Procedures (Coronary Bypass Grafting or Percutaneous Transluminal Coronary Angioplasty)

Cardiac rehabilitation programs are similar after revascularization procedures, such as coronary bypass grafting (CABG) or percutaneous transluminal coronary angioplasty (PTCA). They emphasize secondary prevention, as well as improve cardiac conditioning and overall fitness. Patients can pursue the program immediately after PTCA. In patients who underwent CABG with a sternotomy, arm exercises should be limited until sternal healing occurs.

Cardiac Rehabilitation After Cardiac Transplantation

Transplanted hearts are denervated and have no direct sympathetic or central vagal regulation. The chronotopic response to exercise is mediated by circulating catecholamines, leading to a delayed and blunted HR response to exercise. After transplantation, patients have a lower work capacity, reduced CO, lower peak HR, and lower oxygen uptake, as well as a higher resting HR and SBP, compared with normal individuals. The focus of a cardiopulmonary rehabilitation program after transplantation is on conditioning and education. Target intensity for aerobic exercise is usually approximately 60%–70% of peak effort for 30–60 minutes three to five times per week, with a target intensity "rating of perceived exertion" of 13–14 on the Borg Scale or 5–6 on the modified Borg Scale.

• PULMONARY REHABILITATION

Pulmonary Functional Evaluation

Various pulmonary conditions impose specific physiologic abnormalities and effects on exercise capacity (eSlides 27.5 and 27.6).

Basic static lung volumes and dynamic responses to exercise are helpful in the assessment of exercise capacity in individuals with pulmonary disease. Important values related to pulmonary functional evaluation are listed below:

Total lung capacity: Volume of air in the lungs at full inspiration.

Vital capacity: Volume of air in the lungs between full inspiration and full expiration.

Forced expired vital capacity: Maximum volume expired during a maximal forced expiration.

Forced expiratory volume in 1 second: Maximum volume exhaled in 1 second.

Maximal voluntary ventilation: Measurement of the maximal ventilation in 15 seconds.

Residual volume: Volume of air remaining in the lungs after a full expiration.

Tidal volume: Volume of a regular resting breath.

Diffusing capacity of the lungs for carbon monoxide: Measurement of the diffusion of carbon monoxide (oxygen analog) across the alveolar membrane.

Pulmonary Rehabilitation Programs (eSlides 27.7 to 27.11)

Pulmonary rehabilitation programs are similar to cardiac rehabilitation programs in having both primary and secondary prevention components. Primary prevention strategies involve methods of smoking prevention and cessation. Secondary prevention strategies involve methods to promote medication adherence, smoking cessation, supplemental oxygen use, education, and management of environmental triggers. Mobilization is instituted early during the acute phase. The overall goals of pulmonary rehabilitation programs are smoking cessation, enhanced medical management, medication training, disease-specific training, enhanced pulmonary toilet, improved dyspnea, self-sufficiency in oxygen management, and nutritional counselling. Patients are also taught methods of dyspnea relief, which include exercise training and lifestyle modifications.

Pulmonary Rehabilitation Programs in Specific Conditions

CHRONIC OBSTRUCTIVE PULMONARY DISEASE

Pulmonary rehabilitation is the gold standard management for patients with chronic obstructive pulmonary disease (COPD). The goal of the rehabilitation program is to improve peripheral efficiency and decrease dyspnea. Education on energy conservation, anxiety reduction, and improved endurance all contribute to improved function and decreased dyspnea. Airway clearance and chest physical therapy have a role in the pulmonary rehabilitation of patients with substantial secretions. A combination of external percussion devices, vibration devices, and inhaled saline, in combination with cough training and huffing, may assist in mobilizing secretions.

INTERSTITIAL LUNG DISEASE

Exercise intensity in patients with interstitial lung disease is limited by hypoxemia. Oxygen supplementation may be required to maintain oxygen saturation during activity. Unlike in COPD, airway secretions are usually not problematic in patients with interstitial lung disease.

VENTILATORY FAILURE

Exercise programs for patients receiving nocturnal or intermittent ventilator support aim to improve efficiency and decrease fatigue when the patient is off the ventilator.

Cardiopulmonary Rehabilitation in the Physically Disabled

Individuals who are physically disabled tend to be more sedentary and have lower activity levels. This increases the risk of cardiac and pulmonary disease and presents obstacles for a standard rehabilitation program. Furthermore, mobility of disabled individuals requires greater energy expenditure; thus compromised work capacity from cardiopulmonary disease may impose an even greater degree of impairment in disabled individuals than in able-bodied individuals. A cardiopulmonary exercise prescription for individuals who are physically disabled must be adapted for their individual disabilities.

• RENAL FAILURE

Uncontrolled hypertension, poorly controlled diabetes, and glomerulonephritis are the most common causes of renal failure. Fluid overload with hypertension can occur when the glomerular filtration rate falls below 60 mL per minute. The most important pathologic feature of diabetic glomerulopathy is excessive extracellular matrix. Primary glomerulonephritis can be caused by infection, immune diseases, and vasculitides, with resultant scarring of the nephrons. Renal diseases can be classified based on the anatomic area of the kidney that is affected (eSlide 27.12).

Consequences of Impaired Renal Function

Electrolyte Imbalance (*Hyperkalemia and Hyponatremia*): The ability to maintain normal potassium levels is preserved until the glomerular filtration rate reaches approximately 10% of the normal rate. As the stage of renal failure increases, the rate of potassium excretion declines and the ability to conserve sodium is compromised, resulting in hyperkalemia and hyponatremia.

Uremia: In renal failure, the remaining nephron units increase their capacity through compensatory hyperfiltration and increased glomerular permeability, leading to uremia.

Bone Issues: *Hypocalcemia* can occur because of decreased calcium absorption and stimulation of parathyroid hormone release. *Hyperphosphatemia* is caused by impaired renal excretion of phosphate.

Anemia: *Anemia* can occur because of decreased erythropoietin production and iron deficiency.

Metabolic Issues: *Metabolic acidosis* is caused by reduced ability of the failing kidneys to excrete acid. This is further exacerbated by their decreased ability to resorb bicarbonate, which is the main pH buffer in the body. Anemia and metabolic acidosis may produce physiologic abnormalities and alter exercise capacity (eSlide 27.13).

Factors Leading to Fatigue and Weakness in Renal Failure

Weakness: Anemia of chronic disease results in decreased erythropoietin production and iron deficiency. This contributes to fatigue and weakness.

Debility: A glomerular filtration rate less than 60 mL per minute is associated with reduced well-being and overall function. Patients who are dependent on dialysis have multiple possible sources of debility and often report substantial fatigue following dialysis sessions.

Dialysis-related "residual syndrome": The term "residual syndrome" refers to the syndrome of partially treated uremia. As dialysis cannot fully replace all renal functions, electrolyte imbalances and acid-base abnormalities are responsible in part for the uremic symptoms that are seen in dialysis-dependent patients.

Sarcopenia: Uremic sarcopenia can develop because of the presence of uremia. This causes changes in skeletal muscle fibers, including mitochondrial depletion and atrophy of both slow-twitch and fast-twitch muscle fibers, which contribute to the overall sense of fatigue and weakness.

Rehabilitation for Patients With Renal Transplantation

PRERENAL TRANSPLANTATION

Chronic deconditioning resulting from uremic sarcopenia and a predisposition to chronic pain and gait abnormalities represent areas for substantial rehabilitative intervention. Patients receiving hemodialysis also have an increased risk of substantial sedentary behavior as a result of extended immobility during hemodialysis sessions and postdialysis fatigue following dialysis sessions. Early referral to a rehabilitation professional to establish a home exercise program before starting dialysis is warranted for all patients with uremia.

POSTRENAL TRANSPLANTATION

A comprehensive rehabilitative program will offer numerous benefits following renal transplantation, as reduced mobility, prescribed corticosteroids, and a sedentary lifestyle during recovery can accelerate debility, even in the face of a normally functioning new kidney. Patients deemed appropriate for rehabilitation intervention should be ensured of uninterrupted therapy at least three times per week, with a target intensity of 60%–70% of peak effort for 30–60 minutes. The rate of perceived exertion as described in the Borg Scale is a validated method of regulating intensity. Continuation of posttransplantation outpatient rehabilitation programs must focus on controlled conditioning, as well as education regarding the importance of exercise in maintaining exercise capacity and lifelong function.

• INACTIVITY AND IMMOBILITY

Prolonged immobility has many negative effects (eSlide 27.14).

Sedentary lifestyles result in increased cardiovascular risk, obesity, metabolic syndrome, deep vein thrombosis, elevated insulin levels, and altered insulin resistance. Immobility in the critical care setting poses serious physiologic and pathologic consequences.

• TREATMENT CONSIDERATIONS IN CRITICAL CARE SETTING

Hemodynamic Instability or Orthostatic Hypotension: Majority of patients hospitalized in critical care units experience hemodynamic instability. Constant surveillance of vital signs and gradual early mobilization are necessary.

Ventilator Dependence: Hypoxemic failure can be induced by ventilation-perfusion mismatch, shunting, and altered oxygen exchange. Hypercapnic failure causes decreased minute ventilation relative to the physiologic demand. Ventilator status and oxygen saturation in response to activity must be monitored closely.

Critical Care Unit-Acquired Weakness: Acquired weakness is common following hospitalization in the intensive care setting. Approximately 50% of patients with prolonged mechanical ventilation, sepsis, or organ failure have some degree of neuromuscular dysfunction. Early and aggressive physical therapy intervention is necessary to improve recovery of muscle strength in patients in the intensive care unit.

Psychological Alterations: Posttraumatic stress disorder and delirium can occur.

• FRAILTY SYNDROME

The frailty syndrome is a recognized syndrome of decreased ability to adapt to stressors, which is accompanied by reduced physiologic reserves and energy metabolism. The frequency of frailty syndrome has been reported to vary widely, depending on the population studied; percentages have ranged from 4%–60%. The frailty syndrome is clearly associated with advanced age and becomes more prevalent in older age groups. However, frailty syndrome is not a variant of normal aging; it is considered a separate entity. In addition to functional, psychological, and musculoskeletal changes, there are also altered organ system and homeostatic responses in the frailty syndrome. These include a reduced capacity to maintain homeostasis and an increased vulnerability to stressors because of reduced energy metabolism, sarcopenia, altered hormonal activity, and decreased immune function. Early recognition of the frailty syndrome via screening tools allows for interdisciplinary and multidisciplinary interventions with the common goal of preserving function as long as possible for these patients.

Frailty Screening Tools (eSlide 27.15)

Fried Frailty Phenotype is a rule-based tool that identifies frailty based on a positive score in three out of five phenotypic criteria.

The criteria are as follows:
1. Unintentional weight loss (more than 10 pounds in the last year)
2. Exhaustion ("I felt that everything I did was an effort" and "I could not get going")
3. Slow walking speed (time required to walk 15 feet, measured in seconds)
4. Low physical activity
5. Reduced grip strength

The prefrail stage (one or two criteria) identifies a subset of people at high risk of progressing to frailty. Individuals with none of the phenotypic criteria are considered "robust" or nonfrail.

Canadian Study on Health and Aging (CSHA) Frailty Index (Rockwood Index) is a detailed deficit-based tool. Clinical deficits scores are based on a 70-item index consisting of self-reported functional activities, mood, and motor symptoms, as well as signs and symptoms derived from the medical history and physical examination.

CSHA Clinical Frailty Scale is a descriptive scale with seven categories ranging from "very fit" to "severely frail." It is judgment based, less time consuming, and more applicable in the rehabilitation setting.

Clinical Pearls

1. The best method of evaluating the capacity to exercise in cardiac and pulmonary conditions is the cardiopulmonary exercise test (CPET). The CPET yields diagnostic, prognostic, and exercise prescription guidance for patients with cardiopulmonary disease.
2. Aerobic training is a habitual dynamic physical activity of sufficient intensity, duration, and frequency to produce physiologic adjustments in the cardiopulmonary response to exercise.
3. In pulmonary rehabilitation, weaning supplemental oxygen is not a goal, as pulmonary rehabilitation does not improve lung function.
4. Patients undergoing dialysis have issues with anemia, sarcopenia, debility, bone disease, and electrolyte abnormalities. Despite dialysis, they still experience residual syndrome because of incomplete resolution of uremia by dialysis.
5. Sedentary behavior is distinct from physical activity and has been shown to be a health risk in itself. Meeting the guidelines for physical activity does not make up for a sedentary lifestyle.
6. Consequences of frailty include weight loss, exhaustion, slow walking speed, low physical activity, reduced strength, and an increase in systemic inflammation. Frailty syndrome can be identified by rule-based, deficit-based, or judgment-based tools.

BIBLIOGRAPHY
The complete bibliography is available on ExpertConsult.com.

28 Chronic Medical Conditions: Pulmonary Disease, Organ Transplantation, and Diabetes

Chen-Liang Chou

With an aging population, chronic medical conditions, such as pulmonary diseases, organ transplantations, and diabetic complications, are common, and combining general medicine and rehabilitation principles is necessary to optimize clinical care.

• PULMONARY DISEASE, ORGAN TRANSPLANTATION, AND DIABETES

Pulmonary Rehabilitation

CLASSIFICATION OF PULMONARY DISEASE

Obstructive diseases, including asthma, chronic bronchitis, chronic obstructive pulmonary disease (COPD), and emphysema, are characterized by a reduction in airflow and airflow limitation. Restrictive lung diseases, such as interstitial lung diseases, neuromuscular disorders, sarcoidosis, pleural disorders, and abnormalities of the chest wall, are characterized by a reduction in lung size or an increase in lung stiffness, resulting in a decrease in the maximum volume of air within the lungs.

Epidemiology. COPD, seen mostly in smokers, is the third most common cause of morbidity and mortality worldwide.

GENERAL MEDICAL MANAGEMENT

Medications for COPD include inhaled bronchodilators, inhaled corticosteroids, phosphodiesterase-4 inhibitors, and theophylline. Influenza and pneumococcal vaccines should be administered. α_1-Antitrypsin augmentation therapy is efficacious for α_1-antitrypsin deficiency. Evidence-based treatments for prolonging life include smoking cessation, noninvasive mechanical ventilation, lung volume reduction surgery (LVRS), combined use of long-acting β-agonists and inhaled corticosteroids, and oxygen therapy.

OXYGEN THERAPY

Long-term oxygen therapy (LTOT; administered for ≥15 hours/day) improves exercise tolerance, sleep, cognitive outcomes, survival, and quality of life in people with COPD who have an arterial oxygen partial pressure of 55 mm Hg or below or an arterial oxygen saturation (SaO_2) of 88% or below. LTOT is needed if the SaO_2 is 89% or below in people with pulmonary hypertension, congestive heart failure, or polycythemia.

CHEST PHYSICAL THERAPY (eSlide 28.1)

Breathing retraining for COPD includes pursed-lip breathing, head-down and bending-forward postures, slow deep breathing, and localized expansion exercises or segmental breathing. These strategies maintain a positive airway pressure during exhalation and reduce the likelihood of lung overinflation. Although diaphragmatic breathing is widely taught, it increases the work of breathing and dyspnea. Respiratory muscle endurance training is used to reduce fatigue. Airway clearance strategies can reduce the work of breathing, improve gas exchange, and limit infection. Techniques for airway clearance include postural drainage, chest percussion and vibration, airway oscillation, and incentive spirometry. Head-down positions should be used with caution in people with severe heart disease. Patients can manually assist their cough by compression of the abdomen while controlling their respiratory pattern. Mucoactive medications are administered if necessary. Noninvasive intermittent positive-pressure ventilation (NIPPV) with air stacking or glossopharyngeal breathing (GPB) is used to increase the depth of inspiration. When an upper motor neuron lesion occurs above the midthoracic level, functional electrical stimulation of the abdominal muscles is indicated. Other management strategies include positive expiratory pressure mask followed by huff coughing, autogenic drainage, and a mechanical insufflation–exsufflation cough machine (which is contraindicated in patients with bullous emphysema or a pneumothorax).

EXERCISE PRESCRIPTION FOR PULMONARY REHABILITATION

Cardiorespiratory exercise training is effective for decreasing exertional dyspnea, which is the most frequent symptom of COPD and leads to physical disability and functional impairment. Pulmonary rehabilitation exercises include cardiorespiratory endurance training of larger muscle groups by overground or treadmill walking, leg cycling, and arm cycling. However, many patients have difficulty tolerating arm cycling because it increases ventilatory drive and worsens dyspnea. Resistance and flexibility exercises may improve functional capacity. Initially, individuals supervising the exercise program should monitor the patient closely and adjust the sessions according to the appearance of exertional symptoms.

EXERCISE IN CHRONIC OBSTRUCTIVE PULMONARY DISEASE (eSlides 28.2, 28.3, and 28.4)

An exercise prescription for COPD includes cardiorespiratory endurance exercise therapy (which improves maximum aerobic capacity, timed walk distance, and quality of life) and resistance training (which increases fat-free mass and muscle strength). Continuous positive airway pressure and NIPPV during exercise might reduce the perception of dyspnea.

EXERCISE IN ASTHMA

Aerobic exercise improves overall fitness and health and decreases activation of nuclear factor-kappa B in the lungs, which leads to a reduction in airway inflammation. Exercise-induced bronchoconstriction can be identified by the eucapnic voluntary hyperventilation test, which was reported to identify 90% of athletes with the condition. The severity of exercise-induced bronchoconstriction can be predicted by airway vascular hyperpermeability, eosinophilic inflammation, and bronchial hyperactivity.

EXERCISE IN CYSTIC FIBROSIS

Management of cystic fibrosis includes chest physical therapy and high-frequency chest wall oscillation. A short-term program of anaerobic exercise sessions for 30–45 minutes (with 20–30 seconds for each anaerobic activity) 2 days per week was shown to improve anaerobic performance and quality of life. However, these improvements were not maintained in the long term. Regular aerobic exercise can reduce the rate of expected decline in pulmonary function. Patients with cystic fibrosis are particularly susceptible to infections with *Burkholderia cepacia*.

EXERCISE IN DISORDERS OF CHEST WALL FUNCTION

Many conditions negatively affect the chest wall, including ankylosing spondylitis, pectus excavatum, obesity, sequelae of thoracoplasty or phrenic nerve crush injury, neuromuscular diseases, and Parkinson disease. Ventilatory muscle training can reduce respiratory muscle fatigue.

PSYCHOSOCIAL SUPPORT

Biopsychosocial considerations include education, vocational counseling, and disability evaluation. Occupational therapists can teach patients how to use energy conservation for activities of daily living. Depression and anxiety are common comorbidities of COPD because of the drastic limitations in functional activities and the presence of dyspnea imposed by the lung disease.

• MECHANICAL VENTILATION (eSlides 28.5, 28.6, 28.7, and 28.8)

Respiratory muscle aids include air stacking, maximal insufflations, assisted coughing, and noninvasive ventilation. Diaphragmatic pacing is indicated for congenital central hypoventilation syndrome, acquired central hypoventilation syndrome, and high spinal cord injuries. Cervical implants are used for older individuals, and thoracic implants are used for younger individuals. Other methods include nerve transfer and implanted intramuscular diaphragm electrodes.

• LUNG VOLUME REDUCTION SURGERY

LVRS for emphysema can reduce hyperinflation and improve the volume expired in the first second of a forced expiration (FEV_1), the forced vital capacity (FVC), the 6-minute walk test results, and the quality of life. Combining LVRS with exercise produces greater benefits. Bronchoscopic LVRS is an alternative option to open thoracic surgery.

Long-Term Results of Lung Volume Reduction Surgery

LVRS is most beneficial for patients who have emphysema predominantly involving the upper lobes and a low postrehabilitation exercise capacity.

• LUNG TRANSPLANTATION

Ongoing smoking is an absolute contraindication to lung transplantation. Relative contraindications include previous cancer, psychiatric diagnosis, obesity, correctable coronary artery disease, and individuals who can only transfer from bed to chair. Being able to walk 600 feet during the 6-minute walk test is a minimal requirement.

Long-Term Results of Lung Transplantation

Survival rates for lung transplants have been reported as 78% at 1 year, 50% at 5 years, and 26% at 10 years. The highest mortality rate occurs during the first year. Death is most commonly caused by sepsis and bronchiolitis obliterans.

• SPECIAL CONSIDERATIONS

Obesity-Related Pulmonary Dysfunction

In the United States, 35.5% of adults are overweight or obese. Complications associated with obesity include obstructive sleep apnea, obesity-hypoventilation syndrome, and asthma. Obesity increases metabolic requirements and decreases exercise tolerance and maximal oxygen uptake(VO_{2max}) relative to the body weight.

Spinal Cord Injury and Pulmonary Dysfunction (eSlide 28.9)

Patients with spinal cord injury have diminished cardiopulmonary function, atrophy of lower limb muscles, and reduced bone mass. These patients can learn neck breathing or GPB.

• REHABILITATION IN SOLID ORGAN TRANSPLANT RECIPIENTS

Physiatric Interventions for Enhancing Outcomes

In addition to maintaining rehabilitation goals, the rehabilitation team must also be cognizant of the clinical features of acute and chronic rejection, as well as other medical complications that may be associated with all types of transplantation surgeries. Hypertension, hyperlipidemia, steroid-induced hyperglycemia, post-transplant diabetes, renal insufficiency, and infections are common medical complications. It is important to know how graft rejection and graft-versus-host disease present and the possible pathogens that cause infections during different periods after transplantation.

Immunosuppression (eSlide 28.10)

eSlide 28.10 summarizes the most frequently used immunosuppressive agents. Their side effects should be kept in mind when determining which variables to monitor in patients receiving these medications.

Renal Transplantation Rehabilitation (eSlide 28.11)

In addition to the aforementioned complications associated with organ transplantation, the physiatrist must be able to recognize signs and symptoms of kidney rejection, such as fever, leukocytosis, anorexia, malaise, hypertension, elevated serum renal markers, kidney enlargement with focal retroperitoneal tenderness, edema, weight gain, and reduced urinary output.

Exercise After Kidney Transplantation

Fatigue is a major factor in up to 59% of kidney transplant recipients. Supervised endurance and strengthening exercise programs after kidney transplant can improve peak aerobic capacity, cardiac output, muscle strength, and quality of life.

• REHABILITATION IN CARDIAC TRANSPLANTATION (eSlides 28.12 and 28.13)

Complications After Cardiac Transplantation

The main complications after heart transplant are allograft failure from rejection, problems related to immunosuppression, and multiple types of arrhythmias due to autonomic denervation. One of the leading causes of death in postcardiac transplant patients is infection, such as mediastinitis, pneumonia, urinary tract infection, or intravenous catheter-induced sepsis.

Physiology of the Transplanted Heart

eSlide 28.14 summarizes the effects of cardiac transplantation on various cardiovascular variables. Exercise prescriptions based on target heart rates are not recommended. More useful determinants of exercise intensity include blood pressure reserve, the Borg Scale of Perceived Exertion, and the Dyspnea Index.

Therapeutic Exercise After Cardiac Transplantation

Aerobic cardiovascular conditioning programs and endurance training improve the ability of the heart transplant recipient. Regular exercise training can be effective in improving exercise capacity. Enrollment in a supervised moderate-intensity exercise training program early after cardiac transplantation was shown to improve Vo_{2max}, maximum power output, and body composition when compared with recipients not enrolled in the program, but the overall exercise capacity was still reduced compared with normal patients of a similar age.

• REHABILITATION IN LUNG TRANSPLANTATION

Lung Transplantation and Patient Outcomes

The most common indications for a single lung transplantation are COPD and idiopathic pulmonary fibrosis. Bilateral lung transplantation is often performed for cystic fibrosis and pulmonary hypertension. The prognosis of lung transplant patients is worse than that of recipients of other solid organ transplants because of severe early complications.

Pretransplant Rehabilitation: Assessment, Education, and Conditioning

A dedicated pulmonary rehabilitation program can have positive effects on exercise capacity and functional outcomes. The goal of therapy is to lengthen the exercise duration and decrease the number of rest periods while minimizing adverse symptoms. Energy conservation exercises, such as effective ventilation, expectoration, strengthening, and low-level aerobic endurance, can help patients adjust to the low functional capacity caused by end-stage pulmonary disease.

Medical Complications

Lung transplant recipients require a standard immunosuppressive regimen and are thus highly susceptible to infections. In addition, impairments in the cough reflex, mucus clearance, gas exchange, and circulatory autoregulation may all occur postoperatively because the transplanted lung is denervated. During the immediate postoperative period, maintaining a clear airway and preventing atelectasis, as well as normalizing ventilatory gas exchange, are primary objectives. Modified cough techniques, such as breath stacking and huff coughing, and keeping the patient's head of bed upright can be applied. Daily spirometry, with monitoring of the FEV_1 and FVC, provides objective measurements that can be used to screen for subclinical decrements in pulmonary function. Graft dysfunction or rejection must be considered when otherwise unexplained signs of pulmonary edema or acute respiratory distress syndrome occur.

Postoperative Exercise Considerations

Progressive activity should be initiated on the first postoperative day. Before discharge from the hospital, the patient should engage in stair climbing, which is one of the major milestones of recovery. Lung transplant recipients have an increase in exercise capacity that does not correspond to the improvement in lung function.

• REHABILITATION IN LIVER TRANSPLANTATION

Opportunistic infections caused by the patient's depressed immune system are the greatest risks presenting 1 month after the transplantation. Acute kidney injury may also be observed in these patients. Additional potential complications include prolonged intubation and hyperbilirubinemia. Neurologic dysfunctions, such as cognitive deficits, weakness, or fatigue, can occur secondary to metabolic abnormalities, chronic sequelae of the liver disease, or side effects of multiple transplant medications. Liver graft failure or thrombosis must be high on the list of differential diagnoses.

• REHABILITATION FOLLOWING LIVER TRANSPLANTATION

Resistance training, an isometric exercise regimen, and aerobic endurance training are potential approaches for rehabilitation after liver transplantation. Pretransplant exercise capacity may predict the posttransplant course and survival. Physical and occupational therapies should be initiated immediately after transplantation as long as the patient is medically stable.

Return to Work After Transplantation

Return to employment and even enrollment in additional vocational training after organ transplantation should be integrated into the long-term plan of any rehabilitation program.

• REHABILITATION MANAGEMENT OF DIABETES MELLITUS

Prevention Guidelines

LIFESTYLE MODIFICATIONS

Current recommendations for the prevention of type 2 diabetes mellitus (T2DM) include lifestyle modifications, such as maintaining a healthy weight, following a proper and healthy diet, and participating in aerobic and resistance exercise programs. Preventative guidelines include participation in 2.5 hours per week of moderate-intensity physical activity, which typically consists of 30 minutes per day for 5 days per week for adults with a high risk of developing T2DM.

Treatment Guidelines

ASSESSMENT OF PHYSICAL ACTIVITY

It is important to take into account an individual's overall and incidental physical activity profile.

Objective methods of quantifying physical activity, such as indirect calorimetry, the doubly labeled water method, direct observation, heart rate monitoring, or use of motion sensors (accelerometers and pedometers), may also be used by the clinician, depending on their availability.

Preexercise Assessment

Electrocardiogram stress testing may be indicated for patients with a diagnosis, or risk factors for, coronary artery disease, cerebrovascular disease, peripheral artery disease, autonomic neuropathy, or advanced nephropathy with renal failure.

Exercise Prescription in Type 2 Diabetes Mellitus

It is important to individualize exercise programs to enhance benefits, promote compliance, and reduce the risk of injury. In addition, it is imperative to assess patients for the presence of any T2DM-associated complications, which may limit their ability to participate in a desired exercise program. The potential for delayed hypoglycemia (nocturnal hypoglycemia), a possibly fatal complication of an exercising individual with T2DM, is of particular concern.

Clinical Pearls

1. Pulmonary rehabilitation should focus on a comprehensive individualized rehabilitation protocol that may include strategies to improve pulmonary hygiene, physical therapy, oxygen therapy, and exercise, which can provide the patient with a better overall performance and quality of life.
2. A customized rehabilitation program, including pretransplant assessment, an understanding of posttransplant physiology, and an individualized exercise prescription, is essential to achieve a desirable recovery after solid organ transplantation.
3. Although it is important to individualize exercise programs to enhance benefits, it is imperative to assess people with diabetes mellitus for the presence of disease-associated complications, especially delayed hypoglycemia.

BIBLIOGRAPHY

The complete bibliography is available on ExpertConsult.com.

Cancer Rehabilitation

Vishwa S. Raj

Cancer rehabilitation addresses physical impairments and progressive disablement experienced by patients with cancer. A majority of impairments are directly related to cancer or its treatment; however, many arise from coexistent disease processes, which are increasingly prevalent among the aging cancer population. Successful rehabilitation requires consideration of cancer-specific concerns (limited prognoses, dynamic lesions, heavy symptom burden, and treatment-related toxicities) in the formulation of humane and realistic treatment plans.

• DISEASE CONSIDERATIONS

Phases of Cancer

A primary rehabilitation goal during initial cancer treatment is limiting the functional impact of the main forms of cancer treatment: surgery, radiation, and chemotherapy. Patients treated for recurrent cancer are rendered extremely vulnerable to persistent functional impairments because cancer treatments are often delivered to pretreated tissues, and the cumulative toxicities can be severe. Anticancer therapies are provided when cancers are not deemed curable following recurrence; they are geared toward reducing symptom burden, cancer spread, and the development of medical comorbidities. Patients generally undergo serial chemotherapy trials, which can contribute to progressive deconditioning and disablement. As patients enter the final palliative phase of cancer treatment, the focus is on maximizing patient comfort, psychological well-being, independence in mobility, and the performance of activities of daily living (ADL). Data related to 5-year survival rates may inform rehabilitation goal setting, determine the emphasis placed on symptom-oriented versus disease-modifying treatments, and allow rehabilitation clinicians to gauge the appropriateness of patients' expectations.

The push toward organ preservation in primary cancer care has led to widespread use of combined modality therapy. The trend toward use of combined modality therapy is relevant to rehabilitation because most patients with cancer receive some combination of chemotherapy, radiation therapy, or surgery, contingent on the type and stage of their cancer. This renders the normal tissues of patients vulnerable to cumulative toxicities associated with each modality (eSlides 29.1, 29.2, and 29.3).

• CONSTITUTIONAL SYMPTOMS

Fatigue

Fatigue is the most common symptom experienced by patients with cancer. The mechanisms responsible for fatigue are usually multifactorial. Often, cancer-related fatigue occurs in the absence of anemia or ongoing cancer therapy (eSlide 29.4).

In cases in which reversible causes of fatigue have been eliminated, a multimodal approach is indicated that includes exercise or activity enhancement, psychosocial interventions, and other treatments.

Pain

Pain control might require the integrated use of anticancer treatments, agents from multiple analgesic classes, interventional techniques, topical agents, manual approaches, and modalities. Several factors can contribute to cancer pain (eSlide 29.4), and multiple nonnarcotic medications (such as nonsteroidal antiinflammatories, adjuvant analgesics, corticosteroids, and bisphosphonates [for bone pain]) and interventional techniques may be considered for relieving it.

Opioid-based pharmacotherapy is the current standard of care for the management of moderate to severe cancer pain. The doses of opioids required by many patients with cancer extend far beyond the conventional levels used by physiatrists. Opioids most commonly used in cancer pain management include morphine, hydromorphone, oxycodone, oxymorphone, fentanyl, and methadone. Recognizing that most patients experience constant baseline pain punctuated by transient or incident pain, the combined use of normal-release and sustained-release or continuous-release opioid formulations is recommended. To rapidly estimate initial dose requirements, patients should be provided liberal access to a normal-release opioid formulation. Once the use of this formulation has stabilized, the mean daily or hourly consumption can be calculated and an oral or transdermal sustained-release preparation can be initiated. Ongoing dose titration should be driven by the patient's use of supplemental normal-release "rescue" doses. Typically, rescue doses are 10%–15% of the total daily dose. Current recommendations urge single agent dosing to "effect or side effect," with an adequate trial of each prescribed agent. An alternative opioid should be considered when an adequate trial of a particular agent has failed to control pain or caused refractory side effects. Opioid dose conversion requires calculation of the equianalgesic dose of the novel agent (eSlide 29.5) and reduction by 50% to account for incomplete cross-tolerance between opioids.

Impairments Caused by Tumor Effects

BONE METASTASES

Bone metastases are highly prevalent because bone is the most common site of metastatic spread. Lesions involving the spine and long bones are of greatest physiatric concern. These structures are crucial for weight bearing and mobility; they are the bones most prone to fracture. Bone metastases are managed with medications, radiopharmaceuticals, orthoses, radiation therapy, or surgical stabilization (eSlide 29.6). The choice of intervention(s) will depend on the lesion's location, degree of associated pain, presence or risk of a fracture, radiation responsiveness, and presence of related neurologic compromise. The overall clinical context (e.g., prognosis, severity of medical comorbidities, and operative risk) must also be taken into consideration. Bisphosphonates are the primary medications used to manage bone metastases. In addition to relieving associated pain, use of these agents reduces the spread and progression of bone metastases.

Painful osteolytic lesions are predominantly responsible for pathologic fractures. The incidence of pathologic fracture among all cancer types is 8%. Sixty percent of all long bone fractures involve the femur, with 80% of these located in the proximal portion. Precise quantification of fracture risk has been a persistent challenge in orthopedic oncology; however, rating systems exist to calculate fracture risk (eSlide 29.7).

Rehabilitation approaches can be grouped into the use of orthoses, assistive devices, therapeutic exercises, and environmental modifications. All of these essentially unweight or immobilize compromised bones. Orthoses can be fabricated to stabilize bones in positions that limit potentially damaging forces, as well as protect and unweight sites of fracture or impending fracture. When redistributing weight and loading patterns, extreme caution must be used in patients with diffuse bone metastases. Assistive devices and instructions in compensatory strategies may similarly unload compromised bones. Canes, crutches, and walkers are frequently used to minimize fracture risk. Patients should be instructed to minimize forces by performing activities close to the body, thereby limiting torque on long bones.

A comprehensive exercise program should include postural and balance training, as well as truncal strengthening. Simple environmental modifications may significantly reduce a patient's fracture risk. Throw rugs and other hazards that increase fall risk should be removed. Railings can be added to stairwells and bathrooms as appropriate. The patient's prognosis should inform the decision to implement such modifications.

BRAIN TUMORS: PRIMARY AND METASTASES

Brain metastases are the most common intracranial tumors. The distribution of metastases reflects cerebral blood flow, with 90% situated in the supratentorial region and 10% in the posterior fossa. Brain metastases are multiple in approximately 50%–75% of cases. Presenting symptoms at the time of diagnosis with brain metastases vary significantly (eSlide 29.8).

Corticosteroids are first-line treatment, with dexamethasone being the drug of choice. Corticosteroids reduce peritumoral edema and reverse local brain compression and associated deficits. Treatment generally involves whole brain radiation therapy with stereotactic radiosurgery or surgical resection via craniotomy. Adjunctive chemotherapy can be used contingent on patient performance status, type of cancer, and previous exposure to antineoplastics.

The rehabilitation needs of patients with brain metastases are best determined by understanding their baseline functional status and prognosis, the location and number of metastases, and the antineoplastic treatment plan. Brain metastasis characteristics associated with significant near-term loss of mobility include the following: (1) cerebellar or brainstem location, (2) imaging that reveals new or expanding metastases, and (3) treatment with whole brain radiation therapy.

EPIDURAL SPINAL CORD COMPRESSION

Malignant spinal cord compression (SCC) occurs in up to 5% of patients. Most symptomatic tumors compress the spinal cord or cauda equina from the epidural space. Epidural lesions generally arise from vertebral metastases and rarely breach the dura.

Pain is the most common initial (94%) and presenting (97% to 99%) symptom of malignant SCC. If malignant SCC is detected when pain is the only symptom, efforts to preserve function through surgical decompression or radiation therapy have high success rates. Weakness is present in 74%–76% of patients, autonomic dysfunction in 52%–57%, and sensory loss in 51%–53%. The thoracic spine is the most common site of epidural SCC, followed by the lumbosacral spine and cervical spine in a ratio of 4:2:1. High-dose steroids and surgical decompression are the treatments of choice for operable patients. Radiation is the treatment of choice for nonoperable patients.

Tumors that cause rapid progression of neurologic deficits are associated with poorer functional outcomes following decompression. In general, patients remain ambulatory if they are able to walk at the time of definitive treatment. Motor and coordination deficits rarely resolve if they are present at diagnosis. The recurrence rate for metastatic epidural SCC after successful treatment of the initial compression is 7%–14%.

NERVE PLEXUSES

The brachial and lumbosacral plexuses are commonly compressed or invaded by tumor. The most common sources of brachial plexopathy are tumors at the lung apex and regional spread of breast cancer. Because cancer generally grows superiorly to invade the lower brachial plexus, the inferior trunk and medial cord are most commonly involved. Several clinical signs are associated with brachial plexopathy (eSlide 29.9).

If primary intrapelvic neoplasms are not responsible, then the lumbosacral plexus is generally invaded from lymphatic and osseous metastases. Sacral plexopathies are more common than lumbar plexopathies. Lumbar and sacral plexopathies can also occur concurrently, with varied clinical presentations (eSlide 29.9).

Magnetic resonance imaging (MRI) with gadolinium is the diagnostic test of choice for evaluating the brachial and lumbosacral plexuses. Electromyography can distinguish plexopathies from radiculopathies by defining the distribution of denervation. The presence of myokymia on needle examination is believed to be pathognomonic for radiation plexopathy.

Acute treatment should include corticosteroids for the preservation of neurologic function. Radiation can effectively relieve pain from malignant plexopathies but is less helpful in restoring lost function. Chemotherapy is commonly initiated or altered when plexus involvement heralds cancer progression. Refractory pain requires aggressive coadministration of opioid and adjuvant analgesics and potentially high cervical cordotomy or rhizotomy. Stellate ganglion blockade may relieve pain that is sympathetically maintained.

PARANEOPLASTIC SYNDROMES

Paraneoplastic syndromes are pertinent to rehabilitation because they produce refractory neurologic deficits and severe disability. The incidence of paraneoplastic neurologic disorders (PNDs) is low, occurring in less than 1% of all patients with cancer; several diagnoses are classic for PNDs (eSlide 29.10). Paraneoplastic syndromes are produced when antibodies are made against tumors that express nervous system proteins. Most PNDs are triggered during the early stages of cancer, when primary tumors and metastases may be undetectable by conventional imaging techniques. The emergence of a PND in a patient with known cancer should trigger investigations for recurrent or progressive disease. PNDs are characterized by symptoms that develop and progress rapidly over days to weeks and then stabilize.

CARDIOPULMONARY METASTASES

Malignant pleural effusions should be evacuated when patients become symptomatic. Reaccumulation of malignant effusions can be managed by intermittent thoracentesis or pleurodesis or by placement of an indwelling pleural catheter. Chemical pleurodesis has an overall complete response rate of 64% when all sclerotic agents are considered.

Supplemental oxygen should be initiated as soon as dyspnea becomes function-limiting. If it is tolerated, gradually progressive aerobic conditioning will optimize peripheral conditioning, reducing the percentage of maximum oxygen uptake required for activities. Similar to both cardiac and pulmonary rehabilitation, aerobic conditioning has limited beneficial impact on heart or lung physiology. Improvements in stamina and perceived exertion are attributable to muscle-training effects.

• REHABILITATION APPROACHES

Clinical Considerations

EXERCISE

Studies in breast and other cancer populations during or after cancer treatment have consistently noted improved symptom burden for fatigue, insomnia, nausea, and emotional distress. Aerobic conditioning alone reduces symptom burden and mitigates the physiologic impact of high-dose chemotherapy delivered in the context of bone marrow transplantation as well. Performance of cardiovascular cycling at 50% of heart rate reserve reduced participants' decline in physical performance (e.g., walking distance and speed), physiologic variables, neutropenia and thrombocytopenia, and psychological distress relative to those of controls. Recent randomized and adequately powered trials have consistently demonstrated marked improvements in fatigue, physical functioning, and mental health. Integrated physical training approaches appear to be superior to psychocognitive approaches in enhancing physical well-being and quality of life.

Activities to enhance range of movement (ROM) are crucial for rehabilitation of postsurgical and postradiation soft tissue contractures. The rationale for active and passive stretching is empirical. There is anecdotal evidence that stretching may prevent, reduce, and reverse radiation-induced contractures. Flexibility activities should be optimally tailored to the radiation port and irradiated muscles.

LYMPHEDEMA MANAGEMENT

Lymphedema is a chronic and currently incurable condition that frequently complicates cancer therapy. Following resection or irradiation of lymph nodes and vessels, lymphatic congestion can develop in any region of the body drained by the affected lymphatics. If congestion becomes sufficiently severe, swelling can result from the accumulation of protein-rich fluid.

Complete decongestive therapy is a two-phase, multimodal system that incorporates manual lymphatic drainage (MLD), short-stretch compressive bandaging, skin care, therapeutic exercise, and elastic compression garments. The initial phase (phase I) has decreasing lymphedema volume as its primary goal. Following maximum volume reduction, patients are gradually transitioned to a long-term maintenance program (phase II). In this phase, compressive garments are used during the day, with application of compressive bandages overnight. Patients perform remedial exercises on a daily basis while bandaged and receive MLD as required (eSlide 29.11). Progressive strength training with supervision and gradual progression reduces lymphedema flares and thus strength training should be integrated into the routine management of breast cancer–related lymphedema.

Skin care is stressed in manual approaches to lymphedema. The goals of skin care include controlling skin colonization with bacteria and fungi, eliminating overgrowth in skin crevices, and hydrating the skin to eliminate microfissuring. Daily cleansing with mineral oil–based soap will remove debris and bacteria while moisturizing the skin.

Rehabilitation of Specific Cancer Populations

BREAST CANCER

Functional impairments unique to patients with breast cancer develop after surgical procedures for tumor removal and breast reconstruction. Multimodal physical therapies (i.e., stretching and exercises) and active exercises are effective in treating postoperative pain and impaired ROM following treatment for breast cancer. Physical therapy following surgery for breast cancer offers a number of compelling benefits, including reduced pain, shoulder limitations, and lymphedema, as well as enhanced psychological well-being.

Head and Neck Cancer

Treatment of head and neck cancer continues to produce some of the most challenging impairments within the scope of cancer rehabilitation. Many of the impairments directly undermine a patient's ability to socialize because of factors such as facial dysmorphism, loss of spontaneous or intelligible speech, and the inability to eat normally. Common rehabilitation problems include spinal accessory nerve palsy, radiation-induced xerostomia, soft tissue contracture of the neck and anterior chest wall soft tissues, dysphagia, dysphonia, and myofascial dysfunction. Impairments evolve over the course of head and neck cancer treatment and recovery. Rehabilitative interventions must be adjusted accordingly (eSlide 29.12).

SPINAL ACCESSORY NERVE PALSY

The recognition that comparable cure rates can be achieved with more conservative surgical resection has spurred the shift from radical to functional neck dissections. Functional neck dissections preserve all structures that can be safely left intact, producing dramatically lower rates of postoperative shoulder morbidity.

Important elements of spinal accessory nerve rehabilitation should address prevention of frozen shoulder through active ROM and active-assisted ROM, strengthening of alternate scapular elevators and retractors, instruction in compensatory techniques for activities requiring sustained shoulder abduction and forward flexion, and postural modifications.

CERVICAL CONTRACTURE

Progressive fibrosis of the anterior and lateral cervical soft tissue may be highly problematic for patients with head and neck cancer (eSlide 29.13). Because of the high radiation doses delivered to some patients with head and neck cancer, proactive ROM activities in all planes of neck motion should be initiated as soon as safely possible. Cervical ROM activities can be continued throughout radiation therapy in the absence of significant skin breakdown. Ideally, ROM activities should begin immediately after surgery, before radiation is begun. The delicate balance between flexibility and postsurgical wound healing must be respected.

Manual fibrous release techniques are indicated when ROM is restricted by robust soft tissue fibrosis or tethering of the skin to subdermal tissues (eSlide 29.14). Patients can be taught self-massage to augment the efficacy of ROM activities. Compression of severely fibrotic areas breaks down established scar tissue and inhibits its reformation. Botulinum toxin injection may be tried in refractory cases.

• PRECAUTIONS IN CANCER REHABILITATION

Modalities

Warnings against treating cancer patients with deep heat and massage are ubiquitous in the rehabilitation literature. Precautions regarding heating modalities are largely based on the concern that heat will dilate local blood vessels and increase the metabolic activity in tumor cells, thereby hastening local or systemic spread. Similarly, massage is presumed to potentiate metastasis by encouraging blood and lymph flow or by dislodging tumor cells. This line of reasoning is simplistic. When considering the complex changes associated with other therapeutic interventions, manual dislodgement from a tumor mass or transient exposure to increased blood flow probably has no impact on tumor cells.

Cytopenias

Leukopenia and thrombocytopenia commonly occur following the administration of chemotherapy. The duration and severity of cytopenias have been considerably reduced through the introduction of colony-stimulating factors that accelerate bone marrow recovery.

There are inconsistent guidelines limiting physical activity in the face of chemotherapy-induced cytopenias. Leukopenia is of less concern than thrombocytopenia, given the associated risk of intracranial hemorrhage or bleeding after a fall. However, patients undergoing allogeneic and autogeneic bone marrow transplantation typically spend 7–21 days with platelet counts of 5000–12,000 platelets/µL. During this period, most patients perform ADL independently and ambulate, transfer, and lift greater than 10 pounds repeatedly without developing a hemorrhage. When spontaneous bleeding does occur, it is typically not associated with physical activity. Inappropriate restriction of physical therapy and exercise in this population can contribute to rapid deconditioning, bone demineralization, and contractures.

• CONCLUSION

Cancer rehabilitation is a varied and challenging field of increasing public health importance. A growing evidence base suggests that conventional rehabilitative interventions succeed in preserving and restoring the functional status of patients with cancer. A marked lack of hypothesis-driven research continues to limit the field, as does a lack of experienced and interested clinicians. It is hoped that these deficits will be remedied, given the projections for steadily increasing cancer survivorship.

Clinical Pearls

- Rehabilitation can be provided throughout the cancer care continuum, from the time of diagnosis to the end of life.
- Rehabilitation intervention can help improve constitutional symptoms and functional impairments caused by cancer.
- Therapeutic exercises have been noted to improve symptom burden, physical performance, and mental health.
- Lymphedema management uses complete decongestive therapy to decrease lymphedema volume and provide long-term maintenance for volume control.
- Precaution must be incorporated into rehabilitation prescription; however, inappropriate restriction of therapy may have a detrimental effect on patient outcome.

BIBLIOGRAPHY
The complete bibliography is available on ExpertConsult.com.

30 The Geriatric Patient

Mooyeon Oh-Park

Caring for geriatric patients requires an understanding of the biology of aging, common conditions in older adults, and how these processes affect function. Physiatrists fit well within the geriatric care paradigm because of their experience in working with multidisciplinary teams, treating patients with complex conditions, and focusing on patients' goals and function.

• CHANGES IN THE BODY WITH AGING

Musculoskeletal and Neurologic (eSlide 30.1)

Sarcopenia refers to the loss of muscle mass and strength that occurs with aging. Total body weight may not decrease because of a concurrent increase in fat mass. There is a loss of force per unit cross-sectional area, a decline in muscle power due to lack of rapid force development, and a disproportionate loss of type 2 (fast-twitch) muscle fibers. Men show greater decline in elbow flexors compared to women. Older adults also have a decline in frontal gray matter volume, episodic memory, learning new information, processing speed, task shifting, and executive function.

Cardiopulmonary, Genitourinary, and Endocrinal (eSlide 30.2)

Maximal heart rate decreases at 6–10 beats/min per decade, and maximal oxygen consumption (Vo_{2max}) decreases at 5%–15% per decade after the age of 25 years. Vital capacity is decreased by 50% at the age of 70. The ability to concentrate urine decreases with age, leading to water loss. Urinary incontinence and erectile dysfunction are common; however, they are not normal consequences of aging, and their presence warrants further investigation. Anabolic hormone levels and tissue responsiveness to hormones decrease. The decreased responsiveness to hormones is one reason why hormone replacement therapy may not be a straightforward approach to treating the effects of aging.

Medication Metabolism (eSlide 30.3)

Medication-related adverse effects are more frequent and severe in older individuals. An increase in adipose tissue leads to a larger volume of distribution of fat-soluble drugs and prolongs their biologic half-life. Total body water decreases by 15% between 20 and 80 years of age, which decreases the volume of distribution of water-soluble drugs and leads to higher serum concentrations of these drugs. Hepatic and renal clearance of drugs can be decreased up to 30% and 50%, respectively.

Gait (eSlide 30.4)

Locomotion in older adults is affected by multiple factors, which can be characterized by decreased speed, increased duration of double limb support, and gait variability (which is predictive of falls). Gait speed predicts survival and is a biomarker of health status; a speed of 1.0 m/sec is a guidepost representing relatively good function.

• EVALUATION OF THE GERIATRIC PATIENT (eSlide 30.5)

History Taking, Medication Review, Physical Examination

During an evaluation, questions should be directed toward the patient and not the caregivers. Spending sufficient time with the patient and showing patience will facilitate development of the patient–physician relationship and improve care. Investigation of the origin of the reported symptoms is extremely important. For example, sleep disturbance has several possible causes, such as nocturia, pain, or mood disorders, and if nocturia is responsible for the sleep disturbance, this may be due to urinary frequency or nighttime mobilization of peripheral edema fluid. Patients should be asked about falls, including frequencies, circumstances, and related injuries; activities of daily living; support systems; advance directives; and their goals and wishes regarding the treatment plan. All medications, including nonprescription drugs, should be reviewed and reconciled, with thorough evaluation for possible side effects. High-risk medications in older adults include antidepressants, benzodiazepines, and drugs with anticholinergic effects. In addition, sleeping pills, metoclopramide, tricyclic antidepressants, and antiepileptic drugs may cause cognitive impairment. Geriatric evaluation should also include cognitive screening (e.g., Mini-Mental State Examination) and a functional examination (e.g., tandem stance, Timed Up and Go test for unsteadiness, and rising from a chair five times).

• CONDITIONS AND DISEASES IN GERIATRIC PATIENTS

Frailty and Immobilization (eSlide 30.6)

Frailty is defined as age-related and disease-related loss of adaptation, such that events producing minor stress result in disproportionate biomedical and social consequences. Frail older individuals have three or more of the following: (1) unintentional weight loss of at least 10 pounds over the past year, (2) self-reported exhaustion, (3) weakness (grip strength), (4) slow walking speed, and (5) low physical activity. Bed rest or other immobilization leads to loss of strength, bone, and exercise capacity, as well as increased muscle insulin resistance, orthostatic hypotension, and balance impairment.

Falls

Falls are responsible for 90% of fractures of the upper limb, hip, and pelvis in older adults. Risk factors for falls in the geriatric population (eSlide 30.7) include old age, physical impairments (e.g., gait or balance dysfunction, weakness, dizziness, or visual impairment), cognitive impairment, dementia, depression, previous falls, medications (e.g., psychoactive medications, total number of medications), comorbid conditions (e.g., diabetes, Parkinson disease), chronic pain, arthritis, and poor functional status. Recommendations to prevent falls and fall-related injuries (eSlide 30.8) include fall risk assessment by qualified health care professionals or teams; balance, strength, and gait training exercises (e.g., tai chi); home safety evaluations and modifications; medication review and reduction programs with involvement of the family physician and patient; addressing foot or ankle pain and dysfunction; treating vitamin D deficiency (at least 800 international units per day); cataract surgery; and dual chamber cardiac pacing, if indicated.

Osteopenia, Osteoporosis, and Hip Fractures (eSlide 30.9)

Risk factors for osteoporosis include increasing age, family history, glucocorticoid therapy, and smoking. Hip fractures occur from a fall and osteoporosis. After a hip fracture, only 50% of individuals regain their independence in performing activities of daily living.

Disorders of Cognitive Decline and/or Gait Dysfunction (eSlides 30.10, 30.11, 30.12, and 30.13)

Potentially reversible causes of dementia include subdural hematoma (SDH), normal pressure hydrocephalus (NPH), depression, hormonal imbalance, drug and alcohol abuse, and vitamin deficiency. Irreversible causes of cognitive decline are Alzheimer disease (the most common cause in people older than 65 years), Parkinson disease, Huntington disease, repeated neurovascular insults, and severe or repetitive traumatic brain injuries. Mild cognitive impairment is considered a precursor to Alzheimer disease, with a conversion rate of 12% per year. Delirium is an acute neurocognitive disorder with poor outcomes. Diagnostic criteria for delirium include acute disturbance in attention and cognition, with fluctuation of symptoms. A medical workup, including review of medications, is needed for patients with delirium (including those with baseline dementia). Even minor falls can result in an SDH or spinal cord injury. SDHs may be attributed to age-related brain atrophy, fragile bridging veins within the subdural space, and use of anticoagulant medications. The hallmarks of NPH are dementia, urinary incontinence, and ataxic or "magnetic" gait. In some cases, shunting can reverse the patient's condition. Parkinson disease, with its characteristic gait (shuffling steps, festination, and limited arm swing), affects 2% of people older than 60 years, and 20% of those affected will develop dementia.

Polypharmacy and Medication Management (eSlides 30.3 and 30.14)

Medication side effects (e.g., dizziness, insomnia, confusion, sedation, nausea, change in bowel habits, and balance problems) can be misinterpreted as symptoms of a new illness. Prescribing new medications to treat symptoms of an unrecognized adverse drug reaction to an existing therapy is known as the "prescribing cascade" and may lead to falls and delirium. The physiatrist should partner with the patient and his or her caregivers, geriatrician, and pharmacist to avoid inappropriate prescription.

• NUTRITION AND PHYSICAL ACTIVITY RECOMMENDATION FOR OLDER ADULTS

Possibly modifiable factors for weight loss are depression, swallowing problems, and feeding dependence. Daily protein intake goals for adults older than 65 years are 1.0–1.2 g/kg body weight per day; however, appropriate nutrition should be individualized as per their specific medical conditions.

Activity Recommendations for Older Adults (eSlide 30.15)

It is recommended that older adults participate in moderate-intensity aerobic activity for 150 minutes per week. The intensity should be sufficient to noticeably increase the heart rate and breathing. Older adults should also undergo resistance training (e.g., calisthenics, weight training) for two or three nonconsecutive days per week, with at least one set of 10–15 repetitions of an exercise that trains the major muscle groups. Flexibility is also important, and recommendations include at least 10 minutes of stretching major muscle groups for at least two days per week. The stretching should involve static stretches for 10–30 seconds and three to four repetitions of each stretch. Balance exercises three times per week are also advised.

Modifying the Environment for Older Individuals

Environmental modifications to improve safety include no-slip rugs, appropriate lighting, decreased bed height to prevent fall injuries, and space for accessibility with a walker. Modifying behavior in the environment in public areas includes allowing adequate time for crossing the street at traffic signals and identifying affordable alternative transportation, when needed.

Clinical Pearls

1. Pathologic changes (e.g., loss of arm swing during gait) should be differentiated from physiologic changes of aging.
2. Fall risk factors include previous falls, cognitive impairment, gait and balance abnormalities, certain medications (e.g., psychoactive medications), pain syndrome, and an unsafe environment.
3. Fall prevention includes patient and caregiver education, medication reconciliation, checking environmental safety, exercise programs, nutritional support, and addressing foot dysfunction.
4. The role of the physiatrist includes educating patients and their caregivers regarding the recommended activities for older patients and partnering with local resources to assist individuals in sustaining those activities in the community.
5. Geriatric rehabilitation addresses problems that affect not only the individual patient but also the society at large. Further research and efforts should be directed toward implementing the current knowledge (e.g., regarding recommended exercises) into clinical practice and community-based activities.

BIBLIOGRAPHY
The complete bibliography is available on ExpertConsult.com.

31 | Rheumatologic Rehabilitation

Lin-Fen Hsieh

• INTRODUCTION TO RHEUMATIC DISEASES

Rheumatic diseases manifest as painful conditions typically characterized by inflammation, swelling, and pain in joints or soft tissues. As a result of the associated pain, swelling, decline in functional status, and varying degrees of temporary or permanent disability, patients with rheumatic diseases may form an important aspect of the physiatric practice (eSlide 31.1). Physiatrists can be the primary physicians for diagnosing and coordinating treatment for most of these diseases.

• STRUCTURE AND COMPONENTS OF THE SYNOVIAL JOINTS

The synovial joint is characterized by its mobility, as these joints are able to move freely in multiple planes. A synovial joint consists of two bony surfaces that are encompassed by a fibrous capsule with a synovial lining. The joint contains synovial fluid, which allows the bony surfaces to articulate with each other. The extracellular matrix consists of water and proteoglycans (glycosaminoglycan and hyaluronic acid). The viscoelastic properties of synovial fluid and its inherent function as a lubricant and shock absorber are largely attributed to hyaluronic acid. The fibrous capsule has a rich network of substance P (a neurotransmitter for pain) nociceptive nerve fibers that can potentially generate the sensation of pain. Limb joints are typically synovial joints; these include hip, knee, and shoulder joints.

As inflammation ensues, fluid and polymorphonuclear leukocytes infiltrate the joint space of synovial joints. Vasodilation and venous congestion contribute to pain-provoking capsular distention and neuronal sensitization of substance P nerve fibers. If left untreated, the inflammatory cascade can destroy the integrity of the joint and permanently impair its function. This can lead to chronic pain and disability.

Bursae, tendon sheaths, and entheses are soft tissues commonly located surrounding synovial joints. Bursae are flattened fibrous sacs lined with a synovial membrane, containing a thin film of synovial fluid. Tendon sheaths are elongated bursae that wrap around a tendon that is subject to friction. Entheses are the insertion sites of tendons or ligaments into bones. They are functionally integrated with the synovial joint and can be involved in the rheumatic disease processes.

• OSTEOARTHRITIS

Osteoarthritis (OA) is one of the most common rheumatic diseases, affecting 27 million people in the United States. OA involves failure of the structure and function of synovial joints and is characterized by degradation of articular cartilage, subchondral bone remodeling, meniscal degeneration, synovial inflammatory response, and overgrowth of bone. The risk of developing OA is higher in people older than 45 years; women; individuals with obesity, vitamin D deficiency, estrogen deficiency, bone deformities, or joint injuries; and people engaged in occupations that involve repetitive stress on particular joints. There are various definitions of OA, both symptomatic and radiographic. Symptomatic OA usually includes pain and joint stiffness in the affected joint, along with the presence of radiographic findings. Clinical criteria for diagnosing knee and hip OA include pain, age older than 50 years, stiffness for less than 30 minutes, crepitus, and the radiographic finding of osteophytes. The Kellgren-Lawrence scale is the most common radiologic grading system for OA (eSlide 31.2).

Treatments for OA range from conservative, patient-driven treatments to surgical interventions. The treatment goals are directed toward reducing pain and improving mobility. The initial plan should include education regarding activity modifications, dietary changes, weight loss, and exercise. For acute exacerbations of OA pain, the frontline treatment is pharmaceutical agents. In mild OA, acetaminophen is used as a first-line agent because of its benign safety profile. Nonsteroidal antiinflammatory drugs (NSAIDs) are commonly used as second-line agents in patients with moderate to severe pain; however, long-term use of NSAIDs is associated with adverse effects, particularly involving the gastrointestinal, renal, and cardiovascular (for cyclooxygenase-2 inhibitors) systems. Topical NSAIDs and analgesics have fewer side effects and can be useful as an adjuvant in combination with other therapies. Tramadol and opioids can also be used in patients with severe pain. There are also various injectable medications and techniques, including corticosteroids, hyaluronic acid, proliferant therapy (e.g., dextrose, platelet-rich plasma), and botulinum toxin type A. Joint replacement surgery is a last-resort treatment.

• RHEUMATOID ARTHRITIS

Rheumatoid arthritis (RA) is a chronic, systemic inflammatory disease of unknown etiology that primarily involves the joints. The prevalence of RA varies from 0.3%–1.5% of the population, with a female to male ratio of around 3 to 1. In addition to its primary effect on the joints, RA also often involves soft tissues, such as tendon sheaths and bursae. It may also present with extraarticular manifestations. Inflammation and destruction of the joint and soft tissue may lead to joint deformity and loss of physical function. To facilitate earlier diagnosis of RA and thus early effective treatment, The Joint Working Group of the American College of Rheumatology and the European League Against Rheumatism replaced the American Rheumatism Association revised criteria (eSlide 31.3) with a new classification criteria (eSlide 31.4).Typically, disease onset in RA is insidious, with pain, stiffness, and swelling of the joints being the predominant symptoms. Morning stiffness, or stiffness after prolonged inactivity, often lasts more than an hour in the active inflammatory stage. Up to one-third of patients with RA experience acute onset of polyarthritis associated with systemic symptoms. The most common joints involved in the early stage of the disease are the metacarpophalangeal (MCP) and proximal interphalangeal joints of the fingers, the interphalangeal joints of the thumb and wrists, and the metatarsophalangeal joints of the toes. Other joints, such as the shoulders, elbows, hips, knees, ankles, and atlantoaxial joints of the cervical spine, are also frequently affected. The distal interphalangeal joints are rarely involved in RA. In addition to involvement of the joints, tenosynovitis is also common in RA patients and may cause trigger finger, de Quervain tenosynovitis, carpal tunnel syndrome, tendon rupture, and even compression of the cervical spinal cord.

In the late stage of RA, joint deformities commonly occur. These may include buttonhole deformity, swan neck deformity, ulnar deviation of the MCP joints (eSlide 31.5), palmar subluxation of the wrists, arthritis mutilans, hammer-toe deformity, clawed-toe deformity, flat-feet, hallux valgus (eSlide 31.5), and metatarsal joint subluxation. Management of RA requires a combination of nonpharmacologic measures, medical interventions, and surgery (eSlide 31.6).

• ANKYLOSING SPONDYLITIS

Seronegative spondyloarthropathies (SSAs) are a group of chronic inflammatory arthritides involving the axial structures, which are manifested by chronic back pain and progressive stiffness of the spine. They can also involve the shoulders, hips, and other peripheral joints. SSAs include ankylosing spondylitis (AS), reactive arthritis, arthropathy of inflammatory bowel disease, psoriatic arthritis, undifferentiated spondyloarthropathy, and juvenile-onset AS. In addition to inflammation of the spine and sacroiliac joint, SSA is characterized by the absence of a rheumatoid factor, a tendency for familial aggregation, an association with the human leukocyte antigen (HLA)-B27, inflammation around the entheses, uveitis, urethritis, and psoriatic skin lesion.

The prevalence of AS has been estimated to be 0.1%–1.4% of the population (0.2%–0.5% in the United States), and the male to female ratio is about 2 to 3. The peak age of onset is between 20 and 30 years. The most common presentation is chronic inflammatory back pain. The pain usually starts at the buttock or lower back level and may radiate to the posterior thigh. Morning stiffness usually lasts more than 30 minutes. Pain can be relieved with exercise or activity and worsened with rest (eSlide 31.7). It is usually improved with the use of NSAIDs. Pain and stiffness may ascend from the lower back to the mid-back, upper back, and neck.

Peripheral arthritis occurs in approximately 35%–50% of patients with AS over the course of the disease. The most commonly affected joints, in order of descending frequency, are the shoulders, hips, and knees. Hip involvement is present in 25%–35% of patients with AS and is associated with a high degree of physical disability and poor prognosis. Enthesitis (inflammation of the entheses) occurs in approximately 40%–70% of patients with AS. The most common location of enthesitis is the calcaneal attachment of the Achilles tendon. Anterior uveitis (or iritis) is the most common extraarticular comorbidity in patients with AS (present in 25%–40% of individuals). The prevalence rates of osteoporosis and vertebral fractures in patients with AS are 25% and 10%, respectively.

Laboratory findings are generally nonspecific in individuals with AS. An elevated erythrocyte sedimentation rate or C-reactive protein is present in about 50%–70% of patients with AS during active disease. HLA-B27 is present in 90%–95% of patients of European ancestry who have AS.

In general, radiographic changes of AS need a few years to develop (eSlide 31.8). Magnetic resonance imaging has been shown to be more sensitive than conventional radiography, bone scintigraphy, or computed tomography in the detection of sacroiliitis. Diagnosis of classic AS is based on the 1984 modified New York criteria (eSlide 31.9).

The goals of management of AS patients are as follows: (1) symptom relief, (2) maintenance of function, (3) prevention of spinal disease complications, and

(4) minimization of extraspinal and extraarticular comorbidities. Management includes a rehabilitation program, medications (e.g., NSAIDs), and surgery. For patients with axial disease who are not responsive to NSAIDs, an anti-tumor necrosis factor (TNF) agent is recommended. Anti-TNF agents are very effective for symptom relief, can stop bony destruction, and may have disease-modifying effects. Local corticosteroid injections may be indicated for persistent peripheral arthritis, sacroiliitis pain, or enthesitis at sites other than the Achilles tendon. Systemic corticosteroids are not recommended. In patients with AS whose joints are destroyed, total joint replacement may be necessary. Wedge osteotomy of the spine is reserved for AS patients with severe spinal deformities.

• REHABILITATIVE MANAGEMENT OF RHEUMATIC DISEASES

The goal setting for rehabilitation management should accommodate special considerations of the rheumatic disorder being managed (eSlide 31.10). Rehabilitative interventions include patient education, improvement or maintenance of functional mobility, assessment of the need for orthoses and durable medical equipment, appropriate physical modalities, and exercise. The key components of rehabilitation evaluation of patients with rheumatic diseases may follow the International Classification of Functioning, Disability and Health model; they are described later (eSlide 31.11).

Patient Education

All interventions require teaching the patient and family about the disease, use of adaptive skills, environmental modifications, exercises, weight loss (if obese), stress management or relaxation strategies, and avenues of social support.

Improve or Maintain Functional Mobility

Joint protection is a self-management technique widely taught to people with rheumatic diseases, especially RA (eSlide 31.12). Energy conservation principles are important and should be incorporated in the treatment intervention. To control the effects of fatigue on everyday activities, the therapist teaches the patient to analyze daily activities to determine what causes increasing pain and fatigue. Short rest periods during a prolonged activity are often advised. Many devices and equipment are designed to limit stress on joints and to help patients further achieve functional independence. For patients with limited range of movement (ROM) or pain in the hands, broad key-holders, buttoning and zipping aids, writing aids, and easy-to-hold utensils are suggested (eSlide 31.13). An arthritic crutch with a hand grip and forearm support is highly recommended for arthritic patients to reduce the stress on hand or wrist joints during ambulation. Appropriate footwear or insoles may be considered to enhance comfort during ambulation.

Exercise

The purposes of an exercise program for patients with arthritis include the following: (1) increase and maintain ROM, (2) improve muscle strength and endurance, (3) increase aerobic capacity, (4) increase bone density, (5) improve functional ability (Video 31.1), and (6) improve psychological function. Before the patient begins exercise therapy, it is important to evaluate the condition of the joint and periarticular structures, cardiopulmonary function, and other systemic features of the disease. Common exercise interventions for patients with arthritis include mobilization, strengthening, aerobic exercises (or conditioning), and recreation.

In actively inflamed joints, gentle active or active-assisted ROM through the possible range should be performed. Passive stretching should be applied with extreme caution. As inflammation subsides, the joint should be moved through the full range, possibly with assistance (active-assisted exercise). Aquatic therapy is also useful for mobilizing joints.

For strengthening, isometric contraction has the advantage of producing minimal joint stress during muscle contraction; it is therefore suited for arthritis sufferers with mechanically deranged joints. It may also be useful for an acutely inflamed joint or immediately after surgery. Isotonic contraction is suitable for training isotonic tasks and for patients without acutely inflamed or biomechanically deranged joints; it should be avoided in patients with active arthritis. Isokinetic contraction usually requires a maximal contraction force, which in most cases is not recommended for patients with arthritis.

Aerobic exercises increase aerobic capacity and functional ability in patients with RA, OA, AS, and fibromyalgia. For patients with arthritis, the type of exercise should produce low joint stress. Walking, cycling, swimming, water aerobics, or low-impact aerobic dance are good options. Recreational exercise is usually a group exercise. It may provide social contact and have an antidepressant effect.

Orthoses

Orthotic positioning, especially through the use of hand splints, is usually considered, and it may have different benefits at different stages of a patient's disease. For example, it is very common to prescribe a resting hand splint during the acute stage (eSlide 31.13) and a three-point splint for a swan-neck deformity. Nevertheless, no data have confirmed the effectiveness of splints in decreasing the severity of hand deformities or preserving hand function.

• PHYSICAL MODALITIES

Physical modalities, such as thermotherapy (heat or cold therapy), electric therapy, and low-power laser therapy, are commonly used in rehabilitation practice to relieve pain and increase the flexibility of joints and soft tissues in patients with rheumatic disorders. Most studies have concluded that these modalities may have temporary effects but do not alter the disease process.

• REHABILITATION INTERVENTION FOR RHEUMATOID ARTHRITIS

Rehabilitation intervention for rheumatoid arthritis is based on the patient's disease stage and individual condition (eSlide 31.14).

• REHABILITATION INTERVENTION FOR ANKYLOSING SPONDYLITIS

The main aims of management for patients with AS are pain relief, improvement of posture and mobility, and maintenance or improvement of respiratory function (eSlide 31.14).

• CONCLUSION

With the growing number of patients with rheumatic diseases, research regarding the prevention and treatment of these conditions is evolving. Less invasive surgical options and expansion of conservative treatments to combine allopathic and naturopathic medicine are current trends in disease management. Physiatrists will continue to be an integral part of the management of these diseases. The chronicity and disabling nature of rheumatic diseases will continue to challenge physiatrists to be innovative and creative. Further research may focus on the quality of rehabilitation interventions and the long-term effects of rehabilitation on outcomes.

Clinical Pearls

Control pain and inflammation with medications and/or physical modalities before starting therapeutic exercise. Rehabilitation management of the rheumatic diseases should be multidisciplinary and individualized.

BIBLIOGRAPHY
The complete bibliography is available on ExpertConsult.com.

IV SECTION

ISSUES IN SPECIFIC DIAGNOSES

32 Common Neck Problems

Carl Chen

Successful treatment of painful cervical spine disorders depends on accurate assessment of the underlying tissue injury. Physiatrists can use a range of diagnostic and therapeutic tools to identify and manage these complex disorders (eSlide 32.1).

A working knowledge of the anatomic interrelationships within the cervical spine is important to comprehend the pathomechanisms of cervical spine disorders (eSlide 32.2). The zygapophyseal joints (z joints or facet joints) allow motion within the cervical spine, connect each vertebral segment, and are innervated by medial branches from the cervical dorsal rami (eSlide 32.3).

The lower cervical vertebrae (C3-C7) have unique synovial joint-like articulations known as uncovertebral joints or joints of Luschka, which are located between the uncinate processes. These joints commonly develop osteoarthritic changes, which can narrow the diameter of the intervertebral foramina (eSlide 32.4). The intervertebral disks are located between the vertebral bodies of C2 through C7. Each is composed of an outer annulus fibrosus innervated posterolaterally by the sinuvertebral nerve (comprising branches from the vertebral nerve and ventral ramus) and anteriorly by the vertebral nerve. The inner portions of the disks comprise the gelatinous nucleus pulposus, providing transmission of axial loads to dissipate forces throughout various ranges of movement. Each intervertebral disk is thicker anteriorly than posteriorly, which contributes to the natural cervical lordotic curvature. The normal cervical spine anatomy can undergo degenerative or traumatic changes, leading to various cervical spine disorders.

For a structure to serve as a source of pain, it must be innervated, capable of producing pain similar to that seen clinically, and susceptible to a disease or injury known to be painful. Nonneural structures of the neck, such as intervertebral disks, zygapophyseal joints, posterior longitudinal ligaments, and muscles, can serve as a nidus for pain and produce somatic referral of pain into the upper limb. Pain emanating from the cervical zygapophyseal joints tends to follow relatively constant and recognizable referral patterns. Each joint can produce unilateral or bilateral symptoms (eSlide 32.5).

Cervical radicular pain typically presents with upper limb pain that is more severe than axial pain. Upper limb pain caused by cervical radiculopathy can refer symptoms into the arm, forearm, or hand. However, periscapular or trapezial pain, greater than neck pain, can be caused by involvement of upper cervical nerve roots, such as C4 or C5 (eSlide 32.6). Nerve vulnerability within the intervertebral foramina arises because of changes in one or more of three separate structures: zygapophyseal joints, uncovertebral joints, and intervertebral disks. The most common cause of cervical radiculopathy is a herniated cervical intervertebral disk, followed by cervical spondylosis with or without cervical myelopathy (eSlide 32.6).

Cervical intervertebral disk injury can be divided into two broad categories: herniation and internal disruption. *Disk herniation* is further classified as protrusion, extrusion, or sequestration. *Internal disk disruption* is a phrase used to describe derangement of the internal architecture of the nucleus pulposus, annular fibers, or both, which is accompanied by little or no external deformation. The process of disk degeneration occurs over a spectrum of disk abnormalities. Initially, circumferential outer annular tears secondary to repetitive microtrauma are associated with interruption in the blood and nutritional supply to the disk. Cervical zygapophyseal joint injury can occur because of osteoarthritis or trauma resulting from both macrotraumatic and microtraumatic events. Acceleration-deceleration zygapophyseal joint injuries can result in osseous injury to the articular pillar, articular surface, or subchondral bone; intraarticular hemarthrosis; contusion of the intraarticular meniscus; or tears of the zygapophyseal joint capsule.

• COMMON CLINICAL DISORDERS

Cervical Strain and Sprain

EPIDEMIOLOGY

Cervical strain is a musculotendinous injury produced by an overload injury resulting from excessive forces imposed on the cervical spine. In contrast, a cervical sprain is an overstretching or tearing injury of spinal ligaments. Muscular strains are seen most frequently because many cervical muscles do not terminate in tendons but rather attach directly to bone via myofascial tissue that blends seamlessly with the periosteum. Cervical sprain and strain injuries account for approximately 85% of neck pain resulting from acute, repetitive, or chronic neck injuries. These injuries are the most common type of injury to motor vehicle occupants in the United States and one of the most common causes of pain after noncatastrophic sports injuries. Approximately one-third of motor vehicle accident victims develop neck pain within 24 hours of the injury (eSlide 32.1).

PATHOPHYSIOLOGY

Acceleration-deceleration injuries result in excursions of the cervical spine that result in injury. Tears of the anterior longitudinal ligament have been observed during surgical exploration and identified postmortem. Anatomic studies have demonstrated that the anterior longitudinal ligament merges imperceptibly with intervertebral disks and can be injured during an injury to the cervical disk (see eSlide 32.12) .

DIAGNOSIS

An acute event, such as a motor vehicle accident, sports injury, fall, or industrial accident, can create forces significant enough to injure cervical soft tissues. Details that should be sought are the exact onset of pain relative to a traumatic event, the location of the symptoms, any referral pattern, or the presence of other associated symptoms. Cervical strain and sprain injuries can be associated with headaches. Patients can also report neck fatigue or stiffness that lessens with gradual activity. Aggravating factors include passive or active motion.

Decreased cervical range of movement can be detected on gross examination. Palpation of the involved region is usually uncomfortable or moderately painful. The most commonly involved areas are the upper trapezius and sternocleidomastoid muscles. Neurologic signs are typically absent, and neuroforaminal closure techniques should not elicit referral pain into the distal upper limb. Motor examination may reveal give-way weakness because of pain, but this pattern can be differentiated from true neuromuscular weakness. Further diagnostic testing, such as imaging or electrodiagnostic evaluation, is not indicated unless neurologic or motor abnormalities are detected or significant pain into the limbs is reported. Plain radiography is ordered first to look for bony malalignment or fractures. It is reasonable to examine cervical flexion and extension x-rays to evaluate the possibility of instability before prescribing functional restoration.

TREATMENT

Initial care includes controlling pain and inflammation to curb the injury response, mitigate deconditioning, and facilitate active participation in a functional restoration program. Nonsteroidal antiinflammatory drugs (NSAIDs) and acetaminophen (paracetamol) aid in controlling pain and nurturing restorative sleep patterns. Some clinicians use muscle relaxants for 5–7 days to improve sleep. If patients complain of substantial "spasm" not ameliorated by analgesics and proper positioning, tizanidine or tricyclic antidepressants may be helpful. Physical modalities, such as massage, superficial and deep heat, electrical stimulation, and a soft cervical collar, can be used in the treatment program. Light massage causes sedation, reduction of adhesions, muscular relaxation, and vascular changes. Superficial heat and deep heat with ultrasound produce analgesia and muscle relaxation, help resolve inflammation, and increase connective tissue elasticity. Transcutaneous electrical nerve stimulation (TENS) can also be effective in modulating musculoskeletal pain. A soft cervical collar can be prescribed to ease painful sleep disturbances and reduce further neck strain. The collar can be worn while awake, but its use should be restricted to the first 72 hours after the injury to minimize interference with healing and prevent the development of soft tissue tightening. A gradual return to activities should be initiated by 2–4 weeks after the injury and should include a functional restoration program to address postural reeducation and functional biomechanical deficits.

Cervical Radiculopathy and Radicular Pain

EPIDEMIOLOGY

Cervical radiculopathy is a pathologic process involving neurophysiologic dysfunction of a nerve root. Signs and symptoms of cervical radiculopathy include myotomal weakness, paresthesia, sensory disturbance, and depressed muscle stretch reflex. Cervical radicular pain represents a hyperexcitable state of the affected nerve root. Cervical radiculopathy, by contrast, involves reflex and strength deficits reflecting a hypofunctional nerve root resulting from pathologic changes in nerve root function. Cervical radiculopathy occurs less commonly than cervical axial pain and has an annual incidence of 83 per 100,000 people. The peak age is 50–54 years. Cervical radicular pain differs from usual cervical pain in that the chief complaint of radicular pain is typically upper limb pain (eSlides 32.6 and 32.7).

PATHOPHYSIOLOGY

Cervical nerve root injury is most commonly caused by a cervical intervertebral disk herniation (CIDH) or spondylitic change. Nerve roots are anatomically less resilient than peripheral nerves to both biomechanical and biochemical insults, and they respond to each with the same pathologic sequence of events. Cervical spondylosis (or degenerative osteoarthritic change) is manifested by ligamentous hypertrophy, hyperostosis (bony overgrowth), disk degeneration, and zygapophyseal joint arthropathy. Hypertrophies of the zygapophyseal joints and uncovertebral joints result in intervertebral foraminal stenosis and nerve root impingement. Vertebral body osteophytes and disk material can form a "hard disk" that also compresses the adjacent nerve root (eSlide 32.6).

DIAGNOSIS

History and physical examination. Patients with acute CIDH-related radiculopathy typically report a history of axial cervical pain that is followed by an explosive onset of upper limb pain. In contrast, spondylitic radicular pain presents more gradually. Cervical radicular pain can masquerade as a deep dull ache or sharp lancinating pain. Exacerbating factors include activities that raise the subarachnoid pressure, such as coughing, sneezing, or Valsalva maneuvers. If a significant component of stenosis is present, cervical extension can amplify the symptoms. Alleviation of the radicular pain by elevating the ipsilateral humerus is known as the shoulder abduction relief sign.

Physical examination begins with the clinical observation of neck position, as patients characteristically tilt toward the side of the disk herniation. Atrophy can be detected with more severe or long-standing lesions. Manual muscle testing has greater specificity than reflex or sensory abnormalities and might need to be performed repetitively or with the muscle at a mechanical disadvantage to elicit subtle weakness (eSlide 32.7). Severe weakness is less consistent with a single root lesion; if observed, it should alert the clinician to the possible presence of multilevel radiculopathy, radiculomyelopathy, alpha motor neuron disease, plexopathy, or focal entrapment neuropathy. Light touch, pinprick, and vibration sensations can be altered. Patients should be assessed for the presence of long tract signs, such as the Hoffman sign or Babinski response, to ensure that there is no spinal cord involvement. Provocative maneuvers, such as neuroforaminal closure and root tension signs, help localize the lesion to the cervical spine.

Imaging studies. Although plain radiography is not particularly sensitive in detecting pathologic disk conditions, it remains the initial radiographic examination in almost every assessment of musculoskeletal injury. Plain films of anteroposterior, lateral, open mouth, flexion, and extension views are indicated to evaluate spine stability in patients with rheumatoid arthritis, ankylosing spondylitis, or spondylolisthesis, as well as after fusion surgery or a traumatic injury. Magnetic resonance imaging (MRI) is the imaging modality of choice in investigating cervical radiculopathy because it shows details of the disks and ligamentous, osseous, and neural tissues very well (eSlide 32.6).

Electrodiagnostic evaluation. The American Association of Neuromuscular and Electrodiagnostic Medicine guidelines for the electrodiagnostic examination for a radiculopathy include abnormalities in two or more muscles innervated by the same root but different peripheral nerves, provided that normal findings are observed in muscles innervated by adjacent nerve roots. At least one corresponding motor and sensory nerve conduction study should be performed in the involved limb to ensure the absence of a concomitant plexus or peripheral process. If abnormalities are found, the corresponding contralateral muscle and nerves should be examined to exclude a generalized process, such as a peripheral neuropathy or motor neuron disease. A screening examination of six upper limb muscles, in addition to the cervical paraspinals, can identify 94%–99% of cervical radiculopathies.

TREATMENT

Physical medicine and rehabilitation. The primary objectives of treatment of cervical radiculopathy include resolution of pain, improvement in myotomal weakness, avoidance of spinal cord complications, and prevention of recurrence. Progressive neurologic deficit is a definitive indication for surgery (eSlide 32.7).

Modalities. Patient education, activity modification, and relief of pain are the initial treatment steps. Repetitive and heavy lifting, as well as positioning the cervical spine in extension, axial rotation, and ipsilateral flexion, must be avoided. Severe pain can prohibit continued work or athletic activity and restrict activities of daily living. Mild to moderate symptoms can usually be tolerated by the patient, allowing continued but restricted activities. Thermotherapy is often used to modulate pain and increase muscle relaxation. Deep heating modalities, such as ultrasound, should be avoided in the treatment of cervical radiculopathy because the increased metabolic response and subsequent inflammation can aggravate the nerve root injury.

TENS can be used early in the treatment course of cervical radiculopathy to help modulate pain and enable the patient to engage in other therapeutic modalities. Cervical orthoses function to limit painful range of movement and facilitate patient comfort during the acute injury phase. Soft cervical collars limit flexion and extension by approximately 26% and are prescribed as kinesthetic reminders of proper cervical positioning. The use of a soft collar should be limited to the first week or two of symptoms to minimize adverse outcomes related to further soft tissue deconditioning. Cervical traction applies a distractive force across the cervical intervertebral disk space. It is presumed to work via decompression of cervical soft tissues and intervertebral disks. Superficial heat, massage, or TENS therapy can be performed before and during traction to relieve pain and help relax the muscles (eSlide 32.8).

Medications. NSAIDs are the first line of pharmacologic interventions prescribed to treat cervical radiculopathy. At low doses, they provide an analgesic effect, and at high doses, an antiinflammatory effect. Adjunct medications are often used in conjunction with antiinflammatory medications and include muscle relaxants, tricyclic antidepressants, and antiepileptics. Muscle relaxants sedate and secondarily relax skeletal muscle. They may be used to aid sleep for 5–7 days, if sleep is disrupted by painful muscular guarding. Low-dose tricyclic antidepressant medications, such as amitriptyline or nortriptyline, can be beneficial in decreasing radicular pain and aiding sleep. Antiepileptic medications, such as gabapentin, can be effective in modulating neuropathic pain.

Stabilization and functional restoration. Cervicothoracic stabilization is the functional restoration of spinal biomechanics. It is used to limit pain, maximize function, and prevent injury progression or recurrence. Integral parts of this stabilization include restoration of spinal flexibility, postural reeducation, and conditioning. One of the main goals of the exercise program is to improve muscular balance and flexibility of the cervicothoracic and capital muscle groups. Proper scapulothoracic kinetics and glenohumeral coupling produce a mechanically efficient spinal posture, as well as efficient dissipation of energy by the upper limbs during functional activities.

Diagnostic selective nerve root blocks. A diagnostic selective nerve root block (SNRB) is a functional diagnostic test because the patient's cooperation and understanding is imperative in gaining accurate and valid diagnostic information. The specificity of cervical diagnostic SNRB has been suggested to range from 87% to 100%, and the sensitivity has been reported as 100%.

Therapeutic selective nerve root injections. The goal of selective nerve root injections (SNRIs) is to modulate the inflammatory response to the CIDH by injecting steroids close to the disk–nerve root interface. This is intended to control pain and start the process of nerve root healing while the herniated intervertebral disk naturally resorbs or becomes inert tissue. The natural history of radiculopathy caused by CIDH or spondylosis is a gradual resolution of symptoms with conservative care in 65%–83% of patients. Several studies have examined the use of cervical therapeutic SNRIs to treat cervical radiculopathy after failure of more conservative care, and good to excellent results have ranged from 50% to 83% over follow-up intervals from 6–21 months. Injection of local anesthetic alone has demonstrated efficacy equal to anesthetic and steroid combined and equal reduction in avoiding surgery (eSlide 32.8).

Percutaneous diskectomy/disk decompression. Percutaneous diskectomy has been investigated as a nonsurgical alternative for treating persistent cervical radiculopathy caused by a corroborative focal herniation. Various technologies have been used to achieve cervical intervertebral disk decompression, including laser, enzymatic, and mechanical decompression. Nucleoplasty is a technology that uses coblation energy to vaporize nuclear tissue into gaseous elementary molecules.

Surgery. Indications for surgical treatment of CIDH or spondylotic-related cervical radiculopathy include intractable pain, severe myotomal deficit (progressive or stable), or progression to myelopathy. Surgical outcome studies have demonstrated good or excellent results in 80%–96% of patients.

Cervical Joint Pain

EPIDEMIOLOGY

In patients with complaints of neck pain, the prevalence of pain mediated by cervical facet joints (or zygapophysial, zygapophyseal, apophyseal, or z joints) ranges from 36% to 60%. Cervical zygapophyseal joints are a common source of chronic post-traumatic neck pain. Spontaneous (nontraumatic) cervical zygapophyseal joint pain usually affects one joint and can be caused by spondylosis or improper biomechanics (eSlide 32.5).

DIAGNOSIS

History and physical examination. Traumatic upper zygapophyseal joint involvement, as at the C2-C3 joint, is more likely to cause unilateral occipital headaches than neck pain. Unilateral paramidline neck pain, with or without periscapular symptoms, that is more painful than any associated headaches is suggestive of zygapophyseal joint pain rather than pain arising from a disk or root injury. Physical examination must include assessment of neurologic function and cervical range of movement. Clinicians should suspect zygapophyseal joint injury when the patient can pinpoint a localized spot of maximal pain or define an area of pain typical for the referral distribution of a particular zygapophyseal joint (eSlide 32.5).

Imaging studies. Cervical zygapophyseal joint subluxation can be detected by plain radiography, and computed tomography (CT) can better delineate joint fractures. Soft tissue injury, however, is largely undetected by advanced imaging techniques. Imaging studies, therefore, have a limited role in determining the axial pain generator.

TREATMENT

Physical medicine and rehabilitation. During the acute phase of injury, treatment focuses on analgesia and antiinflammatory modalities. NSAIDs are indicated to provide pharmacologic control of pain and inflammation. If the pain is not controlled with these medications, opiates can be prescribed in the short term to facilitate restorative sleep patterns and participation in functional restoration. Physical modalities should be used in the acute phase of injury to modulate pain and inflammation, and they can be used to reduce or eliminate the need for opiates. Soft cervical collars can be worn for a short period of time, up to 72 hours after the initial injury. These are used for comfort, especially during sleep. Patient education regarding proper positioning to avoid aggravating factors should concurrently occur with analgesic and antiinflammatory medications. The restorative phase encompasses stabilization and functional restoration by normalizing range of movement, soft tissue length, and biomechanical deficits, and strengthening the spinal musculature. Transition to this phase begins after there is a reduction of pain caused by the acute injury. Restoration of cervical spine motion helps achieve a balanced posture that decreases strain on the injured joints and also allows optimal strengthening to occur. Cervicothoracic stabilization addresses flexibility, posture reeducation, and strengthening, all of which reduce pain, improve function, and prevent recurrent injury (eSlide 32.1).

Diagnostic zygapophyseal joint blocks. The close anatomic relationship and overlapping referral patterns of spine structures necessitate the use of fluoroscopically guided diagnostic blocks to confirm a clinically suspected painful joint. Diagnostic blocks offer a definitive means of targeting symptomatic joints. Such blocks historically have been performed via the intraarticular injection of local anesthetic. Anesthetizing the medial branches innervating the suspected joint has been shown to predict treatment outcomes after medial branch neurotomy.

Therapeutic zygapophyseal joint injections. Therapeutic intraarticular cervical zygapophyseal joint injections can be appropriate for individuals who have not improved with pharmacologic and physical modalities.

Percutaneous radiofrequency ablation medial branch neurotomy. If a patient's index neck pain is alleviated by two different comparative medial branch blocks with a local anesthetic, then radiofrequency ablation of the joint's innervating medial branches is indicated.

Cervical Internal Disk Disruption

EPIDEMIOLOGY

Internal disk disruption indicates that an intervertebral disk has lost its normal internal architecture but maintains a preserved external contour; nerve root compression does not occur. In nonlitigation cases, nonoperative and operative outcomes are similar to those for cervical internal disk disruption (CIDD) (eSlide 32.9).

DIAGNOSIS

History and physical examination. The symptom complex of CIDD includes posterior neck pain, occipital and suboccipital pain, upper trapezial pain, interscapular and periscapular pain, nonradicular arm pain, vertigo, tinnitus, ocular dysfunction, dysphagia, facial pain, and anterior chest wall pain. Patients often report a history of preceding trauma, such as a motor vehicle accident, with an acute onset of symptoms. In the absence of a precipitating event, CIDD symptoms can start spontaneously and gradually, or they can begin explosively. If referral symptoms are present, the patient's chief complaint is primarily axial pain associated with nondescript upper limb symptoms. Exacerbating factors usually include prolonged sitting, and coughing, sneezing, or lifting. Lying supine or recumbent with the head supported typically alleviates the patient's symptoms (eSlide 32.1).

Physical examination will show only subtle cervical range of movement restrictions unless there has been previous cervical surgery. A thorough neuromusculoskeletal examination should be performed to exclude myelopathy or radiculopathy. If spondylosis is present, more restriction will be observed during cervical extension and lateral bending than during flexion and axial rotation. Palpation over the cervical spinous processes of the involved level can elicit pain in that region or in an area of the patient's axial pain.

Imaging studies. Distinguishing painful from nonpainful cervical disks solely on imaging characteristics can be difficult. Disk abnormalities have been noted in patients who are asymptomatic. Plain films can reveal hyperostosis and disk space collapse, but these findings frequently do not correlate with pain symptoms. Disk desiccation, loss of disk height, annular fissure, osteophytosis, and reactive endplate changes are markers of disk degeneration. Decreased intradiskal signal on T_2-weighted images correlates well with histologic degeneration of the disk. MRI features are not useful, however, in detecting symptomatic cervical disks. Consequently, functional diagnostic testing, such as provocative discography, is used to diagnose the painful disk level.

TREATMENT

Physical medicine and rehabilitation. Treating cervical intervertebral disk injury without radiculopathy is similar to treating radicular symptoms (eSlide 32.9).

Provocative diskography. Provocative diskography is a functional diagnostic test in which the accuracy of the investigation relies heavily on patient input (eSlide 32.9). Proponents of diskography suggest that healthy disks accept a finite volume of contrast and do not produce symptoms with mechanical stimulation. Diskography should be considered valid only when an asymptomatic control disk injection accompanies a concordantly painful disk injection. Cervical intervertebral disks have been shown to refer pain into the head and face both unilaterally and bilaterally, as well as cause pain referral patterns that overlap those produced by painful zygapophyseal joints.

Transforaminal epidural steroid injections. Instillation of corticosteroids into the anterior epidural space to bathe the posterolateral margins of the annular surface of the intervertebral disks and posterior longitudinal ligament can address biochemically stimulated nociception (eSlide 32.8). Transforaminal epidural steroid injections (TFESIs) can be performed posteriorly via the interlaminar approach, using the loss-of-resistance technique without fluoroscopic guidance. Outcomes have been successful in approximately 40%–84% of treated patients.

SURGERY
Patients who have severe and recalcitrant axial cervical pain thought to be disk-ogenic in origin might be candidates for surgery. The approach to patients with CIDD is to consider cervical diskography if the patient is not relieved of pain after two TFESIs. If the diskogram reveals one or two contiguous levels producing concordant pain, then the patient might be a surgical candidate. If three or more levels are concordant, two levels are noncontiguous, or any concordantly painful disks are lobular, then the patient requires a comprehensive chronic pain-modulation program. The only surgical treatment for CIDD or symptomatic cervical degenerative disks is fusion, which can be accomplished by anterior cervical diskectomy and fusion or by posterior fusion.

Cervical Myelopathy and Myeloradiculopathy
EPIDEMIOLOGY
Cervical spondylitic myelopathy is the most common cervical cord lesion after middle age, but it is not as common as spondylitic cervical radiculopathy. The average age at onset is 50 years or older, and men predominate. Other causes of myelopathy have to be ruled out, including multiple sclerosis, motor neuron disease, vasculitis, neurosyphilis, subacute combined degeneration, syringomyelia, and spinal tumors (eSlide 32.10).

DIAGNOSIS
History and physical examination. Symptom onset is typically insidious, although a minority of patients can experience acute onset with or without a preceding traumatic event. Patients with myelopathy often complain of numbness and paresthesias in the distal limbs and extremities, weakness that is more common in the lower limbs than in the upper limbs, and intrinsic hand muscle wasting. Cervical axial pain can be the primary complaint in up to 70% of patients at one point in the disease course.

Bladder function disturbances occur in approximately one-third of cases and suggest more severe spinal cord injury. Patients can concurrently complain of unilateral or bilateral radicular pain caused by nerve root involvement at the stenosed level. The combination of cord and radicular involvement is referred to as cervical spondylitic myeloradiculopathy (eSlide 32.10). A common examination finding is myelopathic weakness in the lower limbs and to a lesser extent in the upper limbs. The upper extremities will demonstrate intrinsic hand muscle weakness and wasting resulting from anterior horn cell damage. Upper motor neuron signs, such as the Hoffman sign, brisk reflex, and Babinski sign, are often present. Pain and temperature sensation may be affected because of involvement of the spinothalamic tracts.

Imaging studies. Radiographic evaluations typically demonstrate the cervical cord compression, which is usually spondylitic in nature. Other causes include superimposed CIDH impinging on the thecal sac or ossification of the posterior longitudinal ligament. Plain radiography provides information regarding the osseous diameter of the central canal and decreased height of the intervertebral disk spaces, as well as the presence of posterior hyperostosis, foraminal encroachment, and subluxation. A central canal diameter less than 10 mm in a patient who is symptomatic supports the existence of myelopathy. To accurately diagnose cervical spondylitic myelopathy, approximately one-third of the central canal must be compromised, and objective central canal changes should be evident. These include a complete lack of cerebrospinal fluid flow, cord deformation, or intracord signal abnormalities. MRI allows detection of myelomalacia (which reflects progressive cord compression), signal alteration, atrophy, and the amount of cerebrospinal fluid volume surrounding the cord. The preoperative transverse area of the spinal cord at the site of maximal compression tends to correlate with eventual clinical outcomes, whereas the postoperative dimension of the cord strongly correlates with clinical recovery.

Electrodiagnostic evaluation. Electromyography and nerve conduction studies can be performed to diagnose nerve root injury, as discussed in the section on cervical radiculopathy. In cases of cervical myelopathy, the needle electrode examination can reveal rate-coding abnormalities in muscles below the injured segment, in which normal-appearing motor unit potentials are recruited but in a less than full interference pattern at maximal effort; these are indicative of upper motor neuron injury.

TREATMENT
Nonoperative care. Conservative care can include physical therapy and cervical orthoses in patients with mild or static symptoms without definite evidence of gait disturbances or pathologic reflexes. Improvement of sensory and motor deficits occurs in 33%–50% of patients.

Surgery. Surgery is indicated for patients with severe or progressive symptoms, or for those in whom conservative measures have failed.

Cervicogenic Headaches
EPIDEMIOLOGY AND PATHOPHYSIOLOGY
Cervicogenic headaches are a constellation of symptoms that represent the common referral patterns of cervical spine structures. The prevalence of cervicogenic headaches has been reported to range from 0.4% to 2.5% in the general population to as high as 36.2% in patients with a complaint of headaches. Women are more commonly affected (79.1%) than men (20.9%).

Various spinal structures have been implicated in cervicogenic headaches, including nerve roots, spinal nerves, dorsal root ganglia, uncovertebral joints, intervertebral disks, facet joints, ligaments, and muscles. Cervicogenic headaches may be attributed to degenerative changes, resulting directly from trauma, or occurring without any underlying biomechanical insult to the various cervical spine structures subserved by cervical afferent fibers (eSlide 32.11).

DIAGNOSIS

History and physical examination. Support for a structural source within the cervical spine as the etiology of a patient's headache is obtained by eliciting any history of previous head or neck trauma, such as a whiplash event. Whiplash events, such as motor vehicle accidents, have been associated with injury to the cervical zygapophyseal joints, intervertebral disks, or nerve roots, either in isolation or in combination. Cervicogenic headaches have been conceptualized as being primarily unilateral and stemming from the posterior occipital region. The referral of pain is toward the vertex of the scalp, ipsilateral anterolateral temple, forehead, midface, or ipsilateral shoulder girdle. Symptoms can spread to involve the contralateral side, but the side of the initial source of symptoms typically remains the side with the most intense symptoms. The character of pain can vary from a deep ache to sharp and stabbing. The pattern of painful symptoms varies from episodic bouts of pain (seen initially) to more chronic and constant pain. Patients often describe the pain as beginning in the cervical region and traveling to the head and neck as the pain becomes severe. The cervicogenic headache can then become the primary complaint, overshadowing the original cervical axial pain. The duration of the symptoms ranges from a few hours to a few weeks but characteristically lasts longer than symptoms associated with migraine headaches. The pain intensity of cervicogenic headaches is less excruciating than with cluster headaches, and it is usually nonthrobbing in nature. Autonomic complaints, such as photophobia, phonophobia, and nausea, are less apparent than in a migraine attack but can still occur. Physical examination of the patient with complaints of cervicogenic headaches typically reveals reduced active range of movement because of muscle guarding, arthritic changes, or soft tissue inflexibility. If the cervicogenic headache is being produced by a cervical zygapophyseal joint pathology, the patient can usually pinpoint a unilateral area of maximal pain, using one finger or the palm of the hand. Cervical intervertebral disk-induced cervicogenic headache typically begins as midline pain that spreads across the spine and into the head or face (eSlide 32.11).

Imaging studies. A history of trauma requires cervical flexion and extension lateral radiographs to detect abnormal segmental motion. It also requires anteroposterior views, including an open mouth view of the odontoid process, to detect possible fractures. Any suspicion of fracture mandates a subsequent cervical CT scan with multiplanar reformatted images to better delineate the osseous injury. MRI is better than CT for evaluating the intervertebral disks for desiccation, decreased disk height, and frank herniation.

Functional diagnostic tests and treatment. Once the etiology of the cervicogenic headaches has been identified, the offending structure is treated in a manner similar to the strategies outlined earlier.

Whiplash Syndrome

A *whiplash event* is a biomechanical effect incurred by the occupants of one vehicle that is struck by another vehicle. A *whiplash injury* is an impairment or injury to a structure resulting from a whiplash event. *Whiplash syndrome* is the set of symptoms arising from a whiplash injury. During a whiplash event, the head and neck do not suffer a direct blow, but each undergoes an excursion because of the inertial response of the body to the forces imparted on it. Rear-end collisions represent the most common pattern of whiplash-related injury, but injury caused by head-on and side collisions can also occur (eSlides 32.12 and 32.13). The most commonly reported symptoms of whiplash injury include neck pain and headache, followed by shoulder girdle pain, upper limb paresthesia, and weakness. Most patients with whiplash syndrome are destined to recover within the first 2–3 months after the injury, and 82% are free of symptoms within 2 years. Less than 10% remain severely affected 2 years after the injury. Chronicity does not appear to be related to litigation issues (eSlide 32.14).

• CONCLUSION

Neck pain is one of the most common complaints of patients seeking medical attention. Knowledge of spinal biomechanics and pathophysiology helps determine the most likely pain generators in a specific individual. The building blocks for successful therapeutic interventions include controlling pain and inflammation while educating the patient about the injury, treatment objectives, and prognosis. It is important to view the patient as a whole and institute physical, pharmacologic, behavioral, and interventional treatments in the broad context of achieving what is best for the patient's physiologic and psychological well-being.

Clinical Pearls

- The best treatment strategy for neck pain relies on an accurate diagnosis
- A central canal diameter less than 10 mm is the critical spinal canal measurement for cervical spinal stenosis and supports the existence of myelopathy in an individual with symptoms
- In cervical pain, the major indication for surgery is progressive neurologic deficit
- For a structure to be a possible source of pain, it must be innervated, producing pain similar to that seen clinically and susceptible to diseases or injuries known to be painful.

BIBLIOGRAPHY
The complete bibliography is available on ExpertConsult.com.

33 Low Back Pain

Anwar Suhaimi

This chapter elucidates the role of the physiatrist in the prevention, management, and treatment of low back pain (LBP).

• EPIDEMIOLOGY

LBP is a symptom, not a disease, and it has many causes. The lifetime prevalence of LBP approximates 84%. Most attacks are mild to moderate and recur, but they do not limit activities; thus the majority of individuals with LBP do not seek medical care. Ten to fifteen percent of acute LBP becomes chronic; 1% of LBP progresses to permanent disability, consuming up to 90% of health care and social costs for back pain in the United States. Societal acceptance of back pain disability and provision of disability benefits for back pain sufferers contribute to the increasing trend of disabling LBP.

• ANATOMY AND BIOMECHANICS OF THE LOWER BACK

The size and shape of the five lumbar vertebrae confer strength to the lumbar spine for support and protection, while the lumbar lordosis confers flexibility. Intervertebral disks consist of an internal gelatinous nucleus pulposus and an outer annulus fibrosus (with its fibrous layers). The annulus fibrosus is a shock absorber (eSlide 33.1); broken fibers of the annulus result in a herniated nucleus pulposus (eSlide 33.2). Zygapophyseal joints are paired synovial joints with a capsule, which resist vertebral rotation and thus limit torsional stress on the lumbar disks. There are two longitudinal ligaments: the anterior and posterior longitudinal ligaments. There are also segmental ligaments: (1) the paired ligamentum flavum joining adjacent laminae, which are very strong but allow flexion; and (2) the supraspinous, interspinous, and intertransverse ligaments, which resist flexion and prevent excessive shear forces during forward bending. Muscles of the lumbar region can be divided into three functional groups: (1) those originating from the lumbar spine, which are made up of the anterior muscles (eSlide 33.3); (2) the abdominal brace (eSlide 33.4); and (3) the pelvic stabilizers.

• PAIN GENERATORS OF THE LUMBAR SPINE

Structures with nociceptive innervations are potential sources of pain (eSlide 33.5). Innervations of the pain generators are as follows: (1) sinuvertebral nerve, innervating the external annulus fibrosus and posterior longitudinal ligament; (2) medial branch of the dorsal primary ramus, innervating the zygapophyseal joint and multifida; (3) branches of the dorsal primary ramus, innervating the posterior vertebral body and lumbar paraspinal musculature and fascia; and (4) gray ramus communicans (a branch of the lumbar sympathetic chain), innervating the anterior longitudinal ligament.

Aging Spine: The Degenerative Cascade

Kirkaldy-Willis described the degenerative changes in the lumbar spine that result in disk herniation, spondylotic changes, and eventually multilevel spinal stenosis (eSlide 33.6). Axial compression forces on disks anteriorly or torsional stress on zygapophyseal joints posteriorly may affect each other or occur simultaneously, although these structures are anatomically separated. The first change is often an annulus tear, which typically occurs posterolaterally. Internal disk disruption without herniation of the nucleus pulposus may ensue, causing loss of disk height, joint instability, and narrowing of the neural foramina and potential nerve root impingement. Changes at one level place stress on the adjacent levels, causing generalized multilevel spondylotic changes. Synovial hypertrophy of the zygapophyseal joints from repetitive microtrauma results in cartilage degeneration, leading to capsular laxity and joint instability. The laxity, combined with repetitive abnormal joint motion, leads to bony hypertrophy, which in turn causes narrowing of the central canal and lateral recess and potential nerve root impingement.

The disk, the adjacent vertebrae (above and below), and the muscles and ligaments that act across this area form a functional segment. *Segmental dysfunction* can occur when either a segment is too stiff or too mobile. Excessive mobility or functional instability is caused by tissue damage, poor muscle endurance, poor muscle control, or a combination of all three. Sufficient segmental stiffness is required to prevent injury and allow for efficient movement.

• PROGRESSION OF ACUTE LOW BACK PAIN TOWARD CHRONICITY

The experience of nociception is the sum of multiple facilitatory and inhibitory pathways leading to central sensitization; this produces the continued perception of chronic LBP, even when no pain generator is present in the area. Pain is an individual experience influenced by psychosocial factors, which explains the variable clinical presentations that cannot be attributed to biomechanical and neurologic factors alone. Psychosocial factors are linked to transition into chronic pain and disability. Depression is present in up to 40% of people with chronic LBP. A vicious cycle then leads to disability and more pain; depressed individuals tend to develop persistent pain. Depression, anxiety, and distress are strongly related to pain intensity, duration, and disability. Patients' beliefs about pain and their coping mechanisms consistently affect outcomes. *Catastrophizing* is characterized by excessively negative thoughts about pain and high fear of movement and injury or reinjury (kinesiophobia); this predicts more severe or disabling back pain. These sets of maladaptive pain coping behaviors are the target of multidisciplinary pain programs that effectively decrease fear-avoidance beliefs and catastrophizing and improve function.

• CLINICAL APPROACH TO LOW BACK PAIN

A thorough clinical history should be obtained to help determine the cause of the LBP. The history should illicit the features of the pain and identify the presence of serious medical diseases or red flag symptoms (eSlide 33.7). The presence of psychosocial factors (yellow flags) that are prognosticators for developing chronic disabling pain should also be determined (eSlide 33.8). If red flags are present, further diagnostic evaluation is necessary.

The physical examination (eSlide 33.9) should include a detailed neurologic examination. The accuracy of the neurologic examination in diagnosing a herniated disk is moderate, but it can be increased if a combination of findings is present (eSlide 33.10). Special tests for strength and flexibility are performed to detect deconditioning, poor endurance, and muscle imbalances in the abdominal, back, and pelvic stabilizer muscles. Lumbar segmental instability evaluation includes passive intervertebral motion testing and the prone instability test. Assessment of areas above and below the lumbar spine include palpation and evaluation of movement of the thoracic spine, determination of the hip joint range of movement, and screening of the knee and ankle joints. The presence of nonorganic signs should be sought by identifying symptoms out of proportion to the injury during the physical examination. Illness behaviors are learned behaviors and responses used to convey distress, whereas avoidance behaviors are manifestation of anxiety during the examination (e.g., poor effort during muscle strength testing).

Imaging of the low back is warranted only if specific pathology needs to be confirmed. It may include the following: (1) plain radiography after trauma, fractures, or when other bony lesions are suspected; (2) magnetic resonance imaging (MRI) for evaluating degenerative disk disease, disk herniation, and radiculopathy; (3) computed tomography (CT) for bony lesions, especially in patients with excessive hardware that obscure MRI images or implants that preclude MRI (pacemakers and clips); and (4) scintigraphy or bone scan for occult fractures, bony metastases, and infections. Bone scan is a sensitive but not specific imaging modality; single-photon emission computed tomography (SPECT) is best to identify the zygapophyseal joint as a source of pain. Electromyography is used for evaluating neurogenic changes and denervation in radiculopathy, which will help identify which anatomic lesion found on imaging is physiologically significant. Laboratory studies are used as adjuncts in diagnosing inflammatory and neoplastic diseases.

• DIFFERENTIAL DIAGNOSIS AND TREATMENT: BACK PAIN GREATER THAN LEG PAIN

Nonspecific LBP accounts for 85% of LBP with no specific diagnosis. It is multifactorial and may be the result of deconditioning, poor muscle recruitment, emotional stress, injury and aging-related processes such as disk degeneration, arthritis and ligamentous hypertrophy. Risk factors include obesity, smoking, very sedentary lifestyle, very vigorous physical activity, and genetic factors.

Lumbar spondylosis can be caused by degenerative disease of the zygapophyseal joints. In older patients with other sources of LBP, such as degenerative disks and lumbar stenosis, it may be difficult to identify the primary pain generator. Axial back pain is typical, with referred pain extending into the buttocks and legs. Clinically, spondylosis presents with accentuated lumbar lordosis, poor pelvic girdle mechanics, and multiple myofascial sources for pain. Typically the hip flexors are tight, which increases the stress on posterior elements thus increasing back pain. Diagnostic testing includes fluoroscopy-guided zygapophyseal joint injections or medial branch blocks with local anesthetic. According to the results of diagnostic joint injections, the prevalence of facet-mediated pain in people with chronic LBP is 15% in younger populations and 40% in older age groups. Lumbar zygapophyseal joint pain mainly originates from the L4-L5 and L5-S1 zygapophyseal joints.

Lumbar diskogenic causes of LBP can be divided into three categories: degenerative disk disease, internal disk disruption, and disk herniation. Diskogenic pain is typically distributed in a bandlike pattern and exacerbated by lumbar flexion; however, unilateral back pain radiating to the buttock can also be present. Atypically, pain can worsen by extension or side bending, depending on the site of disk pathology. Internal disk disruption occurs when the disk's internal architecture is disrupted, but its external surface remains normal. It is characterized by nucleus pulposus degradation and radial fissures that extend to the innervated outer third of the annulus. Pain is generated through chemical nociception from inflammatory mediators and mechanical stimulation. Disk herniation occurs when disk material extends beyond the intervertebral disk space, either as a disk bulge or herniation (as protruded or extruded, sequestrated or nonsequestrated, or contained or uncontained) (eSlide 33.11). Disk herniation is further discussed later.

Imaging investigations alone are unreliable for diagnosing the cause of nonspecific LBP. Clinicians often combine treatment modalities to provide pain relief and functional improvements. Reassurance and accurate, understandable patient education help improve treatment adherence, reduce anxiety, and counter misinformation about back pain. Patients are advised to continue ordinary activity as normally as possible, leading to quicker recovery and lesser disability. Group classes providing education about back pain (back schools) are effective in reducing disability and pain in people with chronic LBP, but they do not prevent the occurrence of LBP.

Exercise prevents deconditioning in acute LBP and provides modest pain relief in chronic LBP while producing additional health benefits and minimal side effects; thus exercise is a first-line treatment choice. The goals are to strengthen and increase the endurance of muscles to support the spine, improve flexibility, establish normal patterns of muscle activity, and improve biomechanical efficiency. Individualized exercise prescriptions for stretching and strengthening exercises of the abdominal, low back, and hip muscles performed under supervision appear to be most effective. Noncompliance is the main reason for failure of exercise treatments. Exercise progression should be conducted in planned, fixed increments based on goals, with leeway for temporary exacerbations of pain that may occur along the way. Increasing exercise levels benefits pain beliefs and behaviors through decreased fear-avoidance beliefs, anxiety reduction, positive reinforcement for meeting goals, and personal confrontation to reduce fear of movement, reinjury, and catastrophizing. Exercise in patients with LBP should consider general health and fitness goals and include 30 minutes of moderate aerobic activity five times a week, such as walking or aquatic exercises. No specific aerobic activity is superior over another.

There is strong evidence that nonsteroidal antiinflammatory drugs (NSAIDs) provide pain relief for acute and chronic LBP; no particular NSAID is superior. Side effects of these drugs are well established, but the long-term benefits of NSAID use are uncertain. Muscle relaxant use remains controversial, as muscle spasms have not yet been implicated in LBP pathogenesis. Antispasticity medications have been effective for short-term pain relief in acute back pain. Tricyclic antidepressants are effective in chronic LBP, whereas selective serotonin reuptake inhibitors and trazodone are not. Short-acting opioids confer no superior outcomes for pain or function. Long-acting opioids appear to provide better analgesia and are well tolerated. Topical *Capsicum frutescens* (cayenne), *Salix alba* (white willow bark), and *Harpagophytum procumbens* (devil's claw) reduce pain more than placebo.

Anticonvulsants, tramadol, lidocaine (lignocaine) patches, and topical irritant or antiinflammatory creams have not yet been proven effective clinically.

Trigger point injections (dry needling, lidocaine alone, or lidocaine with corticosteroid) are the most studied techniques and are effective in providing long-term pain relief for back pain. The efficacy of acupuncture is doubtful; however, it can supplement other forms of treatment and has a low rate of complications. Botulinum toxin injection and prolotherapy have not yet been proven effective in treating nonspecific back pain. Spinal manipulation has modest effectiveness, whereas traction is not effective. Lumbar support is no more effective than other treatments; compliance is poor and it does not prevent the occurrence of back pain. Transcutaneous electrical nerve stimulation (TENS) provides temporary pain relief and better function; however, long-term efficacy remains to be evaluated. Massage is effective in pain relief and functional restoration, with beneficial results persisting after 1 year in patients with subacute and chronic LBP. Complementary movement therapies effective for LBP include yoga, the Alexander technique, and the Feldenkrais method.

An interdisciplinary pain treatment program with the goal of functional restoration is helpful for severe chronic pain. Treatment of comorbidities, such as depression, anxiety, and sleep disturbances, decreases pain and increases function. A sedentary lifestyle, obesity, noninsulin-dependent diabetes, and cardiovascular disease contribute to greater all-cause morbidity.

Most patients with nonspecific LBP rapidly improve within 1 month, with an approximately slower decline of pain over the next 2 months. Between 3 to 12 months, little change in pain is expected. The risk of recurrence within 3 months can be as high as 34% and within 1 year as high as 84%.

• SPINAL FRACTURES

Spondylolysis is a defect of the pars interarticularis. It is usually due to hereditary dysplasia and repetitive stress on the immature spine, although an acute fracture from a severe hyperextension injury is an uncommon possible cause. Bilateral defects lead to isthmic spondylolisthesis. Spondylolysis commonly occurs at the L5-S1 level. It presents as back pain exacerbated by extension and alleviated by rest, with focal tenderness, a palpable step defect, pain with lumbar extension, and hamstring tightness. Oblique radiographs can show the pars defect, whereas a thin-slice CT through the abnormal level is diagnostic and allows staging to predict healing (eSlide 33.12). Approximate healing rates are 70% for acute defects, 30% for progressive defects, and 0% for terminal lesions.

Conservative management involves relative rest and avoidance of extension for 3 months, which is the shortest healing duration for pars lesions. Bracing can be considered for pain unrelieved by 2 weeks of rest. The treatment goal is a radiographically stable bony union. Deconditioning is a concern and can be addressed through aerobic conditioning, a core stabilization program, training of neuromuscular proprioceptive control, and sport-specific drills. Patients with chronic LBP may benefit from specific training of the lumbar multifidi and deep abdominal muscles. Surgery is rarely indicated except in the presence of spondylolisthesis or radiculopathy. Vigilant monitoring during the adolescent growth spurt or when the listhesis is greater than 50% is recommended to detect progressive slippage; this involves flexion–extension plain x-ray films every 6–12 months until skeletal maturity.

Spondylolisthesis, or anterior slippage of one vertebra on another, can be classified into six groups, according to etiology. The commonest is isthmic spondylolisthesis, which is the result of spondylolysis. Dysplastic spondylolisthesis is caused by congenital facet joint dysplasia. Degenerative spondylolisthesis is due to intersegmental instability from degenerative facet or disk disease, commonly occurring at the L4-L5 level. Traumatic spondylolisthesis is caused by an acute fracture. Pathologic spondylolisthesis is attributable to bone disease that decreases bony strength. Postsurgical spondylolisthesis is the result of extensive spinal decompression.

Typically, spondylolisthesis presents with axial pain, although intermittent radicular symptoms may occur from nerve root irritation caused by instability at the listhetic segment. Clinical findings and treatment are similar to those for spondylolysis; the degree of listhesis can be graded from 1 through 5 on the basis of lateral plain x-ray findings (eSlide 33.13). Risk factors for significant slip progression are the degree of slip, degenerative disk disease at the level of the slip, adolescent age group, and ligamentous laxity. Surgical fusion is only considered for grade 3 or greater slip, recalcitrant pain after rehabilitation, persistent radiculopathy, or progressive instability.

Osteoporotic compression fractures are associated with an increased risk of subsequent fractures, especially hip fractures (which carry high morbidity and mortality rates). Compression fractures contribute to a higher incidence of back pain in older adult women; up to 30% are caused by secondary osteoporosis due to oral corticosteroid use, hyperthyroidism, metastases, or multiple myeloma. Bone mineral density studies are diagnostic and allow assessment of treatment. Treatment includes a combination of medications, lifestyle modifications, and exercises aimed at balancing pain relief and medication side effects. Calcitonin reduces pain with adjunctive use of TENS. Occasionally intercostal nerve blocks are effective. Vertebroplasty is recommended for severe pain unresponsive to conservative management; however, the possibility of spinal nerve roots and cord compression, and pulmonary embolism must be considered.

Other spinal fractures are caused by trauma, with the outcomes depending on concurrent neurologic injury at the time of injury, the time elapsed between the injury and surgery, and the presence of instability. The Denis three-column structural concept is used for the classification of spinal fractures.

Bone metastases from lung, breast, prostate, and renal cell malignancies are common in the spine. Pain is caused by periosteal stretching and the mass effect of the tumor. Metastases should be highly suspected in patients with a previous history of cancer, back pain unrelieved by rest, new onset of back pain after 50 years of age, systemic features (e.g., weight loss), and failure to improve with conservative care. Neurologic deficits occur in 5%–10% of individuals because of mechanical pressure from the tumor or bone extruded from a collapsed vertebra. MRI is a sensitive assessment tool and may show early changes in the bone marrow.

Spinal infections include osteomyelitis, diskitis, pyogenic facet arthropathy, and epidural infections. Prompt treatment is paramount to prevent mortality and morbidity from complications. Hematogenous spread occurs via the spinal artery from urinary tract infections, infected intravenous lines, or endocarditis. Diabetics, hemodialysis recipients, intravenous drug users, and immunocompromised individuals have an increased risk of spinal infections. The lumbar spine is commonly affected, presenting with back pain. A raised erythrocyte sedimentation rate is typically the sole abnormal laboratory finding. Local spread may lead to abscesses in the epidural space and paraspinal or psoas muscles. The first sign is a periosteal reaction on plain x-ray films, followed by irregular endplate erosions and narrowing of the disk space, which are pathognomonic. MRI is the recommended imaging technique. Treatment is usually a 4- to 6-week course of intravenous antibiotics. The choice of antibiotic is determined by blood cultures or bone biopsy, and treatment is guided by the erythrocyte sedimentation rate response. Surgery is indicated in the presence of spinal instability, progressive neurologic deficit, or failure of medical treatment.

Osteomyelitis secondary to a contiguous focus of infection is seen after surgical procedures and with extension of infection from adjacent soft tissues. Risk factors are smoking, obesity, poor nutrition, uncontrolled diabetes, administration of corticosteroids, a history of malignancy, and radiation treatment in the area of surgery. Treatment requires surgical débridement, followed by a course of antibiotics. Diskitis can be the result of contiguous spread of infection or iatrogenic infection after diskectomy and diskography. Although the incidence is low, morbidity from disk infection is significant because of the difficulty with using antibiotics to treat the infection because of the relative avascularity of disks.

Spondyloarthropathies

Spondyloarthropathies are commonly associated with the presence of the *HLA-B27* allele; in genetically susceptible individuals, environmental and immunologic factors interact to produce clinical manifestations. Ankylosing spondylitis is three times more common in men and begins in the late teens or early 20s. It typically presents with morning stiffness and dull low back or buttock ache. These are followed by decreased spinal mobility, decreased chest expansion, and tenderness of the sacroiliac joints. Bony tenderness and enthesitis at the heel, greater trochanter, iliac crest, and tibial tuberosity are common. Systemic disease manifestations include anterior uveitis, heart disease, and inflammatory bowel disease. Radiographic changes include squaring of the vertebral bodies, syndesmophyte formation, and eventually a bamboo spine appearance. Sacroiliitis appears late on plain radiographs. MRI is more sensitive, and its findings are now considered diagnostic of ankylosing spondylitis.

Initial treatment includes exercises that promote spinal extension. Exercise enhances mobility, improves function, and prevents severe deformity. Indomethacin is particularly helpful in reducing pain and inflammation, thereby allowing exercises to be performed and function maintained. Peripheral arthritis necessitates sulfasalazine and methotrexate use. Disease-modifying agents, such as tumor necrosis factor inhibitors, control articular inflammation but do not prevent joint ankylosis. Fluoroscopy-guided sacroiliac joint injections relieve acute symptoms but have no long-term benefits.

• DIFFERENTIAL DIAGNOSIS AND TREATMENT: LEG PAIN GREATER THAN BACK PAIN

Lumbosacral radiculopathy results from mechanical compression or a chemically mediated inflammatory process of the nerve root. Disk herniation exposes the nucleus pulposus fluid and initiates an autoimmune-mediated inflammatory cascade leading to swelling of nearby nerves. This alters their electrophysiologic function, leading to sensitization of these neurons and enhanced pain generation, even in the absence of specific mechanical compression. Mechanical compression induces structural and vascular changes, as well as inflammation. These lead to intraneural blood flow disturbances, causing local ischemia and intraneural edema that triggers an inflammatory cascade. Local structural effects of mechanical compression include demyelination and blockage of axonal transport; mechanical stimulation enhances the production of substance P, which modulates sensory nociceptive feedback.

The commonest cause of nerve root compression is disk protrusion; in less than 1% of patients, compression is caused by an infection, malignancy or fracture. The commonest levels of disk herniation are L4-L5 and L5-S1, commonly affecting the L5 and S1 nerve roots. Posterolateral herniation is the most common type of herniation, affecting the nerve root before it enters the neural foramen. Extraforaminal herniation affects the exiting nerve root, and central disk herniation can affect multiple nerve roots because of the organization of the cauda equina. True cauda equina syndrome occurs in 1% of herniations. It causes bowel, bladder, and sexual dysfunction and is a surgical emergency, with the greatest recovery of neurologic deficits occurring if decompressive surgery is performed within the first 48 hours.

Conservative treatment can decrease pain and improve function in the acute phase of lumbosacral radiculopathy. Favorable outcomes have been reported with aggressive nonoperative care involving an active exercise program and fluoroscopy-guided transforaminal epidural steroid injections, resulting in short-term pain improvement and decreased inflammation; they potentially reduce the need for surgery and facilitate an active rehabilitation program (eSlide 33.14). Surgical management is reserved for significant persistent radicular symptoms, neurologic progression, or cauda equina syndrome. Decompressive procedures significantly improve pain and slightly accelerate the resolution of neurologic deficits.

Lumbar spinal stenosis results from degenerative changes that lead to narrowing of the spinal canal. Spinal venous congestion and radicular artery obstruction cause ischemic neuritis, producing neurogenic claudication. Neurogenic claudication is exacerbated by walking, prolonged standing, or any activity with relative lumbar extension and relieved by forward bending. Foraminal or lateral recess stenosis causes radicular pain in a typical dermatomal distribution.

Electrodiagnostic investigations can differentiate spinal stenosis from peripheral neuropathy and characterize the stenosis. Conservative management is warranted for mild to moderate symptoms, with the goals of pain control and reducing functional limitations. Oral medications, flexion-based lumbar stabilization, and hip mobility and aerobic exercises together with epidural steroid injections have demonstrated short-term improvement in pain and walking tolerance. Decompressive surgery is reserved for intractable pain and profound or progressive neurologic deficit or lifestyle impairment. Fusion is indicated if instability is present. Surgery improves pain but does not affect functional outcomes and is less effective for axial back pain.

Nonlumbar spine causes of "radicular" leg symptoms mimic lumbar radiculopathy because they generate pain referral patterns similar to the lumbosacral dermatomes. Sacroiliac joint disorders are a potential pain generator; however, the exact pathologic structure in these disorders is uncertain. The diagnosis is confirmed by observing pain relief after injecting local anesthetic into the joint. Sacroiliac pain does not radiate above the lumbosacral junction and overlaps substantially with lumbosacral radicular pain patterns. Hip joint pain is typically referred to the groin, posterior pelvis, or anterior thigh, making it easily confused with L1-L3 nerve root involvement. Plain hip radiographs and hip range of movement help differentiate intraarticular hip pain pathology from lumbar radiculopathy. Pyriformis syndrome can cause sciatica from local pressure on the sciatic nerve, producing buttock pain or pain radiating into the posterior thigh to below the knee in a distribution similar to the L5 or S1 dermatomal pattern. Pain can be elicited on palpation of the sciatic notch, through various examination maneuvers, or during electrodiagnostic investigations. Greater trochanteric pain syndrome is a regional pain syndrome around the greater trochanter that is often caused by gluteus medius and minimus tendinopathy or tears. It can also be the result of myofascial pain, causing gluteal muscle inhibition and deconditioning and manifesting as hip abductor weakness. Greater trochanteric pain syndrome and the iliotibial band syndrome can be confused with an L4 or L5 radiculopathy. Myofascial pain syndromes may arise from active trigger points within the surrounding muscle or fascia, with referral patterns mimicking lumbosacral dermatomes.

Peripheral vascular disease presents with vascular claudication, which is similar to neurogenic claudication. Both types of symptoms are exacerbated by walking; however, neurogenic claudication is relieved by forward flexion, whereas intermittent vascular claudication is not (it is only relieved by walking cessation, even when standing erect). Peripheral polyneuropathy causes paresthesias in the lower limbs and often occurs in older individuals with diabetes. Electrodiagnostic studies can differentiate this condition from lumbar stenosis and may be especially indicated in patients with MRI findings suggestive of stenosis. These studies may be particularly useful if epidural steroid injections are contemplated, as the injections will reduce symptoms caused by spinal stenosis but not those due to a polyneuropathy.

LBP in pregnancy is a common problem and needs to be differentiated from pelvic girdle pain. It is caused by increased biomechanical strain from anterior movement of the pregnant woman's center of gravity or from hormones altering the lumbopelvic ligaments and causing instability of the lumbosacral spine. Risk factors include a history of previous back pain or pregnancy-related back pain and LBP during menses. Pain usually peaks at 36 weeks' gestation and decreases afterwards; it is usually substantially improved 3 months postpartum. Persistent back pain may occur in women with both low back and pelvic girdle pain, back pain in early pregnancy, weakness of the back extensor muscles, older individuals, and those with work dissatisfaction. Individualized physical therapy, water aerobics, acupuncture, and massage can be used to decrease pain. Medications should be discussed with the obstetrician.

The prevalence of pediatric LBP is cited between 30% to 51%, with the greatest increase occurring during puberty and the maximal growth spurt. Risk factors for nonspecific LBP include older age, female sex, parents with LBP, hyperlordotic posture, history of spinal trauma, participation in competitive sports, high level of physical activity, and depression. Sitting exacerbates the back pain, and there is a positive correlation between LBP in adolescence and during adulthood. Specific causes of LBP in the pediatric population are listed in eSlide 33.15.

Spondylolysis and isthmic spondylolisthesis in young athletes are common causes of persistent LBP. Scheuermann disease is a painless exaggerated thoracic kyphosis, which causes a compensatory lumbar hyperlordosis; a higher prevalence of degenerative disk changes are present in those individuals with pain. Painful idiopathic scoliosis is indicative of a possible underlying tumor, infection, or spondylolisthesis. The most frequent malignant lesion affecting the pediatric spine is Ewing's sarcoma.

- Low back pain is a symptom of multifactorial etiology that significantly affects function and drains health care resources if poorly managed.
- The annulus fibrosus of intervertebral disks are shock absorbers. Lumbar muscle activities influence intradiskal pressures; lifting a load close to the body decreases forces on the lumbar spine and reduces intradiskal pressure.
- Ankle dorsiflexion weakness, calf muscle wasting, an abnormal ankle jerk reflex, and a positive crossed straight leg test correlate with the presence of a lumbosacral radiculopathy.
- Lumbar spinal stenosis results from narrowing of the spinal canal and causes neurogenic claudication from mechanical compression, venous congestion, and radicular artery obstruction. This type of claudication worsens with lumbar extension (e.g., prolonged standing, walking downhill) and is relieved by forward flexion or sitting.
- Lumbosacral radiculopathy results from annular tears allowing herniation of the nucleus pulposus. Herniation most commonly occurs at the L4-L5 and L5-S1 disks, thereby affecting the L5 and S1 nerve roots. Extraforaminal herniation affects the exiting nerve root, and central disk herniation can affect multiple nerve roots within the cauda equina.
- Spondylolysis is a defect of the pars interarticularis resulting from repetitive extension. It occurs most commonly at the L5-S1 level. Bilateral pars defects lead to isthmic spondylolisthesis. Plain oblique radiographs show the pars defect; computed tomography scans are diagnostic and allow staging to predict healing.
- Spinal metastases should be suspected in patients with a previous malignancy, back pain unrelieved by rest, new onset of back pain after age 50 years, and systemic features. Bone scans are sensitive but not specific for detecting bony metastases.
- Randomized controlled trials have only validated the effectiveness of lumbar stabilization exercises, core strengthening, and motor control exercises in chronic low back pain and spinal manipulation in acute low back pain.
- Treatment modalities are generally combined. Reassurance and patient education are the cornerstones for a therapeutic relationship and successful outcomes. Exercise prevents deconditioning and provides modest pain relief plus additional general health and fitness benefits. Walking is best to achieve aerobic fitness; fast walking results in lower spine loading, while arm swinging facilitates efficient storage and usage of elastic energy.

BIBLIOGRAPHY
The complete bibliography is available on ExpertConsult.com.

34 Osteoporosis

Francesca Gimigliano

Osteoporosis is the most prevalent metabolic bone disease in the United States, and it is a major public health problem. The costs of osteoporosis in the United States are estimated to be more than $14 billion per year, which mainly reflect the costs required for the management of hip fractures. Osteoporosis is a disease characterized by reduced bone mineral density (BMD) and microarchitectural deterioration of bone, leading to increased bone fragility. Osteoporosis is defined as a BMD of at least 2.5 standard deviations (SD) below the mean peak bone mass of young healthy adults. The T-score indicates the BMD of a given individual compared with the BMD of a young adult (at age 35 years) of the same sex with a peak bone mass. The Z-score is calculated in the same way, but the comparison is with the BMD of a person of the same age, gender, race, height, and weight. Normal BMD is characterized by a T-score of –1 SD or greater; osteopenia is a condition defined by a T-score between –1 SD and –2.5 SD. Osteoporosis is considered severe when the T-score is –2.5 SD or less and associated with the presence of a fragility fracture.

• BONE FUNCTION AND STRUCTURE

Bone serves as a mechanical support for musculoskeletal structures, as protection for vital organs, and as a metabolic source of ions, especially calcium and phosphate. There are two types of bone cells: osteoclasts, which are localized in the endosteal bone surfaces and resorb the calcified matrix, and osteoblasts, which synthesize new bone matrix through budding alkaline phosphatase–rich vesicles from their cytoplasmic membrane. Despite its appearance, bone is an active tissue, undergoing continuous renewal to maintain its biomechanical competence: older bone tissue is replaced by newly formed bone tissue. This cyclic process, called bone remodeling, replaces approximately 20% of bone tissue annually. Bone remodeling is a process that removes old bone and replaces it with new bone tissue, promoting maintenance of the biomechanical integrity of the skeleton and supporting the roles of bone in providing mechanical support and acting as an ion bank for the body.

Bone remodeling has five phases:
1. *Activation:* osteoclastic activity is initiated through recruitment of osteoclasts.
2. *Resorption:* osteoclasts erode the bone and form a cavity.
3. *Reversal:* osteoblasts are recruited into the cavity.
4. *Formation:* osteoblasts replace the cavity with new bone.
5. *Quiescence:* the bone tissue remains dormant until the next cycle starts.

This process starts with bone resorption and finishes with bone formation. In adult human bone, each cycle of remodeling lasts 3–12 months. After bone resorption, the reversal phase starts, which involves osteoblastic activity. Osteoblasts start to fill the resorption cavity. During the process of osteoclastic activity, growth factors stored in the bone matrix are released and subsequently stimulate osteoblast proliferation. This process of bone resorption and formation is called *coupling*.

The ideal situation in the coupling process is equilibrated bone formation and resorption.

Peak adult bone mass is achieved between 30 and 35 years of age. The number of active remodeling units in trabecular bone is approximately three times greater than in cortical bone. The physical endurance of any bone is affected by the percentage of cortical bone within its structure. Trabecular bone is more active metabolically than cortical bone because of its considerable surface exposure area. Consequently, more bone loss occurs in the trabecular areas when resorption is greater than formation. The vertebrae consist of 50% trabecular bone and 50% cortical bone, whereas the femoral neck consists of 30% trabecular bone and 70% cortical bone. Thus when bone turnover increases, bone loss and osteoporosis occur in the vertebrae before they occur in the femoral neck.

• PATHOGENESIS AND CLASSIFICATION OF OSTEOPOROSIS (eSlide 34.1)

Osteoporosis can occur primary or secondary to other disorders that result in bone loss. The most common type of osteoporosis is either postmenopausal or age-related. Age plays an important role in the rate of bone turnover. Bone turnover increases in women at menopause but does not increase substantially in men with aging. The secondary causes of osteoporosis are associated with an increased rate of activation of the remodeling cycle.

The rate of bone remodeling can be increased by parathyroid hormone (PTH), thyroxine, growth hormone, and vitamin D (1,25-dihydroxyvitamin D_3) and decreased by calcitonin, estrogen, and glucocorticoids. PTH, secreted by the parathyroid glands, is the major hormone for calcium homeostasis. In general, PTH increases serum calcium concentration and primarily tends to decrease serum phosphate concentration. PTH levels increase with age. The main regulators of vitamin D synthesis are the serum concentrations of 1,25-dihydroxyvitamin D_3 (the active form of vitamin D), calcium, phosphate, and PTH. Vitamin D can also be synthesized through exposure to the sun and conversion in the liver. Reduction in the active form of vitamin D can be the result of decreased consumption of dietary vitamin D, decreased exposure to sunlight, decreased capacity of skin to convert vitamin D, reduced intestinal absorption, and reduced 1-α-hydroxylase activity. The influence of the active form of vitamin D is both a direct effect, through stimulating osteoblastic activity, and an indirect effect, through increasing the intestinal absorption of calcium and phosphorus. Most studies have shown that plasma levels of the active form of vitamin D decrease with age by approximately 50% in both men and women.

Physical strain and mechanical load positively affect bone mass. Exercise stimulates the release of growth hormone and other trophic factors that stimulate osteoblastic activity. A change in physical stress and strain on bone influences bone growth and remodeling. Decreased physical activity with aging and a proportional decrease in muscle strength in women negatively influence bone tissue. Optimal nutrition and physical activity are necessary to achieve the genetic potential for bone mass. The peak bone mass attained by early adulthood is a major determinant of bone mass in later life. Nutrition can also affect both bone matrix formation and bone mineralization. Calcium intake should be increased in men older than 65 years and women older than 50 years.

• CLINICAL MANIFESTATIONS OF OSTEOPOROSIS
(eSlides 34.2 to 34.5)

Osteoporosis is a "silent disease" until fractures occur. Osteoporotic vertebral fractures can go unnoticed until they are incidentally seen on a chest radiograph. The most common areas for osteoporotic fractures are the midthoracic spine, upper lumbar spine, hip (proximal femur), and distal forearm (Colles fracture). Hip fracture is the main clinical issue because it increases the risk of death by 15%–20%. The relationship between bone mass and spinal fractures has been extensively studied, and it is known that fracture risk increases as bone mass decreases. For every 1 SD decrease in BMD, the risk of osteoporotic fracture of the spine increases 1.5- to 2-fold, and the risk of hip fracture increases 2.6-fold. In addition, the risk of fracture from osteoporosis doubles every 5–7 years. It is not clear whether age-related changes in bone density or bone quality are factors that increase the risk of fractures caused by falls.

The incidence of vertebral fractures is unknown, but it has been estimated that 50% of these fractures can be subclinical and the patient might not seek medical attention. Acute pain is usually due to a compression fracture that might not be apparent on radiograph for up to 4 weeks after the injury. Chronic back pain is related to postural changes. The development of a kyphotic posture is the most physically disfiguring and psychologically damaging effect of osteoporosis. Chronic pain can also be attributed to microfractures that are visible only on bone scans.

Pain and skeletal deformities associated with osteoporosis might secondarily reduce muscle strength. Disproportionate weakness of the back extensor musculature relative to body weight or spinal flexor strength considerably increases the possibility of compressing the vertebrae in a fragile osteoporotic spine. Recognition and improvement of decreased back extensor muscle strength can enhance the ability to maintain proper vertical alignment, decreasing both kyphosis and back pain. Vertebroplasty and kyphoplasty procedures can be performed for the management of vertebral fractures. However, they cannot substitute for rehabilitative measures that are needed after a fracture.

Hip fracture should be considered an emergency situation because of its high risk of associated mortality and disability. Hip fractures can be classified as intracapsular (femoral neck fracture) or extracapsular (trochanteric fracture). Surgery is the treatment of choice for both femoral neck and trochanteric hip fractures. In some unusual cases of impacted fracture, however, conservative treatment might be advisable, particularly when the patient is severely debilitated with impaired general health. The postoperative course for all hip fractures, regardless of whether internal fixation or joint arthroplasty is performed, is less eventful if physical therapeutic measures are implemented postoperatively. These include the use of gait aids, with partial weight-bearing on the operative side. Restrictions are placed on weight bearing only in patients with fractures that are severely comminuted or have had an unsatisfactory operative result. There is conflicting evidence as to whether hip protectors can reduce the incidence of hip fractures in older, high-risk individuals. Compliance with the use of hip protectors has been a concern in the nursing home population. Rehabilitation that teaches patients how to fall and land safely can decrease the risk of hip fracture resulting from high-impact contact during a fall.

• DIAGNOSIS OF OSTEOPOROSIS (eSlides 34.6 and 34.7)

The diagnosis of osteoporosis requires a thorough history and physical examination, which should include determining the type and location of musculoskeletal pain, general dietary calcium intake, level of physical activity, current height and weight, and the presence or absence of a family history of osteoporosis. Biochemical markers for bone formation include calcium, phosphorus, PTH, bone-specific alkaline phosphatase, and serum osteocalcin. Resorption markers include 24-hour urinary calcium excretion (corrected for creatinine excretion), hydroxyproline, and pyridinium cross-links (in urine). The gold standard for the diagnosis of osteoporosis is dual-energy x-ray absorptiometry (DXA). BMD evaluation is recommended for the following: women ≥65 years; postmenopausal women <65 years with at least one risk factor for low bone mass and fragility fracture (low body weight, prior fracture, high-risk medication use, disease or condition associated with bone loss); women during the menopausal transition with risk factors for a fracture; men ≥70 years; men <70 years with at least one risk factor for low bone mass and fragility fracture; all adults with a fragility fracture; all adults with a disease or condition associated with low bone mass or bone loss; all adults taking medications associated with low bone mass or bone loss; individuals being considered for antiosteoporotic therapy; people being treated for osteoporosis (to monitor treatment effects); and women discontinuing estrogen therapy. The reference standard from which the T-score is calculated is BMD of a young adult (at age 35 years) of the same sex with a peak bone mass. Osteoporosis can be diagnosed in postmenopausal women and men aged ≥50 years when the T-score of the lumbar spine, total hip, or femoral neck is less than or equal to –2.5 SD. The World Health Organization reference standard for osteoporosis diagnosis is a T-score less than or equal to –2.5 SD at the femoral neck.

MANAGEMENT OF OSTEOPOROSIS (eSlides 34.8 to 34.14)

There are many aspects that should be considered in the prevention and treatment of osteoporosis; therefore a multidimensional approach is always advised. The primary objective of osteoporosis management is prevention, by either increasing the peak bone mass or reducing bone loss. Peak bone mass is achieved at the age of 30 years and is influenced by both nutrition and physical activity. The same strategies, together with a pharmacologic approach, may be applied to prevent bone loss.

The efficacy of exercise in improving bone mass is supported by hormonal and nutritional factors. In postmenopausal women, there is a significant positive correlation between BMD and back muscle strength. To meet the challenge of a mechanical load, skeletal tissue must have enough bone mass and proper architecture to withstand the physical strain that is imposed upon it. Normal musculoskeletal structure is highly adaptable and can meet the challenge of usual mechanical loads. High rates and magnitudes of bone strain are produced during high-impact sports activities, such as gymnastics, badminton, tennis, volleyball, and basketball. The high-impact bone loading results in site-specific increases in BMD. Axial loading of the skeleton during lifting activities at a person's job or while caring for children can be as osteogenic as mechanical loading exercises in a gym.

The challenges imposed by a mechanical load and strain might not be tolerated by individuals with osteopenia and osteoporosis without causing damage to the bone architecture. A supervised, nonstrenuous, progressive resistive exercise program might improve bone mass in inactive individuals. Nonstraining exercises (e.g., walking for 45 minutes three times a week or for 30 minutes daily) are recommended for people with osteoporosis. Aquatic exercises are recommended for patients who are unable to perform antigravity exercises because of pain or weakness. These nonstrenuous, low-resistance exercises can be advanced to antigravity and strengthening exercises as permitted by a patient's musculoskeletal status.

Spinal extension exercises can improve a kyphotic posture and should be prescribed along with exercises to reduce lumbar lordosis. Recent studies showed that progressive resistive back muscle–strengthening exercises can improve back strength, and isometric abdominal muscle–strengthening exercises should be included in order to complement a posture training exercise program. Furthermore, even without pharmacotherapy, patients with osteoporosis who performed back extension exercises had a considerably lower rate of fracture than those who performed spinal flexion exercises or no exercise.

Fractures generally occur with falls; therefore preventing falls decreases the risk of fracture. Falls in older individuals are very common and represent a serious cause of morbidity, severe disability, and death. Impaired mechanisms of postural stability with age (weakness in the lower extremities and kyphotic posture) and the presence of acute and chronic diseases may favor the occurrence of falls in the older population. The spinal proprioceptive extension exercise dynamic (SPEED) program demonstrated considerable improvement in the risk of falls. This program produced a decreased step width, improved steadiness of gait on gait laboratory testing, decreased the risk of falls at obstacles, and increased velocity, cadence, and stride length in individuals. The use of a weighted kypho-orthosis (WKO) and the SPEED program was shown to decrease back pain and increase the level of physical activity.

Acute compression fractures usually produce severe pain and can lead to prolonged immobility and chronic pain if not managed well. Acute pain needs to be actively managed with proper pharmacologic and physical measures. Sedative stroking massage, initial application of cold (followed later by heat), and isometric muscle contractions of the paraspinal muscles can be helpful. Rigid thoracolumbar orthoses to promote extension of the spine are helpful. If thoracolumbar orthoses are not tolerated because of postural changes, a thoracic WKO or a combination of a kypho-orthosis and lower-back support (elastic abdominal support) might suffice. In some cases, long-distance ambulatory activities might require the use of a cane or wheeled walker. Temporary use of a wheelchair with a supportive back cushion is indicated in some patients. Every effort needs to be taken to not only prevent falls but also immobility (including having the patient confined to one room or restricted to prolonged bed rest). Immobility should be limited to avoid resultant bone loss or reactive depression. Safety during ambulation is paramount, and prevention of falls and fractures should be taught in any rehabilitative program for patients with osteoporosis. Implementation of the SPEED program can decrease gait unsteadiness and posture-related back pain and increase the level of physical activity.

An adequate calcium intake is required to permit normal bone development and potentially decrease bone loss. However, adequate calcium and vitamin D intake appears to have only a modest effect on bone loss after menopause. Inadequate intake of calcium and vitamin D is common, especially in older residents of nursing homes. Spinal BMD in women aged 50–60 years is correlated with both calcium intake and back extensor strength. According to the Women's Health Initiative Study, the best strategies for prevention of osteoporosis in women are calcium and vitamin D supplementation and exercise. Recommendations for osteoporosis prevention and treatment in postmenopausal women include nutrient intake of calcium 1000 mg/day, vitamin D 800 IU/day, and proteins 1.0–1.2 g/kg body weight/day, as well as regular physical exercise (3–5 times per week).

Pharmacologic treatment of osteoporosis involves two different types of anti-osteoporotic drugs: antiresorptives (bisphosphonates, calcitonin, denosumab, estrogen, estrogen agonists, and androgens), which decrease the activity of osteo-clasts and inhibit bone loss, and anabolic agents (teriparatide and fluoride), which increase the activity of osteoblasts and stimulate bone formation in bone tissues. Newer medications include anabolics, such as the antisclerostin agent called romo-sozumab, and an antiresorptive, the cathepsin K inhibitor called odanacatib.

• CONCLUSION

Osteoporosis is a progressive and disabling disease with an increasing incidence. The major consequence is a fracture, which may be avoidable with an adequate diet, risk factor avoidance, and pharmacologic treatment. Rehabilitation, especially physical exercise, can reduce bone loss, prevent falls, improve balance, and reduce hyperkyphosis (eSlide 34.15).

Clinical Pearls

1. Osteoporosis is defined as a reduction of bone mineral density, estimated as at least 2.5 standard deviations (SD) below the mean peak bone mass of young healthy adults.
2. The gold standard for diagnosing osteoporosis is dual-energy x-ray absorptiom-etry; osteoporosis can be diagnosed in postmenopausal women and in men aged ≥50 years when the T-score of the lumbar spine, total hip, or femoral neck is less than or equal to −2.5 SD.
3. The primary objective in the treatment of osteoporosis is maintaining bone health and preventing bone loss and fragility fractures. Standard care includes ensuring an adequate intake of calcium and vitamin D, performing regular weight-bearing ex-ercise, avoiding habits that might impair bone health (such as smoking or alcohol) and falling.
4. There are two different types of antiosteoporotic drugs: antiresorptives and ana-bolic agents.
5. Nonstraining exercises are recommended for people with osteoporosis. Aquatic exercises are recommended for those who are unable to perform antigravity exercises because of pain or weakness.

• ACKNOWLEDGMENT

I would like to acknowledge Alessandro de Sire for his contribution to the chapter.

BIBLIOGRAPHY
The complete bibliography is available on ExpertConsult.com.

35 Upper Limb Pain and Dysfunction

Eleftheria Antoniadou

Upper limb musculoskeletal disorders are some of the most common and important sources of pain and dysfunction in all age groups. This chapter reviews the most important and frequent symptoms of, as well as the rehabilitation principles for, upper limb pain and dysfunction.

• REHABILITATION PRINCIPLES OF UPPER LIMB INJURY (eSlide 35.1)

The three broad stages of rehabilitation for all musculoskeletal conditions of the upper limb are the acute, recovery, and functional stages. The acute stage focuses on reducing symptoms and facilitating tissue healing. For these purposes, the most appropriate treatments are rest, ice, compression, and elevation (RICE); cardiovascular fitness; strengthening and flexibility exercises; and avoidance of activities that can aggravate symptoms or be detrimental to tissue healing. Heat and high-frequency electrical stimulation are often used during exacerbations of a chronic injury. Opioid and nonopioid (e.g., nonsteroidal anti-inflammatory drugs [NSAIDs] or corticosteroids) analgesics might be required for pain control. The recovery stage starts when the pain has been controlled and tissue healing has occurred. It involves restoration of flexibility, strength, and proprioception. Muscle substitutions should be corrected in this phase of rehabilitation. Open kinetic chain exercises are used to correct strength imbalances, and closed chain exercises are used to provide joint stabilization. The functional stage of rehabilitation begins when the injured limb has regained 75%–80% of normal strength (compared with the uninjured limb) and when there are no strength and flexibility imbalances. Functional activities should be incorporated into the rehabilitation program with a vocational-specific or avocational-specific progression that eventually leads to a return to normal activities.

• SHOULDER CONDITIONS

Acromioclavicular Joint Sprains (eSlide 35.2)

Symptoms and physical examination findings of acromioclavicular (AC) joint sprains include point tenderness, a positive horizontal adduction test, and a positive O'Brien test. Types 1, 2, and 3 AC sprains are usually treated nonoperatively. Surgical intervention is indicated for type 3 sprains only for persistent pain or poor cosmetic results. Types 4, 5, and 6 sprains require surgical treatment.

Rotator Cuff Tendonitis and Impingement (eSlide 35.3)

Symptoms and physical examination findings of rotator cuff tendonitis and impingement include anterior or lateral shoulder pain with overhead activity and at night, stiffness, weakness (detected during strength testing of the rotator cuff muscles), catching, and possible instability of the shoulder. Evaluation of the cervical spine is necessary to exclude cervical spine pathology, which is the main differential diagnosis. The Neer-Walsh and Hawkins-Kennedy tests should be performed.

Elimination of provoked pain after injection of 10 mL of 1% lidocaine into the subacromial space is useful to establish the diagnosis. Ultrasound and magnetic resonance imaging (MRI) are the preferred diagnostic imaging techniques. In young or active individuals, surgical intervention is required for full thickness tears. All other groups of individuals should receive conservative treatment for 6 months, after which surgery may be considered. Potential alternative treatments include extracorporeal shock-wave therapy or, if calcific tendonitis is present, ultrasound-guided percutaneous lavage and aspiration of the calcification.

Glenohumeral Joint Instability (eSlide 35.4)

Stability of the shoulder is provided by a combination of static and dynamic stabilizers, as well as optimal scapular function. The classification of glenohumeral joint instability includes the degree, frequency, etiology, and direction of instability. Symptoms include pain, popping, catching, locking, an unstable sensation, stiffness, and swelling. Some patients might have a history of glenohumeral joint dislocation or episodes of subluxation with a burning or aching "dead" feeling in the arm.

A full physical examination of the shoulder should be performed, including determination of the glenohumeral joint range of movement (ROM), analysis of scapulothoracic kinesis, assessment of upper limb strength, sensation testing over the deltoid muscle (to determine whether an axillary nerve injury is present), muscle strength reflex evaluation, and special tests (e.g., anterior apprehension and relocation test, posterior apprehension, sulcus sign). The patient should also be examined to assess the possible presence of generalized ligamentous laxity or a connective tissue disorder.

Diagnostic evaluation involves plain radiographs and magnetic resonance arthrography. Nonoperative management is the appropriate treatment for older patients and individuals who have experienced their first episode of traumatic anterior dislocation. In younger patients, there is a very high redislocation rate in those treated nonoperatively compared with those who have undergone surgery.

Adhesive Capsulitis (eSlide 35.5)

Adhesive capsulitis of the shoulder is usually an idiopathic condition, but it can be secondary to many causes. Adhesive capsulitis has been divided into four stages. Stage 1 occurs 1–3 months after onset; pain occurs with movement, but there is no joint ROM restriction. Stage 2, the "freezing stage," occurs 3–9 months after onset; pain occurs with movement, and there is progressive joint ROM restriction in all planes. Stage 3, the "frozen stage," occurs 9–15 months after onset; pain is reduced, but joint ROM is restricted. Stage 4, the "thawing stage," occurs 15–24 months after onset; the joint ROM is gradually improved.

Diagnostic evaluation involves glenohumeral joint arthrography. Up to three intraarticular corticosteroid injections may be administered during stages 1 and 2. Early scapular stability exercises and closed chain rotator cuff exercises can be instituted, together with passive and active assistive exercises. Most patients will have restoration of function over a 12- to 14-month period. In patients who do not improve after 6 months of nonoperative treatment, treatments that are more interventional can be considered. These may include capsular hydrodilatation, manipulation under anesthesia, and arthroscopic lysis of adhesions.

• ELBOW CONDITIONS

Lateral Epicondylitis (eSlide 35.6)

Lateral epicondylitis, or tennis elbow, is a tendinopathy of the lateral elbow, which is especially common in male tennis players. The degenerative changes occur in the origin of the extensor carpi radialis brevis. It can also involve the origin of the extensor digitorum communis in 30% of cases.

Symptoms and physical examination findings include point tenderness over the lateral epicondyle and a positive Cozen test. Entrapment of the posterior interosseous branch of the radial nerve can mimic lateral epicondylitis.

Radiographs might reveal punctuate calcifications in the extensor tendon origin. Treatment includes discontinuation of provocative activities and following the general principles of rehabilitation. Eccentric strengthening of the wrist extensors appears to be the most effective exercise regimen. Peritendinous corticosteroid injections are occasionally used. Newer treatments include ultrasound-guided percutaneous needle tenotomy, autologous blood injections, platelet-rich plasma injections, and extracorporeal shock-wave therapy. Recalcitrant cases can also be treated with surgical débridement.

Medial Epicondylitis (eSlide 35.7)

Medial epicondylitis involves the pronator teres and flexor carpi radialis origins. Risk factors for medial epicondylitis include training errors, faulty equipment, repetitive activities requiring wrist flexion and forearm pronation, and biomechanical abnormalities. Treatment options are the same as for lateral epicondylitis.

Olecranon Bursitis (eSlide 35.8)

Olecranon bursitis can be septic (from a localized or systemic infection) or aseptic (acute hemorrhagic or chronic, caused by repetitive microtrauma). Aseptic bursitis is frequently seen in athletes who participate in football or hockey.

Ulnar Collateral Ligament Sprain Injuries (eSlide 35.9)

Injuries to the ulnar collateral ligament (UCL) of the elbow are the result of valgus stress to the elbow. Ulnar nerve traction and neuritis can occur because of the increased laxity of the elbow.

• FOREARM, WRIST, AND HAND CONDITIONS

De Quervain Syndrome (eSlide 35.10)

De Quervain syndrome is a stenosing tenosynovitis of the first dorsal compartment of the wrist, which contains the abductor pollicis longus and extensor pollicis brevis tendons. Symptoms and physical examination findings include pain over the dorsal radial aspect of the wrist aggravated by activities such as racquet sports, golf, or fly fishing; a sensation of wrist crepitus; mild edema localized to the dorsal radial wrist; and tenderness to palpation over the first dorsal compartment. A positive Finkelstein test is pathognomonic for the diagnosis. Treatment includes RICE and a thumb spica splint. First dorsal compartment peritendinous corticosteroid injections reduce symptoms in 62%–100% of cases.

Scapholunate Instability (eSlide 35.11)

Scapholunate instability is the most common type of wrist ligament injury. It can occur when a person falls on a pronated outstretched hand with the wrist in extension and ulnar deviation. If this injury is not diagnosed early and treated properly, joint stress will ultimately lead to progressive wrist arthrosis and scapholunate advanced collapse.

Triangular Fibrocartilage Complex Injuries (eSlide 35.12)

The triangular fibrocartilage complex is the primary stabilizer of the distal radioulnar joint. It can be injured by falling on an outstretched hand or through repetitive microtrauma, such as during gymnastics.

First Metacarpophalangeal Joint Ulnar Collateral Ligament Sprain (eSlide 35.13)

Ulnar collateral ligament strain of the first metacarpophalangeal joint is frequently seen in skiers and athletes who participate in sports such as basketball and football. Surgical repair is indicated in the presence of a Stener lesion, fracture, or complete tear. If these are not present, then modalities, analgesics, and a spica splint (including during competition) are used for treatment.

Clinical Pearls (eSlides 35.14 and 35.15)

- All conditions are due to repetitive microtrauma or acute trauma with the exceptions of adhesive capsulitis and olecranon bursitis, which can also be secondary to a systemic illness.
- A detailed history and thorough clinical examination, with the adjunct use of special testing (when possible), are usually sufficient to establish the diagnosis. Assessment must be performed at rest and during movement. Always check the cervical spine, as it can be the explanation for pain in the upper limb.
- Radiographic examination (x-rays, magnetic resonance imaging, and ultrasound) can be used to complement the diagnosis and provide more details.
- Conservative treatment should be started 6 months prior to any consideration of surgery if the condition is chronic or when the patient is not a young athlete who needs full movement power.
- Principles of rehabilitation should be used for conservative treatment. Also patients should be instructed regarding the correct posture and ergonomics, to improve function and outcomes.

BIBLIOGRAPHY
The complete bibliography is available on ExpertConsult.com.

36 Musculoskeletal Disorders of the Lower Limb

Elena Milkova Ilieva

This chapter reviews some of the most common musculoskeletal disorders of the lower limb, including soft tissue, bone, and joint pathologies, which are of primary interest to the practitioner of rehabilitation, musculoskeletal, and sports medicine.

• DISORDERS OF MUSCLE–TENDON GROUPS OF THE LOWER LIMB

Trochanteric bursitis involves inflammation of the proximal bursa, which is positioned to decrease friction between the iliotibial band (ITB) and the greater trochanter of the femur. Bursitis usually occurs as a result of improper training techniques or abnormal biomechanics, which leads to imbalance or dysfunction of the hip muscles and abnormal ITB motion. The pain is localized in the lateral hip and sometimes along the path of the ITB in the lateral thigh. On examination, there is tenderness to palpation directly over the greater trochanter or immediately posterior to it. There is often weakness of the gluteus medius, gluteus maximus, and hip external rotators, as well as tightness of the tensor fascia lata. The modified Thomas test is used to assess for inflexibility around the hip girdle. Muscle function along the entire kinetic chain, from the core region to the ankle, should be evaluated by biomechanical assessment while the patient is running or riding. An audible snap (lateral snapping hip syndrome) can be heard as the ITB rubs over the greater trochanter. Treatment involves reduction of exacerbating activities, reduction of pain and inflammation and facilitation of a stretching program by ice application, exercise based on the patient's relevant biomechanical deficits (deficiencies in range of movement, flexibility, strength, endurance, or motor control), and training of the core musculature to stabilize the pelvis. It also includes appropriate training regimens, ITB massage, myofascial release, therapeutic ultrasound (US), and use of off-the-shelf and custom-made foot orthoses for reducing impact and improving subtalar positioning and tibial rotation.

Strains of the hip adductor muscles are usually caused by forceful activation of these muscles while participating in soccer, hockey, and skiing. They occur most commonly at or near the origin of the muscles at the inferior pubic ramus. Physical examination reveals pain during passive stretch and active resistance testing. Radiographs are necessary when looking for avulsion factures. Magnetic resonance imaging (MRI) can show signal changes in the area of injury (eSlide 36.1).

Treatment includes early, gradually progressive range of movement exercises and careful strengthening exercises, with return to sport-specific exercises when tolerated. The entire kinetic chain, the hip adductor–abductor force couple, and the core muscles should be addressed.

Combined Muscle Group Injuries

Pes anserine tendonitis involves acute inflammation and tendinosis (from subacute or chronic irritation) of the tendons of the semitendinosus, sartorius, or gracilis muscles near their insertion at the proximal, anteromedial tibia. Inflammation of the bursa that lies just under the tendons is termed pes anserine bursitis. The patient typically complains of pain, with a history of a sudden increase in activity level. There is local tenderness on palpation. Common biomechanical deficits include a weak core musculature, medial hamstrings, and hip adductors. The rehabilitation program focuses on overcoming the biomechanical deficits of the pes anserine muscles, the entire kinetic chain, and the core muscles, as well as correcting any muscle imbalances. Impaired subtalar motion and abnormal tibial rotation should also be addressed. Running gait and cycling mechanics need to be analyzed; they should be modified if necessary. Running shoes and inserts should be appropriate for each individual's biomechanical characteristics. The pes anserine tendons and bursa can be visualized by both US and MRI. A local corticosteroid injection can help facilitate an active exercise program.

Athletic pubalgia and sportsman's hernia refer to a spectrum of disorders that cause pain in the lower abdomen and groin. These disorders are caused by overload of one or more of the lower abdominal muscles near the superior pubic ramus, strain of the hip flexors or hip adductors, a stress response or stress fracture of the pubic rami, pubic symphysitis, or a defect in the abdominal wall fascia (eSlide 36.2).

They are most commonly seen in football, soccer, and hockey players. Maximizing core stability and restoring full range of movement, strength, endurance, and motor control of the core muscles, hip flexors, and adductors are the keys to successful rehabilitation. As soon as they are tolerated by the patient, exercise movements should be started to retrain muscle groups within the kinetic chain. These exercises should stimulate the muscle groups to function as they normally do during functional or athletic activities. Surgical consultation should be considered if there is suspicion of a fascial defect of the anterior abdominal wall or a true inguinal hernia. Impact or repetitive loading activities should be avoided in the setting of bone overload, such as a pelvic stress response or stress fracture.

Injuries to the Quadriceps Muscle Group

Patellar tendinopathy (jumper's knee) is characterized by a maximum point of pain at the inferior pole of the patella. Individuals at risk for this condition are those who participate in repetitive knee flexion and extension activities, such as basketball players, volleyball players, bicyclists, rowers, and mogul skiers. The muscle groups involved in the jumping motion should be evaluated for eccentric as well as concentric function. MRI and US both provide adequate visualization of the patellar tendon (eSlide 36.3).

Treatment includes ice application, nonsteroidal antiinflammatory drugs (NSAIDs), cross-friction massage, modalities, quadriceps stretching and strengthening exercises, addressing relevant biomechanical deficits, use of a patellar tendon strap, and correction of any errors in training technique. In refractory cases, surgical débridement of the tendon might be of benefit.

Osgood-Schlatter disease presents as pain at the tibial tuberosity that is exacerbated with activities and direct contact. It occurs in young adolescents. Repetitive overload at the patella tendon insertion site can cause inflammation, irregularity, or partial avulsion of the secondary ossification center of the tibial tuberosity. The radiographic hallmark of the disorder is irregularity and fragmentation of the tibial tuberosity (eSlide 36.4).

The rehabilitation program includes ice application, NSAIDs, gently progressive quadriceps stretching, careful pain-free quadriceps strengthening, and activity modification. Symptoms usually resolve spontaneously when the growth plates close.

Quadriceps contusions and myositis ossificans are other knee conditions. Contusions of the quadriceps muscle group resulting from direct trauma to the front of the thigh are fairly common (eSlide 36.5).

The patient typically reports pain, stiffness, and difficulty with weight bearing and knee flexion. Tenderness, ecchymosis, and swelling in the anterior thigh are found. Radiographs are necessary to exclude the presence of a femur fracture. Ice application and early range of movement exercises should be started to decrease muscle stiffness. An intramuscular hematoma can undergo calcific transformation, resulting in myositis ossificans. The quadriceps is the most common location for this to occur. The diagnosis is confirmed by a bone scan and MRI, which are sensitive in the early stages of the condition. First-line treatment includes progressive range of movement and medications. Surgical resection of the calcified tissue is indicated for unresponsive cases that are impinging nerves or restricting functional range of movement, but only after maturation of the mass. Surgery is followed by radiation to prevent recurrence.

Patellofemoral arthralgia (patellofemoral pain syndrome, chondromalacia) refers to pain in the patellofemoral joint. It is the most common cause of knee pain in the younger population. Usually patellofemoral arthralgia is the result of abnormal mechanics along the kinetic chain: a tight quadriceps muscle or ITB, ineffective oblique portion of the vastus medialis, the presence of pes planus, or weak external rotators and abductors of the hip. A mainstay of clinical diagnosis is tenderness to palpation under the medial and lateral aspects of the patella and pain with medial-lateral glide and tilt maneuvers. The differential diagnosis includes infrapatellar or suprapatellar bursitis, synovial plica, quadriceps tendonitis, patellar tendonitis, and intraarticular pathology. Initial treatment protocols include ice application, NSAIDs, strengthening weak or imbalanced muscle groups in the core and lower limbs (especially the quadriceps muscle), stretching tight structures, activity modification, patellofemoral taping techniques, and specific patellofemoral control braces. Patellofemoral forces can be minimized by performing closed kinetic chain quadriceps strengthening exercises between 0 degrees and 30 degrees of flexion. If a patient fails to respond to noninterventional measures, corticosteroid or hyaluronate injections, acupuncture, and arthroscopy should be considered, although evidence of their effectiveness is limited. Surgical intervention includes release of the lateral retinaculum and tightening or reconstruction of the medial patellofemoral ligament.

Injuries to the Posterior Leg Muscle Group and Associated Soft Tissue Structures

Achilles tendon overload is common and is either chronic or acute. In the chronic setting, typical changes of tendinosis can be seen clinically, such as a swollen, nodular, tender Achilles tendon. US and MRI show typical changes that correspond to the microscopic features (breakdown of the normal collagen orientation, vacuole formation, and microscopic tearing) (eSlide 36.6). In addition to usual rehabilitation protocols, eccentric strength training has been shown to be especially effective. Newer treatment modalities, such as platelet-rich plasma injections and extracorporeal shock-wave therapy, should be considered.

Acute rupture of the Achilles tendon occurs as a result of a sudden powerful eccentric force; it is sometimes accompanied by an audible pop. On examination, there will be swelling and a palpable defect in the tendon and difficulty with plantar flexion. Treatment may involve surgical reconstruction, followed by immobilization and then aggressive rehabilitation. The alternative treatment approach involves immobilization for 3 months, followed by aggressive rehabilitation.

Chronic exertional compartment syndrome (CECS) of the lower extremity is a condition in which the pressure within a given muscle compartment is abnormally elevated. It is seen most commonly in high-volume runners. Symptoms can mimic those of tendinopathy or a stress fracture. Patients with CECS complain of recurrent leg cramping or pain with activities. There might be neurologic symptoms, such as temporary foot drop during activities, that are due to compression of the tibial or peroneal nerves. Definitive diagnosis is made by intramuscular compartment pressure testing. Newer MRI imaging techniques that measure increased T2 signal in a specific compartment after exercise might confirm the diagnosis noninvasively. Treatment can be challenging; it includes avoiding inciting activities, massage therapy, fasciotomy, or fasciectomy.

Plantar fasciitis is an enthesopathy at the calcaneus caused by overload of the plantar foot muscles, producing volar heel pain or inflammation and pain in the plantar fascia. Pain is usually worse with the first few steps in the morning. Tenderness to palpation is present at the volar aspect of the heel, slightly medial to the midline. A kinetic chain evaluation might reveal predisposing biomechanical deficits, such as a tight heel cord or tibialis posterior or tibialis anterior deficits. The presence of a calcaneal traction spur correlates poorly with symptoms of plantar fasciitis. The rehabilitation plan should focus on restoring range of movement, strength, endurance, and motor control of the heel cord and foot intrinsic muscles, as well as correction of biomechanical deficits along the kinetic chain. A resting night splint can be very helpful in preventing overnight tightening of the heel cord and plantar structures. Local injection of corticosteroid can relieve symptoms, but creates the risk of rupture of the plantar fascia.

DISORDERS OF THE JOINTS OF THE LOWER LIMB

Osteoarthritis (OA) in the weight-bearing joints of the lower extremities is very common. It is not a purely degenerative condition, but there are various contributing factors, such as biomechanical factors, developmental abnormalities of the femur and acetabulum, local biochemical processes, genetic predisposition, prior joint trauma, and obesity. Pain, functional limitations, and stiffness in the morning lasting not more than 1 hour are the usual complaints in patients with OA. Pain from hip OA can refer to the groin region or into the anterior thigh down to the knee. The differential diagnosis of hip OA includes referred pain from the lumbar spine, anterior hip muscle pathology, and a hernia. Physical examination reveals an antalgic gait, reproduction of groin pain with passive hip internal rotation, and loss of internal rotation (which is one of the earliest findings). Knee OA can affect the three compartments of the joint. The medial compartment is often involved first, causing varus alignment. Other findings are joint line tenderness, crepitus, effusion, and palpable osteophytosis. Ankle arthritis is characterized by pain, swelling, and stiffness in the anterior ankle. Pain from subtalar arthritis is appreciated when walking on uneven surfaces. Osteoarthritis of the first metatarsophalangeal joint results in loss of dorsiflexion, joint swelling, and pain. The radiologic hallmarks of osteoarthritis include joint space narrowing, marginal osteophytosis, subchondral sclerosis, and subchondral cyst formation (eSlide 36.7).

Treatment of OA primarily focuses on symptom management and maintenance or restoration of functional capacity through a combination of nonpharmacologic and pharmacologic interventions. The evidence-based guidelines of the American College of Rheumatology for the treatment of hip and knee OA strongly recommend regular exercise (strength training and aerobic), weight loss, and activity modifications. Strategies aimed at reducing loads on the joints include weight loss, cushioned shoes, and walking aids, such as a cane. Acetaminophen, oral NSAIDs, and tramadol are conditionally recommended to reduce joint pain in hip and knee OA and topical NSAIDs in knee OA. Glucosamine and chondroitin sulfate supplementation are not recommended. Intraarticular corticosteroid injections are conditionally recommended for both hip and knee osteoarthritis. Injections of the foot, ankle, and hip joints are performed under US guidance. There is some evidence that intraarticular hyaluronate injections relieve pain and improve function in patients with mild to moderate knee osteoarthritis and limited evidence regarding their efficacy in other joints of the lower extremity. For patients with recalcitrant pain or severe functional limitations, arthroplasty can provide substantial improvement in pain and function.

Disorders of the Hip Joint

Avascular osteonecrosis is caused by ischemia to a bone, resulting in death of osteocytes and the surrounding marrow. This leads to microfractures and eventual collapse of the affected segment. The femoral head is the area most commonly affected. Avascular osteonecrosis can be caused by various conditions, including trauma, high doses of corticosteroids, alcohol abuse, and systemic illnesses, such as diabetes, systemic lupus erythematosus, and sickle cell anemia. Symptoms are similar to those experienced with hip OA. Radiographs can reveal sclerosis or collapse of the femoral head (eSlide 36.8).

MRI and computed tomography (CT) can detect the condition in its earlier stages. Conservative treatments include keeping weight off the affected joint and use of pain medications. Once collapse occurs, joint replacement surgery is indicated to improve pain and function. Legg-Calvé-Perthes disease is an idiopathic type of osteonecrosis of the femoral head that occurs in children, typically boys between the ages of 4 and 10 years. Because of the potential for revascularization and bone remodeling in children, the prognosis is significantly better than that of avascular osteonecrosis in adults. Good outcomes have been reported in children younger than 6 years of age who are treated nonsurgically with physical therapy, protected weight bearing, and femoral head containment by bracing or casting. Osteotomy is often performed in older children.

Hip dislocation requires significant trauma. In adults, it is often accompanied by fractures of the acetabulum. Most commonly, the head of the femur dislocates posteriorly. The patient presents with severe hip pain and tends to hold the hip in flexion, internal rotation, and adduction. A complete neurologic examination should be performed to assess for lumbosacral plexopathy, sciatic neuropathy, and femoral neuropathy. Radiographs are sufficient to confirm the diagnosis. Hip dislocations are considered an orthopedic emergency, and closed reduction under anesthesia should be performed as soon as possible. Surgery is indicated if closed reduction is unsuccessful. Non-weight bearing is recommended for 3–4 weeks, followed by protected weight bearing for an additional 3 weeks. Gradual, progressive rehabilitation can start a few days to a couple of weeks after reduction.

Disorders of the Knee Joint

In **knee ligament injuries**, the most commonly injured knee ligaments are the medial collateral ligament (MCL) and the anterior cruciate ligament (ACL). MCL sprains are usually caused by a sudden valgus force with the foot planted. The pain is localized to the medial side of the knee. Physical examination reveals tenderness along the course of the MCL and a positive valgus stress test. Medial knee swelling may be present, but an intraarticular effusion is absent in isolated MCL sprains. Radiographs are useful to rule out an associated bony injury. MRI is the imaging study of choice (eSlide 36.9). Initial treatment consists of ice application, elevation of the limb, and use of a knee immobilizer for 1–2 weeks to provide joint stability. Gentle knee flexion and extension exercises are initiated in the first 1–2 weeks after the injury, and gradual return to full activities occurs over 1–4 weeks, as tolerated. Isolated MCL tears rarely require surgery.

Tears of the ACL are the most functionally devastating ligament injury because of the crucial role of the ACL in the dynamic stability of the knee. The ACL courses from the medial wall of the lateral femoral condyle anteromedially to the anterior spine of the tibial plateau. ACL tears can occur as a result of contact or noncontact injuries. The history reveals rotation on a planted foot with the knee in flexion and the quadriceps activating strongly, a "pop" sensation, and a sense of knee instability, especially with twisting activities. When significant pain is present acutely, it can suggest the presence of a bone contusion or meniscus tear. On physical examination, an effusion is usually present, and the anterior drawer and Lachman's tests (most sensitive for ACL sprain) are positive (Video 36.1). Radiographs can show a small capsular avulsion fracture of the lateral tibial plateau (Segond fracture), which is considered pathognomonic for the presence of an ACL tear (eSlide 36.10).

MRI is often obtained to confirm the clinical diagnosis (eSlide 36.11). The management of acute ACL tears includes aggressive use of ice application, elevation, and compression, as well as a knee immobilizer or hinged knee brace. Early, gentle knee flexion and extension exercises can minimize the development of stiffness. Straight leg raises performed in the knee immobilizer promote safe quadriceps activation. Rehabilitation is needed to maximize muscular control of the joint. Young, healthy individuals actively involved in sports should strongly consider ligament reconstruction, which is generally recommended at least 2–3 weeks after the injury to allow time for swelling and stiffness to decrease. The use of functional knee braces provides some benefit in moderate activities but cannot prevent an ACL injury.

A common mechanism for **PCL disruption** is a forceful blow to the proximal anterior leg, typically seen in soccer goalkeepers who get kicked in the shin and in people injured during motor vehicle accidents who sustain a "dashboard" injury. The clinical diagnosis is based on a positive posterior drawer test. MRI can confirm the diagnosis. Acute nonsurgical management is similar to that for ACL injuries. Most individuals with isolated PCL injuries can return to full activities, including athletics, with functional rehabilitation. On rare occasions, surgical reconstruction is performed.

Knee meniscal injuries are common injuries; a sudden or forceful twisting motion on a planted foot is the most common mechanism of injury for acute meniscal tears. The patient typically reports slow onset of swelling after the injury, and pain that occurs with weight bearing and twisting maneuvers. Locking of the knee suggests the presence of a bucket handle meniscus tear (eSlide 36.12). Physical examination reveals medial or lateral joint line tenderness, effusion, and a positive McMurray test. MRI is the study of choice to evaluate meniscus tears. Initial treatments include ice, elevation, NSAIDs, and bracing. Simple tears and those in the outer portion of the meniscus, referred to as the vascularized "red zone," have greater healing potential. In older athletes and in the absence of mechanical symptoms, it is reasonable to allow 3–6 weeks of relative rest and rehabilitation. Referral for arthroscopic intervention is indicated if the patient remains limited in function, has persistent mechanical symptoms, or has recurrent episodes of pain and swelling. Elite and young athletes often proceed earlier to arthroscopy for repair or débridement of the meniscus with partial meniscectomy.

An **osteochondral lesion (osteochondritis dissecans)** is a lesion of subchondral bone that can progress to secondarily affect the overlying articular cartilage. The underlying mechanism is multifactorial. The knee is the most common location for this condition, especially along the lateral aspect of the medial femoral condyle. Adolescent (10- to 15-year-old) boys are most commonly affected. Symptoms include recurrent swelling and pain with activity and a positive Wilson test, which involves extending the knee 30 degrees with the foot internally rotated. Diagnosis usually requires imaging studies or direct arthroscopic visualization. Treatment varies from relative rest to surgery, depending on the grade and severity of symptoms.

Disorders of the Ankle and Subtalar Joints

Ankle sprains are the most common musculoskeletal injury in the lower limb, comprising 25% of all sports injuries. The most commonly injured ligament is the anterior talofibular ligament. Syndesmotic injuries involving the thick ligaments connecting the tibia and fibula are often referred to as "high" ankle sprains. Sprains of the deltoid ligament on the medial aspect of the ankle are often associated with a fracture in the distal fibula or medial malleolus. Ankle injuries are graded from simple distortion or partial tear in the ligament with no instability (grade 1) to partial or complete tear of the ligament with instability (grades 2 and 3, respectively). The anterior drawer test will usually be positive in grade 2 and 3 sprains. A positive squeeze test and external rotation test are suggestive of a syndesmotic injury. When tenderness is present over the distal fibula, ankle joint, syndesmosis, base of the fifth metatarsal, or other bony structures, radiographs should be obtained to exclude the presence of a fracture (eSlide 36.13). Treatment includes ice application, compressive wrapping of the ankle, elevation, early mobilization, bracing, balance and proprioceptive training, dynamic strengthening, and sport-specific functional drills. With a functional rehabilitation program, the patient can return to full activity within a few days to weeks. Medial ankle sprains and syndesmotic injuries require more time to heal (5–10 weeks) and are more likely to require surgical stabilization. Up to 40% of ankle sprains lead to persistent problems with pain and instability. "Functional" instability might be caused by peroneal muscle weakness, proprioceptive deficit, and subtalar instability. Balance exercises and peroneal strengthening can restore functional stability to even mechanically unstable ankles. Surgery can be indicated after failure of an extended period (6 months) of appropriate aggressive ankle strength and stability treatment in patients with symptomatic mechanical instability.

MORTON INTERDIGITAL NEUROMA, METATARSALGIA, AND SESAMOIDITIS

Morton neuroma is caused by irritation of one of the interdigital nerves of the foot and is most commonly located between the third and fourth metatarsal heads. The patient typically presents with pain between the metatarsal heads, as well as pain and paresthesias in the two toes innervated by the interdigital nerve. Pain is exacerbated with forefoot weight bearing, narrow toe boxes, and high heels. The differential diagnosis is metatarsalgia, in cases where pain originates from the second metatarsal head, and there is an injury to the sesamoid bones in the flexor hallucis tendon. First-line interventions aim to unload the forefoot: avoiding high heels, wearing shoes that have larger toe boxes, using gel inserts, and wearing custom-made foot orthoses. Local injection with anesthetic and corticosteroid is often useful both diagnostically and therapeutically for interdigital neuroma, but not for metatarsalgia. For recalcitrant neuroma, surgical excision can be considered.

• BONE INJURIES OF THE LOWER LIMB

Stress reactions and stress fractures are caused by repetitive overload injuries to bones, and they are common in individuals who participate in endurance activities, such as distance running (eSlide 36.14). Intrinsic risk factors include poor dietary habits, altered menstrual status, and biomechanical abnormalities that do not allow for proper distribution of forces along the kinetic chain. Extrinsic factors can include types of training surfaces, footwear, and insoles or training errors. The patient usually provides a history of a recent acceleration in the intensity or duration of training and complains of insidious onset of focal pain that is exacerbated with weight-bearing activities. In some stress fractures, such as femoral neck or navicular fractures, symptoms can be vague, thus increasing the time to diagnosis. The differential diagnosis usually includes tendinopathy, enthesopathy, and CECS. CT provides optimal definition of the bony architecture.

A 6-week period of relative rest with nonimpact rehabilitation and alternative training methods, such as pool running, can be instituted. Most stress fractures heal without complication with activity modification and allow gradual return to sports in 4–8 weeks. Initial treatment includes pain management using acetaminophen (not NSAIDs, which might prevent optimal repair of the stress fracture), ice application, activity modification, strengthening exercises, fitness maintenance, and risk factor modification. Cross-training activities, such as cycling, swimming, water running, rowing, and use of StairMaster, are recommended to maintain cardiopulmonary fitness. A progressive increase in load is necessary to allow the bone to adapt by increasing its strength. Specific treatment is required for some stress fractures that may develop complications: femoral neck, anterior cortex of the middle third of the tibia, navicular, and proximal fifth metatarsal fractures. In femoral neck stress fractures, symptoms are often vague, and an MRI should be obtained to establish the diagnosis and reduce the risk of complications, such as fracture displacement or avascular necrosis (eSlide 36.15).

Fractures on the compression side are more common. If the fracture line extends greater than 50% of the width of the femoral neck, percutaneous fixation should be considered because the likelihood of displacement is increased. In other cases, strict non-weight bearing is necessary for approximately 4–6 weeks until the patient is pain free. This should be followed by functional rehabilitation with progressive weight bearing over the next 4–8 weeks (according to symptoms). Navicular fractures have a higher likelihood of delayed union, nonunion, or avascular necrosis. Therefore, early diagnosis by MRI, bone scan, or CT and appropriate treatment are important. If these fractures propagate across the body of the bone, early surgical intervention should be considered.

Clinical Pearls

Having a sound understanding of anatomy and kinetic chain biomechanics, in conjunction with fundamental history and physical examination skills, permits a practitioner to establish appropriate diagnoses for patients presenting with soft tissue, bone, and joint disorders of the lower limbs. Imaging studies can help confirm clinical diagnoses. The majority of lower limb injuries can be successfully treated with nonoperative measures that include medications, activity modification, and intelligent exercise strategies. The practitioner should be able to recognize injuries that require surgical consultation.

BIBLIOGRAPHY
The complete bibliography is available on ExpertConsult.com.

Chronic Pain

Yung-Tsan Wu

This chapter provides a foundation for comprehensive pain management skills. It discusses our current understanding of both physiologic and pathophysiologic mechanisms of pain, the impact of psychosocial factors on the experience of pain, and the role of these factors in pain assessment and treatment. An interdisciplinary approach appears to be the best model for successful and comprehensive chronic pain management.

• PAIN DEFINED

Chronic pain is defined as an ongoing pain, lasting 3–6 months after the initiating event, without a history of a noxious event or pathologic process (eSlide 37.1). Chronic pain involves a dynamic interplay of additional psychological and behavioral mechanisms (eSlide 37.2). A list of pain terminologies and definitions is included for review in eSlide 37.3.

• PREVALENCE

Prevalence rates of chronic pain vary widely, from 2% to 55% in the general population. Chronic pain is especially common in patients with a primary disability, such as spinal cord injury, amputation, cerebral palsy, and multiple sclerosis (greater than 70%), and its presence can substantially add to the disability.

• PHYSIOLOGY AND PATHOPHYSIOLOGY OF PAIN

The complex interactions involved in the perception of pain can be described by four general processes, known as transduction, transmission, modulation, and perception (eSlide 37.4). Normal pain, or nociception, is primarily characterized by the processes of transduction and transmission, with minimal emphasis on modulation. With a chronic or persistent state of pain, there is a shift of focus to the processes of modulation and perception.

Transduction

The principal receptors for pain are the branched endings of C and Aδ nerve fibers (eSlide 37.5) located in the skin, muscles, and joints. When damaging energy in the cellular environment affects the free nerve endings, the processes of nociceptive transduction occur. There are two broad categories of C fibers: peptidergic and isolectin B_4-binding. Peptidergic fibers (substance P and calcitonin gene-related peptide [CGRP]) appear to be key players in neurogenic inflammation and other chronic inflammatory states. Isolectin B_4-binding is supported by glial-derived neurotrophic factors, which have emerged as potential factors involved in activity-dependent changes at neural synapses and possibly subsequent central nervous system plasticity. Aδ nociceptors respond to noxious, thermal, and chemical stimuli. Type 2 Aδ fibers are responsible for the initial sensation of a burn stimulus. Type 1 Aδ and nociceptive C fibers are more commonly associated with persistent painful sensations.

Transmission

C and Aδ fibers carry noxious stimuli, and Aβ fibers carry innocuous stimuli (touch, vibration, and pressure) (eSlide 37.5). In the skin, the percentage of distribution of nociceptors for these fibers is roughly 70%, 10%, and 20%, respectively. Central neuroplastic changes in Aβ fibers might result in allodynia. Aδ nociceptors, with sensitization, contribute to the process called hyperpathia. Aδ fibers mediate the fast, prickling quality of pain, whereas C fibers mediate the slow, burning quality of pain.

Peripheral Sensitization

Excitatory amino acids and neuropeptides (substance P, CGRP, and neurokinins) are released by peripheral and central nociceptive C fibers, inducing neurogenic inflammation. Neurogenic inflammation involves retrograde release of algogenic substances, which in turn excite other nearby nociceptors, creating local feed-forward loops of sensitization and activation.

Modulation

Aδ and C fibers primarily convey nociceptive information to superficial laminae (I and II) and deep laminae (V and VI) of the dorsal horn. Aβ fibers transmit innocuous, mechanical stimuli to deeper laminae (III-VI). The lamina V cells respond to "wide" stimulus intensities and receive input from mechanoreceptive Aβ fibers and nociceptive (Aδ and C) fibers (eSlide 37.6). Prolonged depolarization of postsynaptic cells allows additional sodium and calcium to enter the cell; this amplified evoked response to subsequent input describes the process of wind-up.

Central Sensitization

Central sensitization describes a complex set of activation-dependent post-translational changes occurring at the dorsal horn, brainstem, and higher cerebral sites.

Ascending and Descending Modulation

The lateral (neospinothalamic) system generally represents sensory-discriminative dimensions, and the medial (paleospinothalamic) system involves more motivational-affective and cognitive-evaluative dimensions of the pain experience. The lateral system projects to the ventral posterolateral and posteromedial thalamic nuclei before projecting to the somatosensory and premotor cortices. The medial pathway projects to the medial thalamic nuclei and limbic cortices, which include the anterior cingulate cortex, orbitofrontal cortex, and amygdala. Descending inhibition includes local endogenous opioids (from the periaqueductal gray), biogenic amines (serotonin and noradrenaline [norepinephrine]), and gamma-aminobutyric acid (GABA), which generally act to inhibit pain signals. Activation of somatosensory cortices (S1-S2) provides information regarding the quality and intensity of pain. Higher processing involves the parietal and insular regions, contributing to an overall sense of intrusion and unpleasantness. Finally, convergence of these pathways with more frontal regions, such as the anterior cingulate cortex, is responsible for attention and emotional valence of the overall pain experience.

Psychological Issues Related to Chronic Pain

The physiatrist must understand the importance of psychological (affective and cognitive) factors that affect the experience of pain. Affective factors usually include relatively negative emotions, such as depression, pain-related anxiety, and anger. Cognitive factors include catastrophizing, fear, helplessness, decreased self-efficacy, pain coping, readiness to change, and acceptance.

Affective Factors
DEPRESSION
Prevalence estimates of major depression in patients with chronic pain vary from 5% to 87%. Predictors of depression in chronic pain include pain intensity, number of painful areas, frequency of experiencing severe pain, and a number of related psychosocial factors. Patients with depression report higher levels of pain, lower levels of activity, greater disability and life interference related to pain, and are more likely to display overt pain behaviors.

ANXIETY
Anxiety related to pain is an important factor involved in maladaptive responses, behavioral interference, and affective distress. In chronic pain, anxiety has been found to be a significant predictor of pain severity, disability, and pain behaviors.

ANGER
Chronic pain is associated with increased levels of anger and physiologic responses to pain, independent of pain intensity. Researchers have reported that 70% of subjects with pain have feelings of anger, most commonly directed toward themselves (74%) and health care professionals (62%).

Cognitive Factors

Many patients with chronic pain demonstrate a reduction in goal-directed activities and assume a more passive, sedentary lifestyle. This further contributes to the downward spiral of inactivity, deconditioning, and increased somatic focus.

Learning Factors
OPERANT LEARNING
Fordyce's operant conditioning primarily focuses on observable behavioral manifestations of pain, which are subject to both reinforcement and avoidance learning.

FEAR OF MOVEMENT
Kinesiophobia, describes an irrational and excessive fear of movement, physical activity, and reinjury. It is exhibited by many patients with chronic pain. Fear of movement can be initially induced by classical conditioning but is reinforced through operant learning.

• BEHAVIORAL TREATMENT APPROACHES

Operant Behavioral Techniques

Operant behavioral therapy refers to interventions focused on the observed behavior of the patient; it can be most useful and practical in patients demonstrating excessive pain behaviors. The goals include encouraging the development and acquisition of more adaptive pain management strategies.

Cognitive Behavioral Techniques

Cognitive behavioral therapy techniques are designed to help patients notice and modify negative thought patterns that contribute to ongoing pain and affective distress. These techniques include cognitive restructuring, problem solving, distraction, and relapse prevention.

• SLEEP AND CHRONIC PAIN

Sleep lasting 8–8.5 hours is considered restorative in adults. Prevalence estimates of disturbed sleep in chronic pain range from approximately 50%–90%. This inability to maintain sleep can be the most important factor in the treatment of disturbed sleep in individuals with chronic pain.

• ASSESSMENT

The assessment of chronic pain involves a thorough physical examination and a comprehensive evaluation of pain intensity and psychosocial factors related to the ongoing pain experience and interference with sleep, daily activities, family life, and employment. A 30% reduction in the numeric rating scale value for pain is considered to represent a clinically important difference. The measurements of pain intensity; psychosocial factors, such as mood (depression, anxiety, and anger), attitudes, beliefs, and personality traits; functional capacity; and activity interference are summarized in eSlide 37.7.

• TREATMENT

The ultimate goals of a rehabilitation-based approach to chronic pain are reduction of pain, maximal restoration of functional mobility, restoration of sleep, improvement in mood, resumption of leisure activities, and return to work.

Pain Treatment Programs

A multidisciplinary program formally refers to a collaboration of members of different disciplines, which is managed by a leader who directs a range of ancillary services. Team members assess and treat patients independently and then share information. Interdisciplinary programs involve a deeper level of a consensus-based collaboration, in which the entire process is orchestrated by the team, facilitated by regular face-to-face meetings, and primarily delivered within a single facility.

Interdisciplinary and Multidisciplinary Approaches

INTERDISCIPLINARY TREATMENT

Interdisciplinary, biopsychosocial, rehabilitation-based programs have been successfully used in the treatment of patients with chronic pain. The scope and intensity vary, with most outpatient-based centers offering part-time (2 days per week) or full-time (5 days per week, 6–8 hours per day) programs lasting 4–6 weeks in total duration.

MULTIDISCIPLINARY TEAM

Physical and occupational therapists use active and passive therapeutic exercises, manual techniques, and passive physical modalities (eSlide 37.8). They also play a primary role in the education of patients, family members, and other caregivers and must be adept in their ability to assess initial levels of functional ability and then monitor and progressively increase the level and complexity of therapeutic exercises. Pain psychology assessment and therapeutic interventions focus on both cognitive and behavioral factors related to pain. Factors involved in the development of, and maladaptation to, chronic pain include anxiety and fear-avoidance behavior, pain catastrophizing, and feelings of helplessness. Factors identified with improvement in adjustment to chronic pain include self-efficacy, pain-coping strategies, readiness to change, and acceptance (eSlide 37.9). Vocational counselors participate in the analysis of current or previous job descriptions, provide suggestions for work accommodation or modification, and, if necessary, facilitate vocational testing and targeted retraining. They should be involved early to ensure identification of employment as a long-term goal for the patient.

Medications

Drug therapy in chronic pain state requires a more comprehensive focus, including mood and sleep disturbances, whereas acute pain treatment primarily focuses on analgesia and control of inflammation.

NONSTEROIDAL ANTIINFLAMMATORY DRUGS (eSlides 37.10 and 37.11)

Conventional (nonselective) nonsteroidal antiinflammatory drugs (NSAIDs) have been a first-line treatment for analgesia and inflammatory conditions. Nonselective NSAIDs are limited by potential adverse effects, such as upper gastrointestinal bleeding and ulceration, renal toxicity, and platelet dysfunction.

OPIOID ANALGESICS (eSlides 37.12 and 37.13)

Opioids work by binding to three types of opioid receptors (μ, δ, and κ). However, because of the potential risk of abuse, misuse, addiction, diversion, and fatal adverse effects associated with these drugs, a "universal precautions" approach should be applied to the management plan for prescribing opioid analgesics on a chronic basis.

ANTICONVULSANT MEDICATIONS

Anticonvulsants have been largely used off-label for chronic pain. However, gabapentin (Neurontin) is approved for postherpetic neuralgia; pregabalin (Lyrica) is approved for postherpetic neuralgia, neuropathic pain associated with diabetic peripheral neuropathy or spinal cord injury, and fibromyalgia; and carbamazepine (Tegretol) is approved for the treatment of pain associated with trigeminal neuralgia. Off-label use of gabapentin includes diabetic peripheral neuropathy (titrated from 900–3600 mg/day) and postherpetic neuralgia. Gabapentin significantly reduces pain and improves sleep, mood, and quality of life at doses between 1800 and 3600 mg/day. Side effects include somnolence and dizziness. Pregabalin is also an $\alpha_2\delta$ ligand and is structurally related to gabapentin, but it has no intrinsic GABA activity. Studies have demonstrated that pregabalin, at doses between 150 and 600 mg/day, is efficacious for postherpetic neuralgia, diabetic peripheral neuropathy, general peripheral neuropathy, and generalized anxiety disorder. Compared with gabapentin, pregabalin might diminish the need for prolonged dose titration. Lamotrigine blocks voltage-dependent sodium channels and N-type calcium channels, and it also inhibits glutamate release. Doses from 50 to 400 mg/day are efficacious for trigeminal neuralgia and central poststroke pain resistant to other therapies. Oxcarbazepine has shown efficacy for postherpetic neuralgia, trigeminal neuralgia, and diabetic peripheral neuropathy at doses averaging between 600 and 1200 mg/day.

ANTIDEPRESSANTS

Antidepressants have demonstrated mixed efficacy in a number of chronic pain-related conditions (e.g., nociceptive, neuropathic, inflammatory, and poststroke pain conditions; central pain states; and headaches) and chronic pain-related disorders (e.g., depression, anxiety, and insomnia). Antidepressants can be divided into several general classes: tricyclic antidepressants (TCAs), selective serotonin reuptake inhibitors (SSRIs), selective serotonin-norepinephrine reuptake inhibitors (SNRIs), and triazolopyridines (i.e., trazodone and nefazodone).

Tricyclic Antidepressants and Selective Serotonin Reuptake Inhibitors. TCAs are effective for a variety of chronic pain conditions. Noradrenergic side effects can include autonomic (e.g., orthostatic hypotension, dizziness, and urinary retention), cardiac (e.g., tachycardia), and ocular (e.g., blurred vision) disturbances. Serotonergic effects can include increased gastric distress, agitation, and headaches. Antihistamine-mediated effects can include decreased gastric acid secretion and sedation. The so-called serotonin syndrome is a rare, reversible, clinical syndrome and medical emergency characterized by mental state dysfunction and autonomic and neurologic symptoms; it can occur with the concomitant use of TCAs and other medications, including SNRIs, SSRIs, and tramadol. Analgesic effects of TCAs can be evident within 1 week of dose initiation, followed later by antidepressant effects with escalating dose titration. Although the use of SSRIs has surpassed the use of traditional antidepressants because of their more tolerable side effect profile, analgesic effects of these compounds have shown mixed results in a number of controlled studies, including diabetic peripheral neuropathy and fibromyalgia.

Serotonin-Norepinephrine Reuptake Inhibitors. SNRIs are the newest class of antidepressants, with a shorter onset of antidepressant effects and fewer side effects because of their relative serotonin and norepinephrine selectivity. Mirtazapine is indicated for depression and can be used to enhance the efficacy of SSRIs and improve sleep. Venlafaxine has analgesic effects for heterogeneous chronic pain conditions, neuropathic pain states, and fibromyalgia. Duloxetine is indicated for major depressive disorder, diabetic peripheral neuropathy, and management of fibromyalgia.

Medications for Insomnia (eSlides 37.14 and 37.15)

The nonbenzodiazepine hypnotics, such as zolpidem, zaleplon, and eszopiclone, facilitate $GABA_A$ transmission by preferential binding to the 1a receptor subunits; therefore they are devoid of the significant muscle relaxant, anxiolytic, and anticonvulsant activities of traditional benzodiazepines. Eszopiclone is approved by the US Food and Drug Administration for treating long-term insomnia. It has a relatively long half-life (5–5.8 hours), and evidence indicates that it has greater sleep maintenance efficacy than zolpidem and zaleplon, which have shorter half-lives. TCAs and trazodone are especially useful for disturbed sleep that is present with concurrent chronic conditions, such as depression or neuropathic pain.

Patients with trouble initiating sleep might require shorter-acting medications, whereas those with fragmented sleep and frequent awakenings could more ideally benefit from medications with an intermediate to long half-life.

Little evidence supports the long-term use of benzodiazepines for the management of insomnia and anxiety in chronic pain. Chronic use might simply prevent rebound insomnia rather than promote restorative sleep. Chronic benzodiazepine use can lead to associated cognitive impairment, increase the risk for falls, produce rebound insomnia with prolonged use, disrupt normal sleep architecture, and promote misuse and abuse in patients with a history of substance-related disorders.

Topical Analgesics

Lidocaine 5% patches act peripherally by blocking sodium channels and are indicated for postherpetic neuralgia and focal peripheral neuropathic pain syndromes. Topical TCAs demonstrate efficacy in a number of neuropathic pain states. Topical capsaicin has demonstrated efficacy for diabetic peripheral neuropathy, HIV-associated neuropathic pain, and painful distal polyneuropathy.

Clinical Pearls

1. Chronic opioid analgesic therapy can lead to counterproductive effects, such as opioid hyperalgesia, impaired psychomotor functioning, and hypothalamic-pituitary-adrenal axis abnormalities.
2. Transduction describes the conversion of energy (thermal, mechanical, or chemical stimulus) into nerve impulses in primary afferents. Transmission is the transfer of this information to higher cortical structures. Modulation describes the activity-induced and signal-induced plasticity that occurs in the dorsal horn of the spinal cord. Perception occurs at the level of the cerebral cortex and involves the emotive aspects of pain.
3. Methadone, an N-methyl-D-aspartate receptor antagonist, is a long-acting opioid agonist with a half-life of 13–47 hours. It is commonly used for detoxification and maintenance of opioid dependence.
4. Hyperesthesia refers to increased sensitivity to stimulation, excluding the special senses. Allodynia describes pain due to a stimulus that does not normally provoke pain. Dysesthesia refers to an unpleasant abnormal sensation, whether spontaneous or evoked. Hyperalgesia is an increased response to a stimulus that is normally painful. Paresthesia is an abnormal sensation, whether spontaneous or evoked, that is not unpleasant.
5. The McGill Pain Questionnaire-Short Form includes 20 descriptors that evaluate the sensory, affective, and evaluative aspects of pain. The Survey of Pain Attitudes evaluates anxiety and coping, the Beck Depression Index evaluates depression, and the 36-Item Short-Form Health Survey evaluates functional capacity and activity limitations.
6. Whirlpool therapy works by convection; it is a superficial heating modality. Ultrasound and microwave are deep-heating modalities that work by the process of conversion. Paraffin baths and hydrocollator packs are superficial heating modalities that act by the process of conduction.

BIBLIOGRAPHY

The complete bibliography is available on ExpertConsult.com.

38 Pelvic Floor Disorders

Clarice N. Sinn

The pelvic floor consists of the muscles, fascia, and ligaments that support the pelvic organs and provide control for bodily functions. Disorders of the pelvic floor are a group of potentially disabling and often painful conditions that lead to the development of pelvic pain, dyspareunia, voiding dysfunction (including urinary incontinence or urgency), fecal incontinence, and pelvic organ prolapse. Women are more likely to develop pelvic floor disorders because of their unique anatomy, biomechanics, and risk of injury to the pelvic floor during pregnancy and childbirth. Abnormal biomechanics of the pelvic floor muscles (PFMs) may lead to changes in muscle contraction, relaxation, strength, and myofascial pain. An interdisciplinary approach to improve function and reduce pain is often beneficial for patients suffering from pelvic floor disorders. The anatomy and physical examination of the pelvic floor, definitions and epidemiology of pelvic floor disorders, and rehabilitation approach to the treatment of these disorders will be summarized in this chapter and accompanying eSlides.

• PELVIC FLOOR NEUROMUSCULOSKELETAL ANATOMY (eSlides 38.1 and 38.2)

The sacrum, ilium, ischium, and the pubic bones form the pelvic ring (Fig. 38.1), with the pelvic floor consisting of muscles, ligaments, and fascia acting as a sling to support the bladder, reproductive organs, and rectum. The anterior sacroiliac ligaments stabilize the joint by resisting upward movement of the sacrum and lateral movement of the ilium, while the posterior sacroiliac ligaments resist downward and upward movement of the sacrum and medial motion of the ilium. The pubic symphysis resists tension, shearing, and compression; it undergoes great mechanical stress as it widens during pregnancy. Somatic, visceral, and central pathways innervate the PFMs. The pudendal nerve arises from the ventral branches of S2-S4 of the sacral plexus and is the most clinically relevant nerve mentioned in this chapter because it contributes to external genital sensation, continence, orgasm, and ejaculation.

• PELVIC FLOOR PHYSICAL EXAMINATION

It is important to perform a thorough musculoskeletal examination of the lumbar spine, hips, pelvic girdle, lower limbs, and PFMs, as well as a vaginal and rectal examination of PFM function and a neurologic examination of the lower sacral segments. The examination should start with an external inspection for swelling, cysts, scars, and lesions, then proceed to visualizing the lift of the perineal body with a voluntary contraction (Kegel) and an involuntary contraction (cough), as

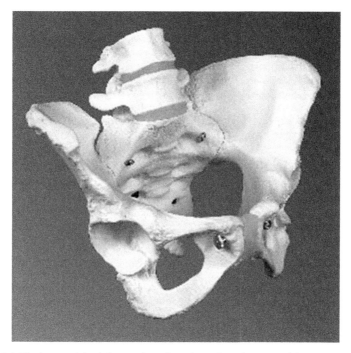

FIG. 38.1 The bony pelvic girdle consists of two innominate bones and the sacrum, which are connected by two posterior sacroiliac joints and one anterior pubic symphysis joint.

TABLE 38.1 Possible Etiologies of Pelvic Floor Pain or Dysfunction by Medical Specialty

Gynecologic	Gastrointestinal/ Genitourinary	Musculoskeletal	Psychological
Vulvodynia	Interstitial cystitis	Low back pain	Anxiety
Dysmenorrhea	Urgency/frequency	Lumbar radiculopathy	Depression
Endometriosis	syndrome	Sacroiliac joint dysfunction	History of abuse
Fibroids	Levator ani syndrome	Coccydynia	
Organ prolapse	Bowel or bladder	Hip disorders	
	incontinence		

well as normal descent of the perineal body with voluntary relaxation and involuntary relaxation (Valsalva maneuver). An external sensory examination of the S2-S5 sacral dermatomes should also be conducted. Checking the anal wink reflex will test the sacral reflex arc.

TYPES OF PELVIC FLOOR DYSFUNCTION

A differential diagnosis of the possible etiologies of pelvic floor dysfunction is listed in Table 38.1.

Urinary Incontinence (eSlides 38.3 and 38.4)

Urinary incontinence is the involuntary leakage of urine and can be divided into three main types: stress urinary incontinence (SUI), urge urinary incontinence (UUI), and mixed urinary incontinence (MUI). SUI is the loss of urine with increased intra-abdominal pressure, such as during coughing, laughing, sneezing, or physical exertion. It is caused by pregnancy, vaginal delivery, pelvic surgery, pelvic organ prolapse, neurologic disorders, active lifestyle, obesity, and aging. UUI is an involuntary leakage accompanied, or immediately preceded, by the sudden onset of an urge to void that cannot be deferred easily. UUI may be caused by neurogenic disorders, such as spinal cord injury, spinal stenosis, multiple sclerosis, or stroke. MUI occurs when a patient experiences symptoms of both SUI and UUI. Urinary incontinence is often discovered during routine screening evaluation for back pain or during the review of systems.

Management of urinary incontinence includes pharmacologic, surgical, behavioral, and exercise-based treatments. Behavioral and lifestyle alterations include dietary changes, regulation of fluid intake, and bladder training. Kegel exercises can be used to strengthen the PFMs to increase support for the bladder and urethra and reduce episodes of SUI. Pharmacologic management of UUI consists of anticholinergic medications to decrease urgency and detrusor instability by blocking parasympathetic innervation of the bladder. Botulinum toxin injections to the detrusor muscle or neuromodulation by stimulating the S3 sacral nerve root can also be used to decrease detrusor muscle contractility. Therapies for SUI include urethral bulking agents and surgery, such as a midurethral sling.

Urinary Urgency and Frequency (eSlide 38.5)

Urinary urgency is defined as "the complaint of a sudden compelling desire to pass urine that is difficult to defer," whereas frequency of urination is considered abnormal when urination occurs more than every 2–3 hours. The symptoms of urgency and frequency are similar to those of UUI and can be associated with or without incontinence, daytime frequency, and nocturia. Patients with *overactive* PFMs may feel that they have a constant or exaggerated urge to void because of increased external pressure around the urethra, and they can have difficulty with voluntary relaxation. Patients can be treated conservatively with pelvic floor physical therapy, biofeedback, urge suppression techniques, and bladder training.

Fecal Incontinence (eSlide 38.6)

Fecal incontinence (FI) is defined as the involuntary loss of liquid or solid stool that is a social or hygienic problem. The physical examination should include a thorough neurologic and spine examination, as well as a digital rectal examination to assess sphincter tone and the PFMs. Treatment includes conservative measures, such as dietary modifications, medications, and pelvic floor rehabilitation, as well as more invasive approaches, such as perianal injectable bulking agents, sacral nerve stimulation, or surgery. Pelvic floor rehabilitation techniques have been successfully used in the treatment of FI and can produce significant functional and quality of life benefits for patients. Incorporating education regarding lifestyle strategies, such as optimal fluid intake and dietary adjustments, into the therapeutic treatment program is of vital importance for patients with FI.

Functional Constipation (eSlide 38.7)

Functional constipation must include two or more of the following: straining during at least 25% of defecations, lumpy or hard stools in at least 25% of defecations, sensation of incomplete evacuation with at least 25% of defecations, sensation of anorectal obstruction or blockage with at least 25% of defecations, manual maneuvers to facilitate at least 25% of defecations, and fewer than three defecations per week. The physical examination should include an abdominal examination and digital rectal examination to assess the sphincter tone and the PFMs. Diagnostic testing for functional constipation includes anorectal manometry to assess dyssynergia, a Sitz marker study to assess colonic motility, and defecography to help distinguish between the many causes of outlet dysfunction constipation. The treatment of functional constipation depends greatly on the cause. *Slow transit constipation* can benefit from increasing fluid intake, fiber supplementation, magnesium supplementation, and stool softener or laxative use. *Dyssynergia* is ideally treated with pelvic floor physical therapy with biofeedback and pelvic floor relaxation training; however, severe cases may require botulinum toxin injections in the puborectalis muscle.

Pelvic Floor Myofascial Pain (eSlide 38.8)

Pelvic floor myofascial dysfunction refers to abnormal muscle activation patterns of the PFMs and is characterized by muscular pain, taut bands, and trigger points that cause pain referral with pressure. It is usually the result of underlying overuse or weakness of the muscles. Patients will report pain that is "deep" and internal, as well as associated symptoms of dysuria, dyschezia, dysmenorrhea, or dyspareunia. Pelvic floor physical therapy is the mainstay of rehabilitation treatment for pelvic floor myofascial pain to restore muscle imbalances, improve function, and reduce pain. Medications, such as nonsteroidal antiinflammatory drugs (NSAIDs), tricyclic antidepressants (TCAs [e.g., nortriptyline]), antiepileptics (e.g., gabapentin or pregabalin), serotonin and norepinephrine reuptake inhibitors (SNRIs [e.g., duloxetine or venlafaxine]), or muscle relaxants (e.g., cyclobenzaprine), can be helpful in reducing pain, treating anxiety, and restoring restful sleep. Trigger point injections, botulinum toxin injections, corticosteroid injections, and dry needling can also be considered.

Pregnancy and Postpartum Pelvic Floor Dysfunction (eSlides 38.9 and 38.10)

During pregnancy there is an increase in body mass, and as the fetus grows, the abdominal muscles lengthen and there is an increase in the lumbar lordosis, anterior pelvic tilt, and pelvic width. Hormonal changes also increase joint laxity. All of these changes lead to increased demands being placed on the hip extensors, hip abductors, ankle plantar flexors, and PFMs, all of which can generate pain. The mainstay of treatment is individualized physical therapy that includes realignment and stabilizing exercises. Pelvic manipulations, sacroiliac joint (SIJ) belts, ice application, acetaminophen, topical lidocaine patches, and cyclobenzaprine can be used for symptomatic relief. Low-dose opioids are generally considered safe and may be necessary. NSAIDs are not thought to be safe for use during pregnancy, but may be resumed in the postpartum period.

Pelvic Nerve Injuries (eSlides 38.11 and 38.12)

Neural injury can be a source of chronic pelvic pain and can coexist with pelvic floor dysfunction and pelvic floor myofascial pain. The iliohypogastric, ilioinguinal, genitofemoral, and pudendal nerves most commonly contribute to pelvic pain symptoms. Electrodiagnostic studies for these nerves are technically difficult to perform; therefore these studies are not routinely used. Diagnostic nerve blocks are a potentially good option for diagnosing iliohypogastric, ilioinguinal, and genitofemoral neuropathies, although they are less useful for pudendal neuropathies. Magnetic resonance neurography of the lumbosacral plexus can also be performed to demonstrate injury to the iliohypogastric, ilioinguinal, genitofemoral, and pudendal nerves. Treatment options for pelvic nerve injuries consist of pelvic floor physical therapy and medications. Medications for neuropathic pain, such as gabapentin, pregabalin, SNRIs, or TCAs, may be beneficial. Corticosteroid injections, radiofrequency ablation, and pulsed radiofrequency treatments have also been found to be useful. A neurectomy is the preferred surgical option for the iliohypogastric, ilioinguinal, and genitofemoral nerves. However, surgical decompression of the pudendal nerve has been less successful.

• OVERLAP OF PELVIC FLOOR DISORDERS AND CHRONIC PELVIC PAIN

Chronic pelvic pain (CPP) is defined as a noncyclic pain, lasting for 6 months or longer, localized to the anatomic pelvis, anterior abdominal wall at or below the umbilicus, lumbosacral back, or buttocks; it is severe enough to cause some disability. Unfortunately, many patients undergo surgical interventions for presumed visceral origins before musculoskeletal causes are considered, which delays diagnosis and treatment of musculoskeletal pelvic pain.

Interstitial Cystitis/Painful Bladder Syndrome (eSlide 38.13)

Interstitial cystitis/painful bladder syndrome (IC/PBS) is a urologic diagnosis characterized by suprapubic pain and urinary urgency and frequency. On pelvic examination, anterior vaginal wall, bladder base, and PFM tenderness is often found, with suprapubic tenderness being a hallmark finding.

Endometriosis (eSlide 38.13)

Endometriosis is defined as the presence of endometrial glands and stroma outside the endometrial cavity and uterine musculature. It is characterized by disabling menstrual cramps, CPP, or low back pain. The diagnostic standard of care is laparoscopic excision of endometrial implants, with histologic confirmation.

Irritable Bowel Syndrome (eSlide 38.14)

Irritable bowel syndrome is defined as a condition with at least 3 months of continuous or recurrent symptoms, including pain relieved by defecation and/or associated with change in frequency of stool or consistency of stool. Physical examination is generally normal.

Vulvodynia (eSlide 38.14)

Vulvodynia is defined as focal chronic nonmalignant urogenital pain characterized by chronic vulvar discomfort without any visual abnormality. Common symptoms include itching, burning, stinging, or stabbing in the area around the opening of the vagina.

Rehabilitation Treatment for Chronic Pelvic Pain (eSlide 38.15)

First-line treatment for IC/PBS should be general relaxation, stress and pain management, patient education, and self-care. Second-line treatment involves manual pelvic floor physical therapy, along with consideration of medications, such as amitriptyline, cimetidine, and hydroxyzine. Patients with IC/PBS are advised to avoid citrus, chocolate, caffeine, sodas, alcohol, and heavily seasoned foods. Medical treatment for irritable bowel syndrome ranges from laxatives and prokinetics to antibiotics, probiotics, and neuropathic pain medications. Vulvodynia treatments have included dietary modifications, physical therapy, and surgery.

• CONCLUSION

In summary, pelvic floor disorders are generally not life-threatening, but they can greatly affect one's quality of life. The prevalence of these disorders is likely to be higher than reported because many individuals are embarrassed by their symptoms and do not report them to health care providers. Diagnosis of pelvic floor disorders can often be made with a history and physical examination. Treatment should include a trial of conservative therapies that can often provide significant symptom reduction and improved quality of life.

Clinical Pearls

- Abnormal biomechanics of the pelvic floor muscles (PFMs) may lead to changes in muscle contraction, relaxation, and strength, and myofascial pain.
- Urinary incontinence is the involuntary leakage of urine, which can be divided into three main types: stress urinary incontinence (SUI), urge urinary incontinence (UUI), and mixed urinary incontinence (MUI).
- SUI is the loss of urine with increased intraabdominal pressure, such as during coughing, laughing, sneezing, or physical exertion.
- UUI is involuntary leakage accompanied, or immediately preceded, by the sudden onset of an urge to void, which cannot be deferred easily.
- The mainstay of pharmacologic management of overactive bladder and UUI are anticholinergic medications that decrease urgency and detrusor instability by blocking parasympathetic innervation of the bladder.
- When prescribing interventions for fecal incontinence, one should consider pelvic floor rehabilitation, biofeedback therapy, and increasing fiber intake.
- Pregnancy-related pelvic floor dysfunction is related to an increase in lumbar lordosis, anterior pelvic tilt, and pelvic width, as well as anterior shift in the center of gravity while the fetus grows.
- When considering pudendal neuralgia as a source of chronic pelvic pain, one should be aware that it does not usually affect anal sphincter tone.
- Interstitial cystitis/painful bladder syndrome is a urologic diagnosis characterized by suprapubic pain and urinary urgency and frequency. It is more likely to occur if there is a history of sexual abuse.

BIBLIOGRAPHY
The complete bibliography is available on ExpertConsult.com.

39 Sports Medicine and Adaptive Sports

Joseph E. Herrera

This chapter is an overview of the key concepts of sports medicine for physiatrists, including the role of a team physician, athletic conditioning and training principles, injury prevention and functional rehabilitation, the biomechanics of sports, performance-enhancing drugs, emergency care, and common medical conditions in athletes. It also presents a review of specific populations of athletes and adaptive sports.

• ROLE OF THE TEAM PHYSICIAN

The team physician has multiple roles when working with the team, individual athletes and their families, the school, and the community. The primary responsibility is caring for the health and well-being of the individual athlete. The principal duties are determining medical eligibility, providing care for the injured athlete, determining appropriateness of return-to-play (RTP) after an injury, giving clearance to play, ensuring emergency preparedness, overseeing the healthfulness of the team's overall training program, supervising the personnel providing health care for the team, and protecting against institutional and personal liability (eSlide 39.1).

Event Administration

The two most common competition venues are on the sidelines of a sporting event and at mass participation endurance events. Establishing and regularly rehearsing an emergency action plan and educating the participant or athlete are important strategies to lessen morbidity, and potentially mortality, during and after a race (eSlide 39.1).

• PRINCIPLES OF CONDITIONING AND TRAINING

Periodization

In a periodization program, training is divided into periods to allow buildup of training stresses, rest and adaptation, and continual progression. These periods include macrocycles (commonly lasting 1 year), mesocycles (commonly lasting 1 month), and microcycles (commonly lasting 1 week). Usually a year-long training program will have three macrocycles: preseason (buildup), competitive season (maintenance), and postseason (recovery).

Overtraining Syndrome

Prolonged, excessive training without sufficient recovery can lead to overtraining syndrome, in which an athlete's performance suffers because of chronic maladaptation. Symptoms include unexplained performance decrement, fatigue, mood disturbance, poor sleep, and increased rates of illness and injury that persist despite more than 2 weeks of rest. The treatment is rest, from weeks to months, followed by a gradual return to training.

Altitude Training

Most scientists agree that the most effective form of altitude/hypoxic training is the "live high–train low" method, whereby athletes "live high" to stimulate erythropoietin and subsequently increase erythrocyte volume, and "train low" at a higher intensity with improved oxygen flux to induce beneficial metabolic and neuromuscular training adaptations.

• INJURY PREVENTION AND REHABILITATION

Kinetic Chain Assessment (eSlide 39.2)

The kinetic chain model is based on the idea that each complex athletic movement is the summation of its constituent parts, and each part connecting in the chain must function well to optimize performance and minimize injury. "Catch-up" is when the person compensates with one segment for a deficiency in a separate segment. The physical examination of the injured athlete should focus on the biomechanical issue and not solely on the painful tissue.

Prehabilitation

Prehabilitation can be viewed as a sport-specific injury prevention program. It addresses the basic components of all athletic movements and potential "breaks" in the kinetic chain: flexibility, strength, and endurance.

Injury Phases and Stages of Rehabilitation (eSlide 39.3)

Injuries can be acute, subacute, chronic, or an exacerbation of a chronic condition. Rehabilitation can be viewed as a three-stage spectrum: from the acute stage to the recovery stage, and then to the final functional stage, resulting in return to full play. Full RTP is achieved when there is no pain, and flexibility, strength, proprioception, and sport-specific skills are normal.

• BIOMECHANICS OF SPORTS

Throwing (eSlide 39.4)

In pitching, the momentum begins with a drive from the large leg muscles and rotation at the hips, progressing through segmental rotation of the trunk and shoulder girdle, transferring energy through elbow extension, on through the small forearm and hand muscles, and finally to the ball. Approximately 50% of the velocity of a pitch results from the step and body rotation (from the potential energy stored in the large leg and trunk musculature). The baseball pitch is composed of six phases. The majority of injuries occur in the late cocking and deceleration phases of throwing (eSlide 39.5).

In late cocking, the injury is caused by the forces needed to stabilize the shoulder in this extreme range of movement (ROM). The dynamic stabilizers of the anterior shoulder (biceps, subscapularis, and pectoralis major) are very active in this phase. The static stabilizers (glenohumeral ligaments, capsule, and labrum) are active as well. The glenohumeral ligaments and capsule increase in laxity because of the extreme ROM in the overhead athlete. This laxity is necessary for performance but increases the potential for injury. During the acceleration phase, shoulder abduction is relatively fixed at 90 degrees. If there is less than 90 degrees of abduction, which can be caused by fatigue, weakness, or poor form, the common observation is a "dropped elbow." Dropped elbow results in a reduced pitch velocity and an increased risk of injury to the rotator cuff and elbow. Another common injury in the acceleration phase is subacromial impingement with internal rotation and adduction of the abducted arm during acceleration. The deceleration phase is manifested by large eccentric muscular forces of the posterior shoulder girdle acting to decelerate the rapid internal rotation of the acceleration phase. Injury is common in this phase because of the large eccentric contractions. The final phase of pitching is the follow-through phase.

Running (eSlide 39.6)

Notable differences are observed between a walking gait cycle and a running gait cycle. In slower running and walking, contact is typically heel to toe. As running speed increases, foot strike occurs with the forefoot and heel simultaneously, or the forefoot strikes initially and is followed by the heel lowering to the ground. Moreover, the third phase in running is called the float phase. This phase is a time when neither foot is in contact with the ground. It occurs at the beginning of the initial swing and the end of the terminal swing. By contrast, the walking gait cycle has a period of double limb support, which is not present in running.

Swimming

Four competitive strokes are used in swimming: freestyle (front crawl), backstroke, butterfly, and breaststroke. Four phases of the swim stroke are common to freestyle, backstroke, and butterfly. The first phase is the entry or "catch." This encompasses hand entry into the water until the beginning of its backward movement. The propulsive phase is divided into two separate phases: pull and push. The pull phase ends as the hand arrives in the vertical plane of the shoulder. During the push phase, the hand is positioned below the shoulder and pushes through the water until its exit from the water, generally at the level of the greater trochanter. The final phase is the recovery phase, which entails the aerial return of the hand. Kick patterns are also an important part of swimming mechanics. In the flutter kick for the freestyle stroke and backstroke, the knees should flex only about 30–40 degrees, and hip flexion should be minimal. The breaststroke kick is a whip-kick that creates a significant valgus moment at the knee. Because of this increased knee valgus, medial knee injuries in breaststrokers are common. General rehabilitation principles have been established for swimmers with shoulder pain. The overarching principle is that most shoulder pain in swimmers (resulting from impingement and rotator cuff tendinopathy) is caused by dynamic muscle imbalances, weakness, and biomechanical faults. A major principle of shoulder rehabilitation for swimmers is scapular stabilization, with a prime focus on endurance training of the serratus anterior and lower trapezius muscles, as well as stretching of the internal rotators and posterior capsule and mobilization of the cervical and thoracic spine.

Jumping and Landing

The biomechanics of jumping and landing in sports are well researched in the setting of noncontact anterior cruciate ligament (ACL) injuries, which occur more frequently with the knee in less flexion. A well-defined gender difference observed in jumping and landing mechanics is likely one reason for the higher rate of noncontact ACL injuries in female athletes. Female athletes land more erect, with less knee and hip flexion and less hip external rotation and abduction. They also generally have muscle imbalance, with an increased quadriceps to hamstrings activation ratio, which creates greater knee extension and lesser knee flexion forces.

• PHARMACOLOGY IN SPORTS

Performance-Enhancing Drugs and Supplements (eSlide 39.7)

ANABOLIC STEROIDS (eSlide 39.8)

Anabolic steroids (ASs) have three general effects that enhance athletic performance. By binding androgen receptors, ASs stimulate messenger RNA synthesis, thereby increasing structural and contractile protein synthesis and producing an anabolic state. ASs also exert anticatabolic effects via competitive inhibition of the glucocorticoid receptor, leading to inhibition of the catabolic effects of cortisol and preservation of muscle mass. Finally, ASs have emotional effects, pushing athletes to train more intensely and more often. Premature deaths have resulted from AS use, most commonly as a result of suicide and acute myocardial infarction. ASs are banned by all major sporting leagues.

ERYTHROPOIETIN AND BLOOD DOPING

Blood doping, blood transfusion, or administration of the drug recombinant human erythropoietin (rhEPO) is used to increase the oxygen-carrying capacity in blood. The risks of artificially elevated hemoglobin or hematocrit include stroke, myocardial infarction, and pulmonary embolism.

STIMULANTS

Common stimulants include caffeine, ephedrine (ephedra or ma huang), pseudo-ephedrine, phenylephrine, amphetamines, and methamphetamines. Stimulants increase arousal, respiratory rate, heart rate, and blood pressure. Side effects include dizziness, insomnia, agitation, restlessness, anxiety, confusion, paranoia, hallucination, dyskinesia, gastrointestinal disturbance, heat intolerance, stroke, myocardial infarction, arrhythmia, and death.

• PREPARTICIPATION EXAMINATION

The primary goals of the preparticipation examination are to accomplish the following: (1) identify life-threatening conditions, (2) identify conditions that can limit competition, (3) identify factors that predispose the athlete to injury, and (4) meet the legal requirements of the institution and state. The lead physician must make the determination to clear the athlete either without restrictions or with recommendations for further evaluation or treatment. Athletes may not be cleared for participation in certain sports or may not be cleared for participation in any sport. A physician might be held liable for malpractice if an athlete is cleared to play despite the presence of a medically contraindicated condition (eSlide 39.1).

• EMERGENCY ASSESSMENT AND CARE

Sudden Cardiac Arrest in Athletes (eSlide 39.9)

The leading cause of death in young athletes is sudden cardiac arrest (SCA), typically as a result of a structural cardiac abnormality. Hypertrophic cardiomyopathy is the most common cause of SCA, accounting for 26% of deaths. In athletes over the age of 35 years, coronary artery disease is by far the most common cause of SCA, being responsible for 75% of deaths.

Exercise-Associated Collapse in Athletic Endurance Events (eSlide 39.10)

The most common cause of collapse in a marathon runner after crossing the finish line is benign exercise-associated collapse (EAC). It is important to keep the athlete walking after crossing the finish line to keep the muscular venous pump engaged. Exercise-associated hyponatremia (EAH) is a hypervolemic hyponatremia causing early symptoms of lightheadedness and a nauseated feeling; these may be followed by a progressive headache, vomiting, confusion, and finally obtundation, seizures, and death. Risk factors for EAH include weight gain during the race, a marathon race time more than 4 hours, and body mass index extremes. Those at risk are runners who ingest too many fluids on the race course and subsequently gain weight. It is appropriate to emphasize individual differences and remind athletes to replace what they need (to compensate for sweat losses) and that more is not necessarily appropriate. The mantra "drink when you are thirsty" is generally safe for slower and at-risk runners. Heat-related illness is another etiology of EAC. Heat exhaustion is the inability to continue to exercise in the heat, but it is not related to an increase in body temperature. In contrast, heat stroke is a medical emergency. Heat stroke is defined as multiorgan system failure secondary to hyperthermia. The rectal core temperature in an athlete with heat stroke is generally more than 39°C. Treatment involves immediate total body cooling. Finally, it is important to note that heat stroke can occur in cool environments; it might reflect more of a genetic predisposition to excessive endothermy (i.e., endogenous heat production) and is not just a factor of extreme environmental conditions.

• SPECIFIC DIAGMNOSES IN SPORTS MEDICINE

Sports Concussion (eSlide 39.11)

Concussions are a subset of traumatic brain injuries (TBIs) resulting from direct blows to the head or forces transmitted through the head and neck. An athlete with a suspected concussion should be removed from play immediately and evaluated on the sideline. The current consensus is that athletes should not RTP on the same day as a concussion. Prognosis after concussion is typically excellent, with 80%–90% of athletes free of symptoms within 7–10 days. No athlete should RTP until all neurologic symptoms of the concussion have resolved. Once the athlete is asymptomatic at rest, a multistep RTP protocol must be completed before competition is resumed (eSlide 39.12).

The athlete will need a 24-hour symptom-free period before advancing to the next step in the protocol.

Stingers

The stinger, sometimes also termed a burner, is probably one of the most common but least understood peripheral nerve injuries in sports. Stingers are nerve injuries that occur within the peripheral neural axis at a specific but variable point, from the nerve root to the brachial plexus. After an initial stinger, if full recovery is demonstrated within 15 minutes, return to same game competition is allowed. If full recovery occurs within 1 week after the initial stinger, then return to competition that next week is allowed. If the athlete has sustained recurrent stingers, a general rule is to hold the player from competition for the number of weeks that corresponds to the number of stingers sustained in a given season (e.g., 2 weeks for a second stinger). If more than three stingers occur in a season, ending the season should be considered.

Exercise-Induced Bronchospasm

Exercise-induced bronchospasm (EIB) describes airway narrowing that occurs in association with exercise. EIB can be present with chronic asthma, but generally is a separate entity. Pulmonary function testing and consultation with an asthma specialist are important to definitively diagnose and optimally treat EIB.

• SPECIFIC POPULATIONS

Female Athlete Triad

The female athlete triad is a constellation of interrelated findings: inadequate eating, menstrual abnormalities, and skeletal demineralization. These do not necessarily occur simultaneously. Skeletal demineralization can lead to premature osteoporosis.

Pediatric and Adolescent Athlete (eSlide 39.13)

Physical activity in children and adolescents prevents osteoporosis, improves self-esteem, and reduces anxiety and depression. Short-term resistance training programs, in which prepubescent athletes are trained and supervised by knowledgeable adults, can increase strength without significant risk of injury. The pediatric skeletal system is distinguished from that of adults by the presence of the active growth plate or physis. The physis is situated between the epiphysis and metaphysis. Injuries involving the traction epiphysis (also called apophyseal injuries) are not usually associated with growth disturbances. Pressure epiphyses are found at the end of long bones, such as the distal femur and proximal tibia. In contrast to apophyseal injuries, injuries to active pressure epiphyses can result in limb-length discrepancies or angular deformities.

Older Athlete (eSlide 39.14)

The benefits of exercise in older people are many, although they are not entirely understood. Higher levels of physical activity are associated with lower rates of many afflictions associated with aging, including coronary heart disease and cancer, although the underlying mechanisms for these findings are largely unknown.

• ADAPTIVE SPORTS MEDICINE (eSlide 39.15)

There are approximately 55 million disabled individuals in the United States, of which about 60% do not participate in any regular physical activity or sports. Sports participation among people with impairments can have significant benefits in terms of general state of health, functionality, life skills, self-esteem, and overall quality of life, similar to any other athlete. There are still only about 2 million recreational and competitive disabled athletes in the United States. The two most limiting factors for participation in athletics are awareness and access. Nevertheless, the growth of the movement exemplified through the phenomenal rise of the

Paralympic Games cannot be ignored. The 1960 Paralympics in Rome had 400 athletes from 23 countries; the 2012 London Games had approximately 4200 athletes from 164 countries.

Classifications

Athletes with impairments are an inherently heterogeneous group with highly variable profiles of sports capacity, depending on the type, location, and severity of the disability. Although many classification systems exist, the common purpose is to determine eligibility for participation and ensure that athletes are not precluded from success in competition on the basis of their disability. To be eligible for paralympic sports, an athlete must have one of the ten types of permanent impairments: ataxia, athetosis, hypertonia, leg-length difference, limb deficiency, loss of muscle strength, loss of ROM, short stature, low vision, or intellectual impairment. Athletes are placed more generally into six main disability categories: amputee, wheelchair user, cerebral palsy, vision impairment, intellectual disability, or "les autres" (a French term meaning "the others"). Athletes are given a specific designation based on their disability category and functional ability. Because there are significant variances among the different sports, the sporting event also greatly influences the classification process. Within each sport, there are different types and severities of disability, which affect the performance to varying levels. Depending on the sport, designations may be condensed into fewer classes, containing a wider range of disability. In addition, some sports may entail competition among athletes who maintain similar functional levels, although they may belong to different general disability categories. Team sports, such as wheelchair basketball, often incorporate a wide range of disabilities in direct competition via the use of point systems, in which athletes with less disadvantageous levels of disability are assigned higher point values, and a team is not permitted to exceed a given total point value for its players in the game. An athlete's classification is always in evolution, since progressive or periodic worsening or improvement of the disease process may occur, and the ability to adapt and overcome impairments may change. Thus, classifications are not permanently assigned. Continued assessment and revisions of these systems can be anticipated in years to come.

Adaptive Sports Equipment

The prosthetic device for an athlete with a limb deficiency has specific considerations when compared with the prosthetic device for everyday use. Aspects to consider include the weight of the prosthesis, limb alignment, prosthetic foot dynamics, shock absorption, and possible need for transverse rotation. The wheelchair-bound athlete also requires adaptions to the traditional wheelchair. Adjustments can be made in seating systems, leg rests, wheel type, wheel position, wheel angulation, and length. Certain frame materials, such as aluminum, titanium, and composite materials, were all first introduced in sports wheelchairs.

Injury Patterns in Adaptive Sports Medicine

Lower limb injuries are more common in ambulatory athletes (e.g., visually impaired, amputee, cerebral palsy), whereas upper limb injuries are more frequent in athletes who use a wheelchair.

Injuries and Complications by Cause of Disability

Disabled athletes are subject to many of the same injuries and complications from physical exertion as the able-bodied population.

WHEELCHAIR ATHLETE

Sports participation by wheelchair users has been found to be associated with improved functional outcomes and fewer physician visits, hospitalizations, and medical complications, while also serving as a powerful means for improving inclusion and equality within society.

SHOULDER INJURIES

Despite increases in repetitive use and high-intensity activity, wheelchair athletes do not have a higher incidence of shoulder pain than nonathletic wheelchair users.

ELBOW INJURIES

The most common sources of elbow pain are lateral epicondylitis, osteoarthritis, and olecranon bursitis.

WRIST INJURIES

The most common sources of wrist symptoms are carpal tunnel syndrome, ulnar nerve entrapment in Guyon canal, osteoarthritis, tendinitis, and De Quervain tenosynovitis.

UPPER LIMB FRACTURES

Wheelchair athletes may be at greater risk for upper limb fractures because of repetitive falls associated with many wheelchair sports, propulsion requiring positioning the hand in a location that is susceptible to injury from nearby wheelchairs or collisions, and the relatively high speeds achieved during certain wheelchair sports.

THERMOREGULATION

Below the level of the lesion, athletes with spinal cord injury have impaired shivering (which produces heat) and impaired sweating and vasodilation (which dissipates heat). These changes lead to greater than usual increases in body temperature with exertion and greater decreases in temperature with exposure to cold weather.

AUTONOMIC DYSREFLEXIA

Autonomic dysreflexia (AD) is a condition resulting from excessive sympathetic outflow in response to a noxious stimulus; the outflow is unregulated because of interruption of neural pathways after spinal cord injury. People with spinal cord injuries at the level of T6 and above are at risk for AD. The most common noxious stimuli that lead to AD include tight clothing, urinary or fecal retention, renal or bladder stones, pressure ulcers, infections, or intraabdominal pathology. In addition, "boosting" is the practice of intentionally inducing AD by athletes for the purpose of improving athletic performance.

SKIN BREAKDOWN

Regardless of the level of the injury, the skin over the sacrum, coccyx, and ischial tuberosities is frequently insensate, increasing the risk of skin breakdown or a pressure ulcer.

HETEROTOPIC OSSIFICATION

The most common site of heterotopic ossification (HO) after spinal cord injury is the hip. Following amputation, HO occurs in the injured tissues within the residual limb. HO typically develops within the first 6–12 months after amputation, during the time when the amputee is undergoing prosthetic training.

SPASTICITY

An increase in spasticity may be an indicator of a systemic or otherwise asymptomatic condition.

OSTEOPOROSIS

Individuals with a spinal cord injury have decreased weight bearing, which predisposes this population to osteoporosis. Other risk factors for osteoporosis, independent of alterations in weight bearing, are related to the severity of the injury, spasticity, and time since the injury.

ORTHOSTATIC HYPOTENSION

Symptoms of orthostatic hypotension include lightheadedness and dizziness; syncope may also occur. Prevention includes the use of lower limb compression stockings and abdominal binders, maintenance of hydration, and salt supplementation. If these measures are insufficient, pharmacologic treatment may be helpful, but it may be banned by antidoping agencies.

LIMB-DEFICIENT ATHLETES

Individuals with partial or full loss of limbs are eligible to compete under the classification of amputee athlete.

SKIN DISORDERS

The best treatment for skin disorders is prevention, which can be achieved through education, close monitoring of prosthesis fit, strategic timing of donning a prosthesis, considering the time out of the prosthesis and liner, and responding to environmental factors.

NEUROMA

A neuroma occurs at the distal end of a transected nerve in the residual limb. Treatment may involve prosthetic modifications to relieve pressure on the neuroma; oral medications, including antiepileptics and tricyclic antidepressants; injection of corticosteroids and local anesthetic into the neuroma; and radiofrequency ablation.

Clinical Pearls

- The traveling team physician presents a unique issue, given that licensure and malpractice coverage are state-specific.
- Medicolegal liability related to the preparticipation examination is not covered by Good Samaritan laws. A physician might be held liable for malpractice if an athlete is cleared to play despite the presence of a medically contraindicated condition.
- Concussions are a subset of TBIs that may result in neuropathologic changes. However, the acute clinical symptoms largely reflect a functional disturbance rather than a structural injury, and as such, no abnormality is seen on standard structural neuroimaging studies.

• ACKNOWLEDGMENT

I would like to thank Gerardo Miranda-Comas, Eliana Cardozo, and Svetlana Abrams for their contributions to the chapter.

BIBLIOGRAPHY

The complete bibliography is available on ExpertConsult.com.

Motor Neuron Diseases

40

Lydia Abdul Latif

The objective of this chapter is to provide an overview of the spectrum of motor neuron diseases (MNDs), predominantly focusing on the impact of amyotrophic lateral sclerosis (ALS) and the general rehabilitation approach to the evaluation, diagnosis, and management of this disease.

• CLASSIFICATION

MNDs can be broadly grouped into inherited and acquired causes. The main acquired or sporadic causes include poliomyelitis, ALS, and ALS variants. The most common inherited causes include spinal muscle atrophy (SMA), familial ALS, and X-linked bulbospinal muscular atrophy (Kennedy disease [KD]). MNDs can also be divided into groups of disorders based on selectivity for loss of upper motor neurons (UMNs; the corticospinal and corticobulbar tracts) or lower motor neurons (LMNs; the spinal anterior horn cells and cranial nerve LMNs) (eSlide 40.1).

Amyotrophic Lateral Sclerosis

ALS has an incidence of 1.4 per 100,000 people. It typically begins in the sixth to seventh decade of life. Men are affected somewhat more commonly than women, with a ratio of 1.6 to 1. An important and distinctive feature of ALS is the selective degeneration of both UMNs and LMNs, with relative sparing of other neurons in most cases. Pathogenic mechanisms underlying the disease remain surprisingly undefined. ALS, by definition, involves both UMNs and LMNs, but some ALS variants may involve only UMNs or LMNs, or certain body regions. Such variants include primary lateral sclerosis (PLS) and progressive muscular atrophy (PMA), in which neuron loss is restricted to the UMNs or LMNs, respectively. Similarly, regional variants include progressive bulbar palsy (PBP), affecting the cranial nerve nuclei of the bulbar musculature; brachial amyotrophic diplegia (BAD), affecting the upper limbs in a proximal predominant manner; and leg amyotrophic diplegia (LAD), predominantly affecting the distal lower limbs. All restricted variants, with the unfortunate exception of PBP, have a better prognosis than the more typical ALS. Typically, these are referred to as the flail limb syndrome (i.e., flail arm syndrome and flail leg syndrome).

Primary Lateral Sclerosis

PLS is a disorder associated with progressive spasticity and weakness of limb and bulbar muscles secondary to degeneration of UMNs, which is mainly seen in the fifth decade. The etiology is unknown. PLS is defined as having little or no LMN involvement, observed clinically or by electromyography (EMG). PLS progresses much more slowly than ALS; studies show an average life span of between 8 and 15 years after diagnosis. The diagnosis of PLS is established clinically, but testing can be helpful to exclude other possible diagnoses.

Progressive Muscular Atrophy

PMA is an MND causing progressive weakness and muscular atrophy, which is attributable to LMN degeneration. It is thus the LMN analogue of PLS. By definition, patients with PMA have no clinical evidence of UMN dysfunction at onset, but it is important to note that as many as 70% of patients with PMA will eventually demonstrate signs of UMN degeneration. Treatment is supportive and similar to the treatment for ALS. Prognosis is better than for ALS, with a 5-year survival rate of more than 50% and patients living an average of 1 year longer than those with ALS.

Amyotrophic Lateral Sclerosis-Plus Syndromes

ALS-Plus syndromes meet clinical and electrodiagnostic criteria for ALS, but they also have associated nonmotor neuron features, which may include Parkinsonism, frontotemporal dementia, ocular motility abnormalities, extrapyramidal signs, autonomic dysfunction, or sensory loss.

Spinal Muscular Atrophy

SMA is a group of genotypically and phenotypically diverse disorders associated with features of LMN loss. The most common form, proximal SMA (also called SMN-related SMA, 5q-SMA, or simply SMA) is an autosomal recessive LMN disorder with a frequency of 1 in 11,000 births. Carrier frequency is approximately 1 in 50. Importantly, proximal SMA is the most common genetic cause of death in infants. There is a spectrum of diseases associated with SMA, which differ in onset and severity of the disease. Proximal SMA can be classified into five subtypes of disease (eSlide 40.2). The most severe form, type 0, is characterized by very severe weakness, which begins before birth; joint contractures are often present because of diminished intrauterine movement. Type 1 is the most common form of the disease, representing 60%–70% of patients with SMA. It is characterized by onset before 6 months of age and an inability to sit independently. Approximately 95% of patients with type 1 die by the age of 2 years unless they receive ventilatory and nutritional support. Onset in patients with type 2 occurs between 6 and 18 months of age, and the ability to sit upright independently is achieved but ambulation is not. Patients with type 3 have an onset after 18 months of age and are able to walk independently. Type 4 is the mildest form, with onset in adulthood and relatively mild proximal limb weakness. The clinical presentation of SMA is that of proximal predominant weakness and hypotonia. Reflexes may be absent or reduced in the setting of milder weakness, mimicking a muscle disease. Sensory examination is normal. The most efficient strategy for diagnosis is gene testing for homozygous deletion of the SMN1 gene, which is seen in 95% of patients with SMA.

Some forms of SMA are associated with a distal predominant pattern of weakness, and therefore have been described as distal SMA (eSlide 40.3). A more rare form of SMA, called scapuloperoneal SMA or Davidenkow syndrome, is associated with features of motor neuron and axonal loss in a periscapular and distal leg distribution, mimicking the pattern of defects in facioscapulohumeral muscular dystrophy (eSlide 40.4). There are no effective therapies for any form of SMA, but supportive care can effectively reduce disease impact and burden. A recent study now shows that nusinersen may be effective in children especially and has been approved by the Food and Drug Administration. Pulmonary disease is the main source of mortality and involves primary complications of muscle weakness, such as impaired ventilation and secretion management, or secondary complications, such as pneumonia related to aspiration. Scoliosis is common in SMA, and progression of scoliosis and the associated impact on pulmonary function is less severe in patients with SMA type 3 compared with type 2.

X-Linked Spinobulbar Muscular Atrophy (Kennedy Disease)

KD is an X-linked recessive disorder that leads to progressive limb and bulbar weakness, testicular atrophy, gynecomastia, muscle cramps, and fasciculations. KD typically has an onset of more overt symptoms by the fourth or fifth decade and is a slowly progressive disorder; therefore life span is not usually dramatically reduced. Patients with KD often have prominent bulbar involvement, with profound atrophy and perioral fasciculations (eSlide 40.5).

Poliomyelitis and Postpolio Syndrome

Poliomyelitis is an MND caused by a viral infection of the central nervous system, resulting in loss of anterior horn cells and cranial nerve nuclei. It results from an infection with the poliovirus, a human enterovirus of the Picornaviridae family. There has been a dramatic reduction in the annual number of cases of polio as a result of the development of vaccination strategies in the 1950s. Symptoms of asymmetric flaccid paralysis and subsequent atrophy are typically more common in limb muscles, but they may also affect bulbar muscles. Approximately 50% of patients with poliomyelitis develop late features of declining motor function, known as postpoliomyelitis syndrome. This usually occurs 30 or more years after the initial infection and can have a gradual or abrupt onset. Thorough evaluation is critical to exclude other disorders that may contribute to a decline in function, and treatment is designed to maximize and maintain function.

Hirayama Disease

Hirayama disease is a relatively benign disorder associated with muscle weakness and atrophy of the distal upper limb muscles. The disorder primarily affects males during the teenage years or early twenties, and the onset of weakness is insidious and gradual. The natural history of the Hirayama disease is associated with initial progression for several years, and spontaneous arrest is also known. Involvement may be unilateral or bilateral, but it is usually more prominent in one limb (eSlide 40.6).

Rare or Less Well-Defined Etiologies of Motor Neuron Disease

Disorders of the motor neuron are rare. Beyond the more common forms of MND, there are myriad other unusual and atypical forms that are less well defined and preclude a detailed description within this chapter. Some of the uncommon forms have been attributed to paraneoplastic and idiopathic immune dysregulation, other infectious agents, hereditary metabolic disorders, electrical injuries, and other idiopathic processes.

• DIAGNOSTIC EVALUATION

History

A thorough history is vital when assessing a patient with a possible MND. A detailed family history is essential to look for any clues of an underlying hereditary process, and examination of family members is sometimes necessary to identify similar but previously unrecognized clinical features. Associated features, such as prominent sensory symptoms or complaints attributable to sphincter or autonomic dysfunction, are unusual in pure motor neuron processes and should prompt consideration of an alternative diagnosis. Respiratory or bulbar involvement may be subtle and may require some probing by the provider to identify the involvement; features such as orthopnea or morning headaches may suggest diaphragm paralysis or nocturnal hypoventilation, respectively. The past medical history and review of systems can identify a systemic process that may be related to motor neuron dysfunction. The functional and social history will provide critical information when prescribing orthotics, assistive devices, and therapy, and when recommending modifications for the patient's living situation (which will eventually be needed as the disease progresses). The presence of focal painless weakness and atrophy without sensory loss should immediately raise red flags, and ALS is an important consideration. The initial location of weakness in ALS is roughly divided into thirds: one-third in the bulbar region, one-third in the upper limbs, and one-third in the lower limbs. Dysphagia is a rare presenting complaint in ALS but is expected during the course of the disease.

Physical Examination

A detailed neurologic examination is mandatory in the evaluation of a patient suspected of MND. Focal atrophy, weakness, and fasciculations are the primary features of LMN injury that should be sought. Evidence of UMN degeneration in the upper limbs includes spasticity, clumsiness, increased muscle stretch reflexes, and UMN signs. Findings of fasciculations in a patient with weakness and denervation on EMG are suggestive of MND.

Laboratory Studies

Genetic testing can effectively confirm the diagnosis of hereditary MNDs, and other testing may not be warranted. Muscle biopsy is not normally necessary in patients with a suspected MND. Imaging studies may not be required in the evaluation of patients with suspected MND, but they are very useful and sometimes of vital importance to help exclude mimicking or confounding diagnoses with UMN or LMN involvement.

Electrodiagnosis

Electrodiagnostic testing is the primary diagnostic modality to confirm loss or impaired function of the peripheral nervous system. Studies in patients with suspected MND are designed to identify LMN involvement and exclude other mimicking disorders of the peripheral nervous system. Needle EMG is the most pertinent aspect of the electrodiagnostic examination for identification of LMN loss, but nerve conduction studies are equally important to help exclude other diagnostic possibilities within the peripheral nervous system.

Amyotrophic Lateral Sclerosis: Diagnosis and Criteria

The revised El Escorial criteria with the Awaji modification form the diagnostic criteria generally used today (eSlide 40.7). Three main clinical features are required to make the formal diagnosis of ALS: evidence of LMN degeneration, evidence of UMN degeneration, and involvement of different regions (bulbar, cervical, thoracic, and lumbar). EMG, pathologic, or neuroimaging evidence of another disease process excludes the diagnosis of ALS (eSlide 40.7). Findings of UMN and LMN dysfunction are grouped into four regions: bulbar, cervical, thoracic, and lumbar (eSlide 40.8).

• TREATMENT

General

Currently, there are no treatments that can dramatically counteract the effects or stop the progression of most MNDs. Treatment strategies are generally designed to reduce the symptomatic impact of MNDs.

Medication

No medications with major disease-modifying capacities are available in the field of MNDs. Riluzole is the only medication shown to slow the progression of ALS. Riluzole reduces mortality 23% at 6 months and 15% at 12 months and appears to prolong survival by around 4 months.

Rehabilitation

Strategies for rehabilitation must be tailored to the targeted patient population and depend on the impact and natural history of the disease. Stage 1 includes patients who are ambulatory and fully independent, with mild weakness or clumsiness. These patients need to only maintain active range of movement and continue their normal activities of daily living, but they can benefit from strengthening of the unaffected muscles. Strengthening all (including affected) muscles is reasonable, with precautions taken to avoid overwork damage.

Patients in stage 2 remain ambulatory and independent but have moderate weakness. Functional impairment may be severe in some areas despite preserved overall function (eSlide 40.9). An opponens splint can be used to accommodate lack of thumb opposition due to thenar muscle weakness (eSlide 40.10). Stage 3 includes patients who remain ambulatory but have severe weakness in selected muscle groups. Stage 4 includes patients who are nonambulatory but remain independent. In stage 5, patients are no longer independent. Stage 6 patients are completely bedridden and dependent, and require maximal assistance.

Exercise

Exercise in ALS and other progressive neuromuscular diseases is a subject of controversy. Despite theoretical concerns of worsening weakness from overtaxing already struggling motor units, no controlled outcome study has shown worsening after exercise in patients with ALS. Range of movement and stretching are considered safe and should be prescribed for all patients with ALS. Some form of exercise should be discussed with every patient with ALS.

Specific Disease-Related Impact

SPASTICITY

Treatment of spasticity in patients with ALS is similar to spasticity treatment in other disease states but with some important differences. Not all patients with ALS would be appropriate candidates, especially patients with rapid progression or very advanced disease. Botulinum toxin may be useful, but it can lead to generalized weakness that can be more problematic.

COMMUNICATION

Effective communication is a major factor in the quality of life of patients with ALS and should be managed aggressively. As verbal communication becomes more limited, augmentative and alternative communications systems are useful.

DYSPHAGIA AND NUTRITION

Dysphagia contributes to malnutrition, poses a risk for aspiration, and can be a major source of anxiety. Improved nutritional status can have major impact on various MNDs. Malnutrition is proportional to the degree of dysphagia and is a major predictor of death in patients with ALS. A nasogastric tube can provide greater nutrition but is uncomfortable and can lead to aspiration if improperly placed. A percutaneous endoscopic gastrostomy (PEG) tube is a permanent feeding solution. Indications for placement of a PEG tube in a patient with ALS include decreased caloric intake with weight loss greater than 10% of baseline, dehydration, and meals limited by dysphagia or taking longer than 30 minutes to consume.

SIALORRHEA

Sialorrhea in patients with ALS can be socially disabling and encourage oral infections. A home suction machine is helpful for most patients. Treatments include amitriptyline, nebulized or intravenous glycopyrrolate, oral or transdermal scopolamine, and benztropine. Botulinum toxin type A, injected every 3 months at a dose of 7.5–20 units into each parotid gland, has been used effectively. Radiation treatment is a fast, safe, inexpensive, and effective option, but it is not frequently used. Surgical treatments are available but not generally recommended.

RESPIRATORY INSUFFICIENCY

Respiratory muscles may be affected by motor neuron loss similar to other muscles. In addition to respiratory insufficiency being the main source of mortality in patients with ALS and other MNDs, the choices and methods of compensating for respiratory insufficiency may ultimately have the most impact on the lives of patients. Patients who choose tracheostomy and long-term ventilation will generally survive much longer, but they must consider the eventual possibility of a locked-in, noncommunicative state.

Symptoms of respiratory insufficiency are noted at initial presentation in around 25% in ALS. These symptoms can include fatigue, dyspnea, orthopnea, and morning headaches. Although many patients have no symptoms, subclinical respiratory insufficiency is frequent. Up to 85% of patients with ALS will have an abnormal forced vital capacity (FVC) at presentation. Experts recommend routine assessment of respiratory physiologic measurements every 2–4 months.

Noninvasive ventilation (NIV) has many advantages to offer. It has been shown to improve quality of life measurements, including energy, vitality, dyspnea, somnolence, depression, sleep quality, physical fatigue, concentration problem, and cognitive function. A typical initial prescription for NIV would include the International Classification of Diseases, 9th Revision, code (335.20) for the diagnosis of ALS and documentation of an FVC <50%, maximal inspiratory pressure ≤60 cm H_2O, or arterial carbon dioxide partial pressure ≥45 mm Hg. Despite the benefits of NIV, eventually all patients will require more respiratory support and secretion management, and the decision regarding whether to undergo a tracheostomy and invasive ventilation (IV) with a mechanical ventilator will be faced. Triggers for considering IV on a nonurgent basis include use of NIV >12 hours in a day or intolerance of NIV in a person with an FVC <50% or symptoms of dyspnea.

Oxygen therapy should almost never be used in patients with ALS. It worsens respiratory symptoms, as well as hypercapnia, and can lead to hypercapnic coma or respiratory arrest. Bronchial secretions are often problematic in patients with ALS and a major source of anxiety. First-line treatments include a portable home suction device and room humidifier. Mucolytics, such as N-acetylcysteine, 200–400 mg three times daily, can also be helpful. Nebulized saline, beta-antagonists, anticholinergic bronchodilators, and mucolytics have been used in various combinations with success. The combination of NIV and a mechanical insufflator–exsufflator has been shown to reduce hospitalization and improve oxygen saturation in patients with neuromuscular disorders, including ALS.

MOOD AND COGNITIVE DISORDERS
Mood disorders are common in ALS. It is important for treatment providers to discuss symptoms of mood disorders with patients (and families of patients) with ALS, as these disorders are associated with a lower quality of life. Approximately 50% of patients with ALS will develop at least mild-to-moderate impaired cognition, and around 15% of patients develop features of frontotemporal dementia.

PSEUDOBULBAR AFFECT
Pseudobulbar affect refers to pathologic weeping, laughing, and yawning that is inappropriate or excessive for the emotional state of the patient. Pseudobulbar affect is seen in more than 50% of patients with ALS, with or without bulbar motor signs.

PAIN AND CRAMPS
Cramps are common in patients with various forms of MNDs .Cramps are a common source of discomfort in patients with ALS and are fairly common early in the disease.

PROGNOSIS AND END-OF-LIFE CARE
End-of-life issues need to be addressed early in the management of every patient with ALS and other severe MNDs. Delaying uncomfortable end-of-life conversations may be tempting for both the provider and patient alike. The alternative to a potentially uncomfortable conversation is critical decisions made during a crisis by family members who may be unaware of the patient's true wishes. The prognosis for ALS is grim (eSlides 40.11, 40.12, and 40.13).

• CONCLUSION (eSlide 40.14)
MNDs represent a diverse group of disorders with the common feature of motor neuron loss and associated deficits within the motor system. The effects of MNDs are often devastating, and there is generally no cure. A multidisciplinary approach is usually the most effective way to address the complexities of diagnosis, prognosis, and management of these disorders, and physiatrists have key roles in the detailed evaluation, accurate and timely diagnosis, and treatment of patients with MNDs.

Clinical Pearls

1. MND is associated with dysfunction and degeneration of motor neurons and has heterogeneous clinical spectrum of conditions with inherited and acquired causes.
2. ALS is the main acquired or sporadic cause, presenting with UMN and LMN features, and is more common in men.
3. Diagnostic evaluations for MND include thorough history, detailed neurologic examination, and electrodiagnosis as the primary diagnostic modality.
4. Treatment strategies are generally aimed to reduce the impact of MND because no treatment is available to treat or stop progression of most MNDs.
5. Rehabilitation strategies are tailored to individual patients depending on the stage of the disease progression.
6. Specific disease-related impacts, including respiratory insufficiency, dysphagia, spasticity, communication, pseudobulbar affect, pain, and mood and cognitive disorders, need to be treated accordingly.
7. End-of-life issues need to be addressed early in the management of ALS and other severe MNDs.

BIBLIOGRAPHY
The complete bibliography is available on ExpertConsult.com.

Rehabilitation of Patients With Neuropathies

41

Yi-Chian Wang

This chapter provides an understanding of peripheral neuropathies (PNs) to allow physiatrists to diagnose these conditions, offer a prognosis, and provide rehabilitative therapies.

• CLASSIFICATION OF NEUROPATHIES

PNs can be caused by systemic processes or focal injuries and described in three axes: (1) axonal or demyelinating; (2) motor or sensory fibers; and (3) distal, proximal, asymmetric, or multifocal pattern. For example, alcoholic neuropathy tends to be axonal, sensorimotor, and symmetric. Localized nerve injuries are classified according to the Seddon system and the Sunderland system (Table 41.1 and eSlide 41.1).

• EVALUATION OF GENERALIZED NEUROPATHIES

History

History taking should cover symptoms (duration, rate of progression, and distribution); functional impairments; medical comorbidities; toxic exposures; family history (e.g., gait problems or pes cavus); and sensation changes, including small fiber symptoms (pain, temperature, and pressure) and large fiber symptoms (vibration and proprioception). Motor symptoms can manifest as gait difficulties, impaired balance, repeated falls, or decreased fine motor skills. Neuropathies in children often have an insidious onset and present with delayed developmental milestones and clumsiness during normal childhood activities (eSlide 41.2).

Physical Examination

The limbs should be inspected for the presence of atrophy and fasciculations. Weakness without significant atrophy suggests a demyelinating etiology, whereas atrophy in proportion to the weakness is more consistent with an axonal neuropathy. Foot findings include pes cavus, hammertoes, collapse of the midfoot architecture, "hot foot" (small fiber neuropathy), and skin lesions (insensate foot). Sensory testing includes light touch, pinprick, proprioception, and vibration. Physical findings predictive of electrodiagnostic confirmation of a PN are loss of the Achilles reflex, inability to perceive 0.5- to 1.0-cm movements of the great toe during at least 8 of 10 trials, or inability to detect a vibrating 128-Hz tuning fork for at least 8 seconds at the great toe. Detection of weakness is improved by repeated testing

TABLE 41.1 Classification of Nerve Injury: Seddon and Sunderland Systems

Seddon	Sunderland	Description
Neurapraxia	First degree	Focal conduction block without axonal damage
Axonotmesis	Second degree	Axon damage with Wallerian degeneration; supporting structures intact
Neurotmesis	Third degree	Damage to axon and endoneurium
	Fourth degree	Damage to axon, endoneurium, and perineurium
	Fifth degree	Damage to axon endoneurium, perineurium, and epineurium

and observing the patient during functional tasks, such as performing a unipedal stance test or buttoning without visual input (eSlide 41.3).

Electrodiagnostic Studies

Electrodiagnostic studies are an extension of the physical examinations. A decrement of the sensory nerve action potential (SNAP) and compound muscle action potential (CMAP) usually suggests axon loss. In a demyelinating process, the conduction velocities slow down, and the SNAPs show temporal dispersion. Acquired demyelinating neuropathies often present with nonuniform demyelination and focal conduction block, whereas hereditary neuropathies usually result in uniform demyelination without focal block. Late responses (F waves) are useful for assessing more proximal segments; they are particularly sensitive for detecting demyelinating processes, such as early Guillain-Barré syndrome (GBS). Needle electromyography (EMG) signs of denervation, such as positive waves and fibrillation potentials, are seen when there is ongoing axonal loss. As collateral sprouting begins, the motor unit shows early reinnervation signs of increased duration and polyphasia and late reinnervation signs of increased motor unit amplitude or giant waves (eSlide 41.4).

• COMPLICATIONS OF NEUROPATHIES

Foot Complications

Foot ulceration manifests a lifetime risk of 15% in diabetic patients. The presence of neuropathy is associated with a 2- to 15-fold greater risk of amputation. Patients with neuropathy should be educated regarding proper shoe wear, nail and callus care, and signs of infection (for self-monitoring). Charcot neuroarthropathy is a pathologic fracture, often in the midfoot region. Acute Charcot foot can present similarly to cellulitis, as a warm, erythematous, and swollen foot, which can be diagnosed by bone scan but not radiographs. Strict immobilization with a total contact cast should be ordered until clinical inflammatory signs and bone scan findings subside.

Pain

Large fiber neuropathies often manifest with a dull, deep, aching, or cramping pain. Small fiber neuropathies frequently manifest as superficial, burning, and hypersensitive pain. Topical capsaicin or lidocaine can be applied in patients with a discrete distribution of pain. Transcutaneous electrical stimulation might be of benefit. Medications for neuropathic pain include tricyclic antidepressants (e.g., amitriptyline and nortriptyline), gabapentin, duloxetine, pregabalin, tramadol, and opioid analgesics. Second-line medications for the treatment of neuropathic pain include lamotrigine, carbamazepine, other selective serotonin reuptake inhibitors, and clonidine.

Functional Impairment

Patients with PN are approximately 20 times more likely to fall than those without a neuropathy. Neuropathy impairs proprioceptive sensation at the ankle, and people with this neuropathy are less able to rapidly develop ankle torque to correct for lateral lean. Recently, the ratio of hip strength to ankle proprioceptive precision has been used to predict unipedal stance time, falls, and fall-related injuries in older patients with diabetic neuropathy. Proximal hip strengthening, eyewear to correct distant vision, proper lighting, proper shoes, walking devices, and Tai Chi exercises might reduce the risk of falling. Bifocals, however, have been shown to increase the risk of falls.

• SPECIFIC NEUROPATHIES

Diabetic Neuropathies

Diabetes is one of the most common causes of neuropathy, which is symmetric, exhibits features of both demyelination and axon loss, and affects sensory fibers more than motor. Diabetes mellitus mononeuropathies can also occur, primarily in cranial nerves III, VI, and VII, as well as in median, ulnar, and peroneal nerves (eSlide 41.5).

DISTAL SYMMETRIC SENSORIMOTOR POLYNEUROPATHY

Risk factors for diabetic neuropathy include the severity and duration of hyperglycemia, as well as the presence of hypertension, elevated triglycerides, tobacco use, obesity, and cardiovascular disease. Large fibers are involved early, causing impaired proprioception. When small C fibers are involved, significant pain, hyperalgesia, loss of sweating, and vasomotor changes occur. Among routine studies, sural sensory studies show the earliest changes. In younger patients, medial plantar nerve conduction studies may be even more sensitive, given the nerve's more distal location. Tight glycemic control has been shown to reduce the prevalence of PN by almost 70% and autonomic dysfunction by more than 50%, but it has not yet been shown to reverse PN. Therefore it is important to initiate strict sugar control as soon as diabetes is diagnosed.

PROXIMAL NEUROPATHY

Diabetic proximal neuropathy, or *diabetic amyotrophy*, is thought to be an immune-mediated microvasculitis affecting the nerve roots and plexus. It causes acute and severe pain for months, which is later followed by weight loss and muscle atrophy. The atrophy primarily involves the quadriceps, adductors, and iliopsoas muscles, with relative sparing of the hamstring and gluteal muscles. Corticosteroids, plasmapheresis, and intravenous immunoglobulin (IVIG) have not been shown to be efficacious treatments. The prognosis is good, and it typically takes 12–24 months for the patient to recover.

AUTONOMIC NEUROPATHY

Autonomic neuropathy is a significant cause of morbidity, and even mortality, in diabetic patients. Patients with cardiac autonomic neuropathy have a 40% greater mortality compared with people without this neuropathy; the increased mortality is due to silent ischemia, lethal arrhythmias, and prolongation of the QT interval. Clinical signs of autonomic neuropathy include a resting tachycardia >100 bpm and a decrease in systolic blood pressure >20 mm Hg on standing, without an appropriate heart rate response (orthostasis). Management involves education regarding slow postural changes, use of compressive stockings and abdominal binders, and use of medications, such as fludrocortisone or midodrine. Autonomic dysfunction can also affect the gastrointestinal and genitourinary systems, leading to erectile dysfunction and neurogenic bladder.

Guillain-Barré Syndrome

The etiology of GBS has been suggested to involve pathogen-triggered autoimmune damage of the peripheral nerves. The most common subtype is the acute inflammatory demyelinating polyradiculoneuropathy (AIDP), which affects both motor and sensory nerves and is responsible for 95% of GBS cases. Purely axonal forms (<5%) can occur as acute motor axonal neuropathy or acute motor and sensory axonal neuropathy; they are more common in Asia and South America. The Miller Fisher variant, manifesting as a triad of ataxia, areflexia, and ophthalmoplegia, is rare (eSlide 41.6).

CLINICAL FEATURES AND DIAGNOSIS

GBS is a progressive, symmetric weakness of the limbs, with or without sensory abnormalities. Maximal weakness occurs at 2–4 weeks. Ventilatory support is required in 25% of cases because of respiratory muscle weakness. The cranial nerves and autonomic nervous system can also be affected. Deep aching pain might precede weakness and affects the back, buttocks, and posterior thighs. Typical clinical features, high protein concentration in the cerebrospinal fluid, and typical electrodiagnostic findings constitute the diagnosis of GBS. Nerve conduction studies are initially normal. Prolonged F-wave latencies are often the earliest abnormality, followed by an acute acquired demyelinating pattern of temporal dispersion and focal conduction block.

MANAGEMENT

Mortality for GBS is 10%. Both plasma exchange and IVIG have been shown to be effective, but IVIG is more convenient and readily available. Rehabilitation of patients begins in the acute phase with contracture prevention, aggressive pulmonary hygiene, and early mobilization. Inpatient rehabilitation commences when neurologic deterioration has reached its nadir, the patient is autonomically stable, and pulmonary status is stabilized. Fatigue is common but can be relieved by exercises (e.g., those involving correcting orthostasis, ambulating with or without orthoses, and weight training for the upper extremities) and the use of assistive devices for self-care activities. Only 20% of patients remain nonambulatory or require an assistive device to walk at 6 months. Poor outcome is associated with advanced age, male gender, axonal involvement, antecedent diarrhea, and cytomegalovirus (CMV) infection.

Chronic Inflammatory Demyelinating Polyneuropathy

Chronic inflammatory demyelinating polyneuropathy (CIDP) progresses over at least 2 months. Its course is recurrent and remitting (polyphasic) in younger patients and progressive in older adults (monophasic). The classic form is a symmetric neuropathy mainly affecting proximal and distal motor fibers. Reflexes are reduced, and muscle atrophy is not significant. Cranial involvement can occur in 10%-20% of cases. Sensory involvement typically affects large fibers responsible for vibration and proprioception. The diagnosis is made by the presence of typical clinical features, electrodiagnostic studies showing segmental demyelination, nerve biopsy findings, cerebral spinal fluid study results, and magnetic resonance imaging (MRI). In addition to IVIG and plasma exchange, CIDP is also responsive to corticosteroids. Corticosteroids are most likely to produce disease remission in the demyelinating form, but they may be ineffective or detrimental in pure motor variants of CIDP. After the patient is neurologically stabilized, appropriate physical and occupational therapy, orthotic management, and treatment of neuropathic pain should be addressed (eSlide 41.7).

Infectious Neuropathies (eSlide 41.8)

LEPROSY (HANSEN DISEASE)

Leprosy is the most common cause of neuropathy in the world. It is caused by the bacterium *Mycobacterium leprae*. Tuberculoid leprosy is caused by excessive cell-mediated immunity, which not only destroys the bacillus but also damages the nerves, leaving granulomatous skin macules. In the lepromatous form, deficient immune responses allow the bacillus to proliferate, and the nerve damage is caused by direct invasion of Schwann cells by the bacteria.

LYME DISEASE

Lyme disease is a tick-borne illness caused by *Borrelia burgdorferi*. Meningitis is the most common neurologic abnormality. The typical PN is an irregular axonal neuropathy. In stage 2 of Lyme disease, cranial neuropathy, radiculoneuritis, mononeuritis multiplex, or plexopathy may occur. In stage 3, 50% of patients develop a distal symmetric neuropathy with stocking-glove paresthesia and sensory loss. After ceftriaxone treatment, acute PN recovers fairly well, but chronic PN does not.

CYTOMEGALOVIRUS-RELATED PROGRESSIVE POLYRADICULOMYELOPATHY

CMV infection is a severe neurologic emergency that rapidly progresses to polyradiculomyelopathy over days; death would ensue within weeks if left untreated. Initially there is low back pain with unilateral lower limb radiation and urinary incontinence, which is followed quickly by progressive leg weakness and saddle anesthesia. Lumbar puncture is mandatory to identify the pathogen. Electrodiagnostic studies are consistent with axonal loss in the lumbosacral roots.

HUMAN IMMUNODEFICIENCY VIRUS-ASSOCIATED NEUROPATHIES

Early in the course of human immunodeficiency virus (HIV) infection (at the time of seroconversion), immune-mediated neuropathies are most common. These are similar to AIDP, CIDP, and vasculitic neuropathies. In mid-to-late disease, HIV itself causes neuropathies. In late-stage disease, opportunistic infections, nutritional deficiency, diffuse infiltrative lymphocytosis, antiretroviral (ARV)–related immune reconstitution inflammatory response, and ARV drugs themselves can all cause PN. The distal sensory polyneuropathy caused by antiretroviral drugs (ARV-DSP) leads to distal axonal degeneration of small unmyelinated fibers; ARV treatment may be discontinued.

TABLE 41.2 Features of Toxic Neuropathies

Type of Neuropathies	Causative Drugs and Toxins
Distal sensorimotor neuropathies without conduction slowing but with predominant axon loss	Chronic alcohol abuse, as well as chronic arsenic, carbon monoxide, and mercury poisoning **Drugs:** metronidazole, amitriptyline, lithium, nitrofurantoin, phenytoin, vincristine, hydralazine, isoniazid
Motor-predominant neuropathies without conduction slowing	Organophosphates **Drugs:** vincristine
Pure sensory axonal neuropathies	Alcohol, pyridoxine (vitamin B₆), thallium **Drugs:** cisplatin, nitrofurantoin, thalidomide
Motor-predominant demyelinating neuropathy resembling AIDP	Acute arsenic poisoning, hexacarbons **Drugs:** amiodarone
Sensory-predominant demyelinating neuropathy	Saxitoxin (shellfish poisoning associated with red tide), tetrodotoxin (puffer fish)
Mononeuritis multiplex	Trichloroethylene **Drugs:** dapsone
Subacute motor neuropathy with segmental demyelination and axonal degeneration	Chronic lead intoxication

AIDP, acute inflammatory demyelinating polyradiculoneuropathy.

Toxic Neuropathies

Toxic exposure is often suspected when the results of standard history taking and laboratory testing in the workup of PN are unrevealing; establishing the diagnosis is important because prompt withdrawal of the causative agent might lead to improvement. Common features of toxic neuropathies are summarized in Table 41.2 and eSlide 41.9.

Toxic neuropathies also frequently present with other systemic effects, and symptoms vary according to exposure dose and duration. Gastrointestinal complaints are reported in arsenic, lead, and thallium poisoning. Mees lines in the fingernails can be found in lead and arsenic poisoning. Gingival abnormalities manifest in phenytoin, lead, and mercury exposure. Irritant dermatitis occurs with acrylamide, thallium, and toluene exposure. Exposure to organophosphates causes symptoms of cholinergic excess. Chronic alcohol abuse can cause midline cerebellar degeneration and a triad of ataxia, dementia, and ophthalmoplegia, known as Wernicke-Korsakoff syndrome. Lead poisoning has a predilection for the radial nerve, and patients can present with a wrist drop. Cognitive, learning, and behavioral impairments may be seen in children with blood lead levels around 10 μg/dL. Many chemotherapeutic drugs can cause treatment-limiting neuropathies. Dose reduction, longer infusion times, or longer periods between doses may improve symptoms, but recovery can be incomplete. Amiodarone can cause encephalopathy, basal ganglia dysfunction, optic neuropathy, pseudotumor cerebri, and action tremor. Concomitant myopathy is present with colchicine-induced neuropathy.

Vasculitic and Connective Tissue Disease Neuropathies

The prototypical vasculitic neuropathy is a mononeuritis multiplex, which is commonly seen with polyarteritis nodosa, Churg-Strauss syndrome, microscopic polyangiitis, and Wegener granulomatosis. Typical presentation begins with vasculitic ischemia and pain in the affected nerve, followed by side-to-side asymmetric sensory loss and weakness. The peroneal nerve is involved in 63% of the cases, followed by the tibial, ulnar, and median nerves. Involvement is greater proximally than distally, at areas that are not typical sites of anatomic compression. Electrodiagnostic testing shows an axonal pattern in the affected sensory and motor nerves. Needle EMG shows a chronic denervation pattern. Prompt management with corticosteroids and cyclophosphamide can halt progression.

Apart from asymmetric mononeuritis multiplex, rheumatoid arthritis (RA), systemic lupus erythematosus (SLE), and Sjögren syndrome more frequently cause a diffuse symmetric distal neuropathy involving sensory, motor, and autonomic fibers, which occurs late in these diseases. RA can progress to rheumatoid vasculitis, causing typical mononeuritis multiplex. Compression neuropathies, such as carpal tunnel syndrome (CTS), are also more common in SLE, RA, and Sjögren syndrome.

CHARCOT-MARIE-TOOTH DISEASE

Charcot-Marie-Tooth (CMT) disease, also called hereditary motor and sensory neuropathy (HMSN), is the most common inherited PN. It is subclassified as HMSN types I–VI (eSlide 41.10). HMSN I/CMT1, the most common subtype (74% of cases), is characterized by slow conduction velocities and diffuse demyelination. HMSN II/CMT2 is the axonal form. HMSN III is now more commonly known as Dejerine-Sottas neuropathy and is characterized by an early disease onset and severe "hypertrophic" demyelination. HMSN IV, HMSN V, and HMSN VI describe various motor-only forms, which are now referred to as distal hereditary motor neuropathies. The typical pattern for CMT is a slowly progressive weakness starting before 20 years of age. Foot drop and steppage gait might be the earliest signs because of marked peroneal weakness and relatively preserved plantar flexor strength. Although gait is affected, loss of independent ambulation is rare. Skeletal deformities, such as pes cavus and hammertoes, are seen in 66% of all CMT patients. Progressive strengthening of the hip flexors can improve walking duration, and strengthening the ankle musculature results in improved muscle strength, leading to improved walking speed, cadence, and stride length.

• MONONEUROPATHIES

Mononeuropathies are usually caused by local trauma or compression of a specific nerve, often in an anatomically vulnerable location. "Double crush" refers to the concept that proximal compression of a nerve, or a systemic disease injuring the nerve, will predispose its distal portion to being vulnerable to a minor insult (such as cervical radiculopathy predisposing to CTS). CTS is 3 times more common in diabetic patients than in the general population.

Brachial Plexopathy

Trauma is the most common cause of brachial plexopathy, affecting multiple roots, trunks, cords, or distal nerves, and needle EMG is necessary for localization. Milder plexus injuries cause a sharp burning pain in the shoulder with transient weakness. Erb palsy occurs in newborns during a difficult delivery, with the upper trunk being most commonly affected. Management includes proper positioning, range of movement and strengthening exercises, medications for neuropathic pain, neurolysis, nerve repair or grafting, and tendon transfer (eSlide 41.11).

ACUTE BRACHIAL NEURITIS

Acute brachial neuritis (Parsonage-Turner syndrome) typically presents with acute, severe pain in the shoulder and neck area, followed by weakness of the shoulder girdle muscles. Antecedent events include immunization, infection, surgery, and pregnancy. The upper trunk is preferentially affected. Systemic corticosteroids might relieve the pain but do not alter the disease course. Prognosis is generally good, with 85% of patients recovering within 3 years.

THORACIC OUTLET SYNDROME

The brachial plexus travels between the medial and anterior scalene muscles, runs between the first rib and the clavicle, and then passes beneath the pectoralis tendon and the coracoid process; all of these areas are common compression sites. The lower trunk is most commonly affected, and needle EMG might demonstrate abnormalities in the T1-innervated thenar muscles. Treatments include postural therapy and botulinum toxin injection to the scalene, subclavius, and pectoralis minor muscles.

NEOPLASTIC-INDUCED AND RADIATION-INDUCED PLEXOPATHIES

Lung, breast, and lymphoma are the most common metastatic tumors that cause brachial plexopathy; early symptoms include severe pain and weakness involving muscles supplied by the lower plexus (C8-T1). The pain may be relieved with pharmacologic treatment, radiotherapy, or regional blocks. If the mass is adjacent to the first thoracic vertebrae, it may affect the sympathetic ganglia, causing a Horner syndrome. Radiation-induced plexopathy is a late effect of radiotherapy, presenting 6 months to 20 years after the treatment with reduced sensation and weakness of muscles supplied by the upper plexus. EMG may show characteristic myokymia. Management of both neoplastic and radiation plexopathy is largely supportive.

Median Mononeuropathies (eSlide 41.12)

PRONATOR SYNDROME

Pronator syndrome occurs when the median nerve is compressed as it passes between the superficial and deep heads of the pronator teres, beneath a fascial band from the flexor digitorum superficialis, or under the biceps aponeurosis. Patients present with easy fatigue and pain after repeated elbow flexion, forearm pronation, and finger flexion, as well as paresthesias in the first three fingers and the skin over the thenar eminence; the latter is usually spared in CTS. Needle EMG can demonstrate abnormalities in all muscles supplied by the median nerve except for the pronator teres. Improvement with conservative treatment is reported in more than 50% of patients, and in those who do not improve, surgical decompression has been reported to have a high success rate.

ANTERIOR INTEROSSEOUS SYNDROME

Distal to the pronator teres, the median nerve gives off the anterior interosseous nerve, a pure motor nerve innervating the flexor digitorum profundus, flexor pollicis longus, and pronator quadratus, which can be compressed at the fibrous arch formed by the flexor digitorum superficialis. This prevents patients from making the "OK" sign; they make a key pinch posture instead. Patients often complain of an aching pain in the forearm but no sensory loss. Treatment starts with avoidance of repetitive elbow flexion, pronation, or forced gripping. A trial of nonsteroidal antiinflammatory drugs (NSAIDs) and a posterior elbow splint can be applied. Spontaneous improvement has been reported 3–24 months after symptom onset. Surgical decompression can be indicated if there is no motor recovery.

MEDIAN MONONEUROPATHY AT THE WRIST (CARPAL TUNNEL SYNDROME)

CTS is the most common focal neuropathy. Repetitive hand and wrist movement, diabetes, hypothyroidism, RA, obesity, and pregnancy are predisposing factors. The typical presentation of CTS includes paresthesias over the first four fingers, which worsens at night or when driving or holding objects, and improves after flicking the hands. Weakness or atrophy of the thenar eminence muscles can be seen. Both the Tinel sign and Phalen sign are sensitive tests. EMG studies are useful in confirming the diagnosis of CTS and assessing its severity. Prolonged median sensory latencies may be the earliest abnormality, and mid-palmar stimulation might be more sensitive because it records over a shorter segment across the carpal tunnel. Motor fibers are affected in more severe disease and can show decreased compound motor amplitude and prolonged distal latency. Needle EMG can demonstrate acute or chronic denervation in the abductor pollicis brevis or opponens pollicis and is useful in differential diagnosis. Treatment includes activity modifications, the wrist splinted in 0–5 degrees of extension, oral NSAIDs, local corticosteroid injections, and surgical decompression.

Ulnar Mononeuropathies (eSlide 41.13)

ULNAR NEUROPATHY AT THE ELBOW

Ulnar neuropathy at the elbow (UNE) is the second most common focal neuropathy. Risk factors include repetitive elbow flexion, repetitive gripping, external pressure over the ulnar groove, older age, male gender, and smoking. Patients with UNE typically present with dysesthesias and sensory changes over the ulnar aspect of the hand and forearm. As the disease advances, patients lose hand dexterity and grip strength. A Tinel sign might be elicited at the retroepicondylar region, where the nerve dives between the twin heads of the flexor carpi ulnaris. Interossei weakness, atrophy, and claw hands may be noted in severe cases. Electrodiagnostic studies are able to differentiate UNE from radiculopathies and lower trunk plexopathy. When assessed by needle EMG, the first dorsal interosseous is the muscle most likely to be affected, followed by the abductor digit quinti and flexor carpi ulnaris. If there is still diagnostic uncertainty, ultrasonography may provide more information, as it may show nerve enlargement. Therapies include avoiding powerful grip, preventing prolonged or repetitive elbow flexion, cushioning of the posterior-medial elbow to prevent compression, stopping smoking, and undergoing surgical release of the fascia of the flexor carpi ulnaris; however, the response to both nonsurgical and surgical therapy is variable.

ULNAR NEUROPATHY AT THE WRIST

The ulnar nerve enters the Guyon canal in the wrist between the hook of the hamate and the pisiform bone. When the nerve is compressed within the Guyon canal, the patient has altered sensation in the fourth and fifth digits and weakness of all the ulnar-innervated hand muscles. With injury distal to the Guyon canal, sensation in the fourth and fifth fingers would be spared. With a more distal injury, the hypothenar musculature is also spared, with weakness occurring only in the interossei. Needle EMG can help lesion localization. Although this disease can respond to activity modification, hand surgeons might be consulted if there is possible wrist bone disease.

Radial Mononeuropathies (eSlide 41.13)

RADIAL NEUROPATHY AT THE SPIRAL GROOVE

Radial neuropathy at the spiral groove is seen in fractures of the humerus or with external compression of the nerve (e.g., tourniquet use, honeymoon palsy, and

Saturday night palsy). Radial injury at the spiral groove typically presents with wrist or finger drop and mild weakness of elbow flexion due to brachioradialis involvement. Sensation is abnormal in the dorsum of the hand and first four digits. Motor nerve conduction studies may show conduction block at the spiral groove. Neuropathy caused by external compression is typically a neurapraxia, which usually recovers spontaneously within 2 months. Any response recorded from the extensor indicis at an early stage indicates a good prognosis. If there is no recovery within 8–10 weeks, surgical exploration is indicated. If there is no return of function after 1 year, tendon transfer is considered. During the recovery period, a "cock-up" splint may be needed.

POSTERIOR INTEROSSEOUS NEUROPATHY

Posterior interosseous neuropathy can occur with entrapment of the radial nerve at the arcade of Frohse (supinator syndrome) or as a result of elbow fractures or external compression. Weakness is seen in the finger extensors, supinator muscle, and extensor carpi ulnaris, sparing brachioradialis function and hand sensation. EMG needle examination typically localizes the lesion. Treatment involves avoidance of provocative activities, use of oral NSAIDs, and splinting; up to 80% of patients will recover.

Lumbosacral Plexopathies

Lumbosacral plexopathies can be seen in pelvic or hip fractures, in which the sacral plexus is preferentially affected; concurrent root avulsion can occur in cases with sacroiliac joint separation. Metastatic plexopathy presents with neuropathic pain as the predominant symptom, with weakness and sensory loss occurring later. In contrast, radiation-induced plexopathy typically presents years after radiotherapy, presenting with painless, progressive weakness. Other causes of lumbosacral plexopathy include retroperitoneal hemorrhage and obstetric injury.

Femoral Neuropathy

The femoral nerve supplies the iliopsoas muscles before emerging under the inguinal ligament, after which divides into branches to supply the quadriceps, sartorius, and pectineus muscles, the anterior aspect of the thigh and medial aspect of the leg. The femoral nerve is usually injured within the retroperitoneal space or under the inguinal ligament after iatrogenic injuries and presents with unilateral thigh weakness and numbness of the anterior thigh and medial leg. If the nerve is compressed within the pelvis, hip flexion can also be affected. Needle examination of the iliopsoas muscle can assist in localizing the lesion site as proximal or distal to the inguinal ligament. CMAP preservation at >50% of the normal value is a sign suggesting a good prognosis. With mild-to-moderate weakness, an ankle-foot orthosis with a dorsiflexion stop can create an extension moment at the knee to compensate for quadriceps weakness. If the weakness is severe, a knee-ankle-foot orthosis may be indicated.

Lateral Femoral Cutaneous Neuropathy

The lateral femoral cutaneous nerve is a purely sensory nerve innervating the anterolateral thigh. Neuropathy involving this nerve is known as "meralgia paresthetica," which presents as numbness or hyperesthesia in the nerve's territory. Potential causes include compression at the anterior superior iliac spine (ASIS) and the inguinal ligament, obesity, pregnancy, diabetes, wearing tight waistbands, or surgery within proximity of the nerve. The Tinel sign might be elicited by percussing just medial and inferior to the ASIS. Diagnostic tests include nerve conduction studies, ultrasound examination, and local anesthetic nerve blocks. Treatment involves eliminating exacerbating factors, weight reduction, topical capsaicin or lidocaine, drugs for neuropathic pain, and local corticosteroid injections. The prognosis is generally good.

Fibular (Peroneal) Mononeuropathies (eSlide 41.14)

Fibular neuropathy is the most common nerve injury in the lower extremity. Etiologic lesions include prolonged compression at the fibular head due to bedrest, improper splinting, or tumor; prolonged squatting that causes nerve traction; knee trauma; and anterior compartment syndrome. The most striking clinical finding is weakness of ankle dorsiflexion, resulting in a premature foot slap or steppage gait. Sensation is diminished in the lower two-thirds of the lateral leg and dorsum of the foot. A Tinel sign may be produced by tapping over the common fibular nerve as it courses around the fibular neck. The most specific electrodiagnostic finding is conduction block, with a greater than 20% drop in CMAP from above the fibular head to below the head. The extensor digitorum brevis or anterior tibialis should also be tested for motor response, and the presence of any CMAP is associated with good recovery. Assessment of the short head of the biceps femoris muscle is particularly useful for excluding a sciatic lesion. Treatment starts with offloading the lateral aspect of the knee, avoiding prolonged knee flexion and habitual leg crossing, and fitting the patient with an ankle-foot orthosis to improve the gait. Surgical management includes neurolysis, decompression, nerve repair, and nerve or tendon transfers.

Tibial and Plantar Mononeuropathy

Proximal tibial neuropathies are unusual but can result in weakness of plantar flexion and ankle inversion. Lesions under the flexor retinaculum, referred to as tarsal tunnel syndrome, can be caused by ankle trauma, arthritis, heel deformity, and vascular or mass compression; they present with paresthesias and pain in the sole. A Tinel sign might be elicited by percussion over the flexor retinaculum at the medial malleolus. The interdigital nerves can become entrapped under the second and third intermetatarsal ligament and form a Morton neuroma. X-ray, ultrasound, and MRI can be used to assess any structural abnormalities. Needle EMG can examine the abductor hallucis to detect injury to the medial plantar nerve and assess the abductor digiti quinti to identify dysfunction of the lateral plantar nerve. Treatment consists of NSAIDs, local corticosteroid injections, and an ankle-foot orthosis with a dorsiflexion stop to compensate for weakness of the medial gastrocnemius.

Sciatic Mononeuropathy (eSlide 41.14)

The sciatic nerve contains tibial and fibular components, which run as distinctly separate nerves that do not interchange fascicles. The fibular division is much more susceptible to injury. Common causes of sciatic nerve injury include hip fractures, posterior hip dislocations, and hip surgeries. In severe sciatic neuropathy, the tibia, fibular, and sural nerves will all show abnormalities during EMG studies. In mild cases, only the fibular division is injured, in which case sampling of the short head of the biceps femoris is useful to differentiate this from a more common distal fibular lesion. Treatment of sciatic nerve injury is largely supportive.

Other Common Mononeuropathies (eSlide 41.15)

Lower abdominal neuropathies refer to injuries to ilioinguinal, iliohypogastric, and genitofemoral nerves, causing pain affecting the lower abdomen and genital region. A Tinel sign can sometimes be elicited near the ASIS. Frequent areas of entrapment include the psoas muscle, transverse abdominis muscle, and inguinal ligament. *Obturator neuropathy* may be associated with pelvic trauma or iatrogenic injuries and presents with sensory loss of the medial thigh and weakness of hip adduction and internal rotation. A circumducted gait may be noted. EMG is most useful for detecting this injury. Most obturator injuries recover well with conservative management. *Sural neuropathy* presents with paresthesias at the posterolateral aspect of the distal calf and lateral aspect of the foot. It might be caused by a Baker cyst in the popliteal fossa, a gastrocnemius mass, or ankle surgery. Treatment involves symptomatic management and alleviation of the sources of compression.

Clinical Pearls

- PNs can be described in three axes: (1) axonal or demyelinating; (2) the motor or sensory fibers; and (3) distal, proximal, asymmetric, or multifocal pattern.
- Electrodiagnostic studies (EDS) can add confirmative or exclusive information to physical examinations. Please pay attention to conduction velocities, the dispersion and amplitude of the action potentials (APs), late responses (F waves), and needle EMG signals
- Complications of PNs include neuropathic pain, functional impairment, foot ulceration, Charcot foot, and foot deformity.
- Diabetes is the most common cause of neuropathy, which is symmetric and involves motor, sensory, and autonomic systems. Diabetic proximal neuropathy is an immune-mediated microvasculitis affecting the nerve roots and plexus.
- Both AIDP (also called Guillain-Barré Syndrome) and CIDP are responsive to steroid therapies.
- Common pathogens to trigger PNs include leprosy, Lyme disease, CMV, and HIV.
- HMSN, also called Charcot-Marie-Tooth disease, can affect gait, but loss of independent ambulation is rare.
- Common mononeuropathies in the upper limb include brachial plexopathy and median, ulnar, and radial neuropathies.
- Common mononeuropathies in the lower limb include lumbosacral plexopathy and peroneal, tibial, sciatic, and femoral neuropathies

BIBLIOGRAPHY
The complete bibliography is available on ExpertConsult.com.

Myopathy

42

Ziad M. Hawamdeh

Myopathies encompass a large group of motor diseases characterized by symmetric, proximal greater than distal weakness and preserved reflexes and sensations, which result from structural or functional abnormalities of muscle fibers. Sensory or autonomic involvement occurs in a small number of myopathies. Successful identification and classification of a myopathic disease entails obtaining a detailed history and physical examination, accompanied by the judicious use of diagnostic strategies (eSlide 42.1).

• EVALUATION OF THE PATIENT WITH A SUSPECTED MYOPATHY (eSlides 42.2, 42.3, 42.4, and 42.5)

A detailed medical history is essential for diagnosis. Weakness and hypotonia in an infant are common presenting concerns for parents. Early feeding, respiratory difficulties, and the timing of developmental milestones may provide insight into disease progression. An adolescent or adult is more likely to have symptoms that include weakness, pain, muscle cramps, decreased endurance, difficulty keeping up with peers, and muscle atrophy. A comprehensive physical examination should be performed. Evaluation of the musculoskeletal system may start with the assessment of muscle bulk. Manual muscle testing is not reliable in patients with myopathy; a handheld myometer provides much more reproducible results. Spine examination for the presence of scoliosis and kyphosis is essential. Cognitive impairment may be present. After 5 years of age, most cognitively intact children will be able to fully participate in manual muscle testing. Myopathies with pelvic girdle weakness may demonstrate a Gower sign, in which the upper limbs are used to generate hip extension moments by "walking" up the lower limbs. Gait may be altered for many reasons in myopathic diseases. Hip extension weakness may result in a lordotic posture and gait. An equinus gait pattern is seen with weak knee extensors. Hip abductor weakness may contribute to a drop of the pelvis, which is compensated by swaying the body toward the weak side (a compensated Trendelenburg gait pattern).

Diagnostic Workup

Initial laboratory screening tests include determination of serum creatine kinase (CK), alanine aminotransferase (ALT), aspartate aminotransferase (AST), and aldolase levels. CK levels, however, may be elevated after strenuous exercise in normal individuals.

Electrodiagnostic testing may be useful when the underlying pathologic process is unclear. Sensory and motor nerve conduction studies are normal in myopathic diseases; however, with disease progression, the compound motor action potential amplitude may be reduced. Needle electromyography will provide the greatest information. Many myopathies will have normal insertional activity that is reduced with muscle fibrosis. The motor unit morphology may demonstrate short duration, low amplitude, polyphasic potentials with increased or "early" recruitment. Muscle fiber necrosis may generate fibrillation potentials and positive sharp waves. Myotonic dystrophies may show "dive bomber" sound from myotonic discharges.

Muscle biopsy may be needed. A weak muscle is typically selected; however, one with marked atrophy or profound weakness is best avoided. Biopsies are commonly obtained from the biceps, triceps, deltoid, and quadriceps muscles.

• SPECIFIC MYOPATHIC DISORDERS

Inflammatory Myopathies (eSlide 42.6)

Inflammatory myopathies are rare. They include dermatomyositis, polymyositis, and inclusion body myositis.

Dermatomyositis may affect adults and children. Clinical findings include a heliotrope rash around the eyelids, an erythematous macular rash, Gottron papules, and nailfold telangiectasias. The juvenile form may have multisystem involvement. Interstitial lung disease is possible; cardiac involvement is common and the adult form may be associated with malignancy.

Polymyositis affects individuals over 20 years old and has a female predilection. It is characterized by neck flexor and symmetric proximal limb involvement, which can be associated with myalgia and muscle tenderness. Cardiac involvement may be seen; interstitial lung disease and malignancy may also occur but less frequently than with dermatomyositis.

Sporadic inclusion body myositis is the most common inflammatory myopathy in individuals older than 50 years. Patients often have asymmetric weakness, which includes the knee extensor and finger flexor muscles. Weakness of the latter produces the "intrinsic positive" hand posture, with marked difficulty in making a fist.

In inflammatory myopathies, the serum CK is usually elevated, but it may be normal. Electromyography demonstrates a myopathic pattern. Muscle biopsy reveals a characteristic inflammatory pattern. Pharmacologic treatment involves immunosuppressive agents.

Muscular Dystrophies (eSlides 42.7, 42.8, and 42.9)

DYSTROPHINOPATHIES

Dystrophinopathies are X-linked recessive muscular dystrophies caused by mutation of the dystrophin gene, which is found at locus Xp21; the dystrophin gene is the largest identified human gene. Dystrophin protein functions as a plasma membrane stabilizer. Duchenne muscular dystrophy (DMD) may be suspected in male children with hypotonia, delayed developmental milestones, and progressive limb-girdle weakness resulting in loss of ambulation between 7 and 12 years of age and death at the start of the third decade. Examination typically reveals calf pseudohypertrophy, compensatory toe walking, and use of the Gower maneuver. Contractures due to prolonged static positioning are common. Scoliosis and kyphoscoliosis may be seen, with reported incidences of up to 100%. Becker muscular dystrophy (BMD) is much less common and less severe than DMD. In BMD, ambulation is preserved until 16 years of age or later. BMD shares with DMD a similar limb-girdle weakness pattern, and it often presents after 7 years of age. Joint contractures occur less frequently with BMD.

Monitoring of respiratory function is critical in patients with DMD. Individuals with BMD usually do not exhibit the rapid changes in scoliosis and decline in respiratory muscle strength noted in DMD. Cardiac involvement occurs in up to 90% of patients with both muscle dystrophies.

CK is elevated up to 100 times the normal level in both types of dystrophinopathies (up to 20,000 IU/L). AST and ALT may also be elevated. Dystrophin gene mutation testing is indicated. Steroids have been shown to slow the rate of functional decline and prolong ambulation ability in DMD.

LIMB-GIRDLE MUSCULAR DYSTROPHIES

Limb-girdle muscular dystrophies (LGMDs) are a large group of myopathic diseases with predominantly proximal limb-girdle weakness. They are classified into dominant (LGMD1) and recessive (LGMD2) types. Most cases are slowly progressive, presenting from early childhood with LGMD2 to the start of the third decade of life with LGMD1.

CK is generally elevated. Electrodiagnosis reveals a myopathic pattern. Muscle biopsy may demonstrate myopathic changes. DNA analysis for mutations is the mainstay of diagnosis.

FACIOSCAPULOHUMERAL MUSCULAR DYSTROPHY

Facioscapulohumeral muscular dystrophy is an autosomal dominant myopathy. Most patients exhibit asymmetric weakness by 20 years of age. Individuals may first notice facial weakness more in the lower face. Nearly 5% of patients have cardiac conduction abnormalities. Most patients have symptomatic sensory neural hearing loss. Retinal telangiectasias are present in more than half of individuals and, in rare cases, may cause retinal detachment.

Serum CK levels range from normal to moderately elevated, and electromyography is consistent with a myopathic process. Muscle biopsy may exhibit inflammatory findings, but the findings are generally nonspecific. Molecular genetic testing allows quantification of D4Z4 repeats.

EMERY-DREIFUSS MUSCULAR DYSTROPHY

Emery-Dreifuss muscular dystrophy encompasses mutations of the EMD and LMNA genes, which encode the emerin and lamin proteins, respectively. The X-linked type is less common than the autosomal dominant type, which may present earlier; however, both types demonstrate weakness, atrophy, and elbow flexion and ankle plantar flexion contractures. Both forms produce humeroperoneal weakness with marked biceps atrophy, whereas the autosomal dominant type also has scapular involvement. Cardiac involvement, which is more severe in the autosomal dominant form, may lead to arrhythmias and cardiomyopathy.

CK levels are mildly elevated. Electromyography may show a myopathic pattern. Muscle biopsy rarely demonstrates necrotic fibers and increased connective tissue. Type I fibers may be slightly reduced in size and exhibit an increased predominance. Gene sequencing will detect most mutations.

Myotonic Muscular Dystrophy(eSlide 42.10)

Myotonic muscular dystrophy is an autosomal dominant disorder that includes genetically and clinically different entities. Myotonic muscular dystrophy type 1 (DM1) is the most common adult-onset muscular dystrophy. It is characterized by genetic anticipation between generations, which is related to expansion of the cytosine-thymine-guanine (CTG) sequence during cellular replication. The clinical picture depends on the number of CTG repeats. Individuals with classic DM1 have predominantly distal muscle weakness, facial weakness with a tented upper lip, frontal balding, temporal muscle atrophy, and cognitive impairment. Clinical myotonia may be observed. Patients may demonstrate the "warm-up phenomenon." Cardiac conduction abnormalities are common. Insulin insensitivity is observed; however, the incidence of diabetes mellitus is not increased. Cataracts can occur.

Myotonic muscular dystrophy type 2 (DM2) does not demonstrate anticipation like DM1. Individuals typically exhibit symptoms in adulthood consisting of proximal muscle weakness associated with pain, along with clinical myotonia, mild cognitive impairment, and daytime somnolence. DM2 can be associated with cardiac arrhythmias, cataracts, dysphagia, hypogonadism, and insulin insensitivity. The number of CTG repeats exceeding 75 confirms the diagnosis of DM2.

Congenital Myopathies (eSlide 42.11)

Congenital myopathies are rare myopathies associated with autosomal dominant or recessive genetic mutations. They include central core myopathy, nemaline myopathy, centronuclear myopathy, multiminicore myopathy, and congenital fiber-type disproportion. In congenital myopathies, serum CK is normal or mildly elevated and electrodiagnostic findings are nonspecific.

Central core myopathy initially presents as a floppy infant with proximal weakness. Individuals may have cardiac involvement, skeletal abnormalities, and facial weakness without ophthalmoplegia. Muscle biopsy demonstrates the presence of unstained "cores" found in the center of type I muscle fibers.

Nemaline myopathy can be mild, moderate, or severe. Patients may have extraocular and facial muscle weakness. Cardiomyopathy is associated with nemaline myopathy. Muscle biopsy reveals threadlike inclusions.

Patients with centronuclear myopathy may have symptoms neonatally, such as a poor cry, weak suck, and hypotonia. In childhood, a milder form of myopathy is seen. Muscle biopsy includes findings of centrally located nuclei, type I fiber predominance, and atrophy.

The classic phenotype of multiminicore myopathy includes proximal and axial muscle weakness, progressive respiratory decline, scoliosis, and spinal rigidity. Affected individuals may have arthrogryposis, external ophthalmoplegia, or predominantly distal weakness. Most patients achieve and maintain ambulation ability. Multiple small, unstructured cores and sarcomeric disruption of type I and type II fibers are found in muscle biopsy specimens.

Congenital fiber-type disproportion is a diagnosis of exclusion, which has a good prognosis. Patients often have symptoms in childhood, including proximal greater than distal weakness, hypotonia, delayed developmental milestones, facial weakness, and ophthalmoplegia. Muscle biopsy results are notable for type I fiber predominance on histologic examination.

Metabolic Myopathies (eSlide 42.12)

Metabolic myopathies are rare autosomal recessive disorders. They include acid maltase deficiency (Pompe disease) and myophosphorylase deficiency (McArdle disease). Pompe disease can occur as infantile or late-onset forms. The infantile form presents with cardiomegaly, hepatomegaly, hypotonia, weakness, and death by 1 year of age. The late-onset form presents after 1 year of age with slowly progressive proximal more than distal muscle weakness. McArdle disease patients present late in childhood with symptoms of myalgia, weakness, and reduced exercise intolerance. In extreme cases, rhabdomyolysis may occur. "Second wind" phenomenon, in which muscle stiffness, cramps, and exercise tolerance improve after a brief rest, is seen in some individuals.

Mitochondrial Myopathies (eSlide 42.12)

Mitochondrial myopathies represent a rare group of myopathies that result from mitochondrial abnormalities. They include Kearns-Sayre syndrome (KSS); mitochondrial encephalomyopathy, lactic acidosis, and strokelike episodes (MELAS); and myoclonic epilepsy with ragged-red fibers (MERRF).

KSS has an onset before the age of 20 years. Patients have progressive external ophthalmoplegia and pigmentary retinopathy. They may develop ataxia, cardiac abnormalities, diabetes mellitus, myopathy, and sensorineural hearing loss.

MELAS has symptom onset generally in childhood but may occur as late as 40 years old. In addition to the encephalopathy and strokelike episodes, individuals may have ataxia, cardiomyopathy, deafness, diabetes mellitus, migraines, myopathy, seizures, and, rarely, progressive external ophthalmoplegia.

MERRF generally begins in childhood. Ataxia, generalized seizures, cardiomyopathy, and occasionally progressive external ophthalmoplegia may be noted.

• REHABILITATION OF INDIVIDUALS WITH MYOPATHIES (eSlides 42.13, 42.14, and 42.15)

The use of progressive resistive exercise in people with myopathies has been a controversial issue. Studies have demonstrated that low-to-moderate intensity exercise may increase strength, with little to no muscle injury. Guidelines for exercise prescription include avoiding muscle damage, avoiding exercising to the point of exhaustion, and not overworking the muscles. Overwork weakness may present with muscle pain, hyperthermia, and severe muscle cramps. Aerobic training exercises are also recommended.

Braces and adaptive equipment are used to maximize the independence of an individual with a myopathy. Nighttime bracing of the wrists, fingers, and ankles may be of benefit to minimize the progression of flexion contractures. Although spinal bracing has been recommended, research has not demonstrated its efficacy in limiting progression of neuromuscular scoliosis curves.

Cardiac involvement may exhibit a vast array of presentations. Management of cardiac conduction abnormalities and heart failure by a cardiologist is mandatory. Heart transplantation may be considered in patients with end-stage heart failure. In some myopathies, the respiratory muscles may be weakened and fibrosed, resulting in a functional restrictive lung disease. Symptomatic hypoventilation will often be reported as snoring, insomnia, daytime somnolence, fatigue, drowsiness, depression, impaired cognitive function, and morning headaches. Once hypoventilation has been identified, determination of the most appropriate management strategy becomes the focus of care. Patients should also be encouraged to receive appropriate vaccinations, including annual influenza vaccinations.

Nutritional inadequacy may develop. Progressively impaired mobility, impaired respiratory mechanics, and dysphagia may limit the ability of the patient to self-feed. A gastrostomy tube for supplemental nutrition and hydration may be needed. A nutritionist should be incorporated in the health care team. Disease severity, pain, fatigue, depression, and anxiety have demonstrated a high level of association with and impact on the quality of life in myopathic patients. Psychiatric consultation and initiation of antidepressant medications may be indicated.

• CONCLUSION

Myopathies encompass a large heterogeneous collection of diseases defined by muscle abnormalities and characterized by proximal muscle weakness. Appropriate diagnosis is important for prognosis and medical and rehabilitative services. Patient and family integration in decision-making is essential to achieve optimal functional outcomes.

Clinical Pearls

1. Acquired myopathies include inflammatory myopathies, toxic myopathies, and systemic disease–associated myopathies.
2. Hereditary myopathies involve genetic mutations that compromise muscle fiber structure, physiology, or both.
3. Myopathies with muscle fiber destruction are classified as muscular dystrophies.
4. Congenital myopathies are symptomatic at birth or in the perinatal period. Metabolic and mitochondrial myopathies are classified by the mechanism underlying the physiologic dysfunction of the muscle fibers.
5. Rehabilitation of myopathic individuals should include exercise of mild-to-moderate intensity, frequent breaks, and avoidance of fatigue and overwork weakness. Bracing is used to maximize independence.
6. Cardiopulmonary evaluation and early diagnosis and management of related complications are essential in most myopathic individuals.
7. With disease progression, most myopathic individuals may have nutritional and psychosocial problems that should be adequately addressed.

BIBLIOGRAPHY
The complete bibliography is available on ExpertConsult.com.

Traumatic Brain Injury

43

Mazlina Mazlan

The pathophysiology, types, risk factors, consequences, evaluation, and management of traumatic brain injury (TBI), along with brief updates on the current relevant clinical trials, will be discussed in this chapter and the accompanying eSlides.

• DEFINITION

TBI is defined as "an alteration in brain function, or other evidence of brain pathology, caused by an external force." The diagnosis of TBI is often established through an evaluation of clinical symptoms, as well as positive neurologic signs and neuroimaging findings.

• SEVERITY

TBI is categorized as mild, moderate, or severe based on certain parameters: (1) the initial Glasgow Coma Scale (GCS) score (eSlide 43.1), with a GCS score of 13–15 classified as mild TBI, GCS score of 9–12 as moderate TBI, and GCS score of 3–8 as severe TBI; and (2) the duration of loss of consciousness (LOC) or coma, including the duration of posttraumatic amnesia (PTA). Individuals sustaining moderate to severe TBI often have a more prolonged LOC or coma and continue to exhibit symptoms of PTA for a significant period of time.

• EPIDEMIOLOGY

The overall worldwide incidences of TBI are as follows: 80% are mild, 10% are moderate, and 10% are severe. Individuals who survive moderate to severe TBI generally require significant medical care and hospital stays. Many are left with long-term disability as a result of these injuries, with 40% of individuals hospitalized because of TBI reporting at least one ongoing issue 1 year after their injury.

• CAUSES

The leading causes of TBI in the United States are falls (35%), traffic-related crashes (17%), "struck by or against" events (sports) (17%), assaults (10%), and other injuries (21%). However, these statistics vary by age, gender, and geographic location within and between countries. In Europe, for example, 60% of TBIs are caused by road traffic injuries, 20%–30% are caused by falls, 10% are due to violence, and 10% are sports-related or work-related.

• ASSOCIATED COSTS

The costs associated with TBI can be divided into direct and indirect costs. Direct costs involve the financial requirements for medical care. Indirect costs refer to costs associated with lost productivity of the individuals with TBI, as well as the family members caring for them, and costs associated with reduced participation in complex leisure or recreational activities.

• RISK FACTORS

Age and Gender

The three age groups most at risk for sustaining a TBI are 0- to 4-year-olds, 15- to 19-year-olds, and adults over the age of 75. Motor vehicle accidents result in the greatest number of TBI injuries for people 15–19 years of age, whereas fall-related injuries are highest among adults over the age of 75. Men are twice as likely to sustain a TBI as women, although in the older population with TBI (age >65 years), women are increasing in number.

Socioeconomic Status

People with a lower socioeconomic status have an increased risk of injury because of several factors, such as unhealthy lifestyle, risk-taking behavior, high-risk occupation, and personal violence.

Violence

Assault or violence-related injuries account for 11% of TBIs. People who sustain a TBI caused by a violence-related injury are more likely to be younger, single, male, and a member of a minority group. They are also more likely to have a history of alcohol abuse.

Child Abuse

Infants are at greatest risk for sustaining a TBI as a result of shaken baby syndrome (SBS). One-third of SBS victims survive with no consequences, one-third sustain permanent injury, and one-third die. Risk factors for the occurrence of SBS include maternal factors (mothers younger than 19 years), education less than 12 years, single marital status, African American or Native American race, limited prenatal care, or newborns less than 28 weeks old.

Psychosocial Factors

Factors such as substance use, a prior psychiatric history, and affinity for high-risk behaviors are related to TBI incidence.

Members of Military

Military members who sustain a TBI are more likely to be male, with approximately 88% of TBIs classified as mild injuries and the remaining 12% as moderate to severe. The leading causes of military TBIs are blasts (72%), falls (11%), vehicular incidents (6%), injuries caused by fragments (5%), and other injuries (6%).

Country Income

Low- and middle-income countries have more risk factors that contribute to TBIs, including poor road design, substandard vehicles, higher rates of violence because of war, and fewer prevention measures.

• PATHOPHYSIOLOGY (eSlide 43.2)

The pathophysiologic processes associated with TBI are complex.

Primary Injury

Primary injury occurs immediately, in conjunction with the mechanical forces that disrupt the brain tissue. The two main forces are contact forces that occur when the head is prevented from moving after it is struck and inertial forces that occur when the head is set into motion and result in acceleration. Focal contusions, coup and contre-coup injuries, and epidural hematomas (EDHs) result from contact forces in TBI, whereas diffuse axonal injury, subdural hematomas (SDHs), and traumatic subarachnoid hemorrhages result from inertial forces in TBI.

Secondary Injury

Secondary injury develops over the hours and days after the initial impact. Elevated intracranial pressure (ICP) and decreased cerebral perfusion pressure may result from brain swelling, focal extra-axial lesions (such as SDH and EDH), or global mechanisms occurring on a cellular level that lead to brain edema. An excess of excitatory amino acids, such as glutamate and aspartate is seen in the extracellular fluid and cerebrospinal fluid (CSF) after TBI. This contributes to excitotoxic injury, which eventually leads to acute neuronal and astrocytic swelling, delayed cellular damage, or cell death via cellular necrosis and apoptosis. More severe TBIs are often associated with multiple other injuries. These concomitant injuries can directly affect secondary injury and the associated pathology. Experimental models show greater hippocampal injury with TBI and hemorrhagic shock than with TBI alone, a phenomenon likely associated with increased secondary ischemia.

Long-Term Degeneration, Neurotransmission Repair, Regeneration, and Recovery

The chronic period after injury is characterized by multiple neurotransmitter deficits and cellular dysfunction. During this period, the brain is amenable to neuroplasticity, repair, and recovery. Early TBI recovery occurs through resolution of cerebral edema and blood flow regulation. At a later stage, recovery occurs through reversal of diaschisis, which involves factors such as synaptic plasticity, axonal sprouting, and cortical reorganization. Late recovery can also be manipulated by relevant rehabilitation strategies and pharmacologic interventions.

Military Blast Injury

Many active combat military personnel sustain a TBI from blast injury, resulting in specific types of primary, secondary, tertiary, and quaternary injuries. Explosives are categorized as high-order explosives (HEs) or low-order explosives (LEs). HEs can result in both primary and tertiary blast injuries, whereas LEs can produce tertiary blast injury from the person being physically thrown by a blast wind. In many patients, the TBI is produced by more than one facet of a blast injury.

• EVALUATION AND TREATMENT OF TRAUMATIC BRAIN INJURY

Mild Traumatic Brain Injury (Concussion)

Concussion produces significant alterations in brain physiology; grading systems have been developed for injury characterization and management (eSlide 43.3).

Patients with mild TBI complain of associated symptoms, including memory loss, poor concentration, impaired emotional control, posttraumatic headaches, sleep disorders, fatigue, irritability, dizziness, visual acuity, depression, anxiety, personality changes, and seizures. For most patients, symptoms resolve over time. Persistent symptoms of mild TBI are also referred to as postconcussion syndrome. Special issues arise with the management of mild TBI in athletes with regard to "on-site" concussion screening tools, determination of the most effective algorithm for return to play (RTP), use of safety equipment, management and prevention of recurrent injuries, and academic performance. Several RTP protocols are being developed for athletes, but in general, athletes should be free of postconcussive symptoms before returning to competition.

Acute Medical Management of Moderate to Severe Traumatic Brain Injury

The care of the patient with TBI begins in the field, where issues such as prehospital care, triage, and direct transport of a patient with a severe TBI to a level 1 or 2 trauma center are addressed. Recommendations include complete and rapid physiologic resuscitation; correction of hypoxia, including endotracheal intubation if necessary; and the use of sedation and neuromuscular blockade to optimize conditions during transport of the patient. ICP monitoring is appropriate for patients with a GCS of 8 or less after resuscitation, a head computed tomography (CT) scan showing contusions or edema, or a systolic blood pressure (SBP) less than 90 mm Hg. It can also be considered in patients with severe TBI and negative head CT findings if they are older than 40 years, are posturing, and/or have a SBP less than 90 mm Hg. Surgical treatment of TBI is indicated when there is a significant mass effect or a depressed skull fracture greater than the thickness of the skull. Decompressive craniectomy surgery may be a management option for increased ICP. Prevention and treatment of secondary complications in the intensive care unit, such as abnormal electrolyte and glucose levels and infections, are started early. Adequate and early initiation of nutrition is important in a patient with TBI; replacing 140% of the resting metabolism expenditure via the gastrointestinal tract is preferred to maintain a positive nitrogen balance. As a part of the acute medical care, early consultation with a physiatrist can result in improved mobility, improved functional outcomes, and decreased acute care length of stay.

Physiologic Measurements During Acute Care

Some physiologic measurements are beneficial as clinical predictors and tools to determine the injury severity and depth of coma, as well as to detect clinical deterioration. Commonly used measurements are somatosensory-evoked potentials (SSEPs), continuous electroencephalography, and pupillary reflexes. In severely injured patients, SSEPs, including the central somatosensory conduction time, have been associated with long-term functional outcome measures.

Neuroimaging for Medical Management

The head CT scan is the current standard neuroimaging modality for the initial evaluation of patients with suspected moderate to severe TBI. The CT scan can identify mass lesions that constitute a neurosurgical emergency, as well as other findings that correlate with the severity of the TBI (eSlides 43.4, 43.5, 43.6, and 43.7). CT has the advantages of being relatively low cost, rapid, and noninvasive, and it can accurately detect facial and skull fractures, as well as acute hemorrhages and mass effects. The use of CT in cases of mild TBI is still debatable because the head CT is often negative. Magnetic resonance imaging (MRI) is the second method of structural neuroimaging in TBI. Compared with CT, MRI has superior resolution and provides much higher soft tissue detail, which is useful for detecting brainstem and frontal area injuries, small hemorrhages, and nonhemorrhagic white matter injury. However, MRI takes longer to complete, is more susceptible to motion artifacts, and is less able to detect skull fractures and acute bleeding than CT.

Traumatic Brain Injury Patients With Disorders of Consciousness

The different states of disorders of consciousness (DOC) are classified into coma, vegetative state (VS), and minimally conscious state (MCS). Coma is defined as a state of pathologic unconsciousness in which the eyes remain closed, and there is no evidence of purposeful motor activity. Patients in a VS show some evidence of wakefulness in the form of eye opening but no sustained or reproducible responses to the environment. In an MCS, patients exhibit definite, reproducible responses that provide evidence of self or environmental awareness. Current evaluation of patients with DOC includes a thorough neurologic examination, including brainstem reflexes and observation of spontaneous activity and responses to environmental stimuli. Behavioral observation should consider family observation of behaviors performed in an optimal environment and in the absence of sedating medications. Standardized rating scales are available to differentiate among the DOC states.

A variety of interventions have been studied in patients with DOC to promote arousal and behavioral persistence. These include multimodal sensory stimuli, pharmacology, and implantation of electrodes within the brainstem and thalamus.

Behavioral Measures of Responsiveness and Cognition

EMERGENCE FROM COMA

Evaluation of emergence from coma involves a serial assessment of a patient's ability to respond to external stimuli, often conducted through the use of a standardized measure of responsiveness, such as the 11-item Coma/Near Coma scale and the 23-item JFK Coma Recovery Scale-Revised.

EVALUATION OF POSTTRAUMATIC AMNESIA

PTA involves a period of time before injury, during injury, and after injury. The Galveston Orientation and Amnesia Test and the Orientation Log are commonly used to measure symptoms of disorientation or confusion and amnesia in PTA. The Neurobehavioral Rating Scale has items to measure psychiatric symptoms, and the Confusion Assessment Protocol measures delirium associated with TBI. The Ranchos Levels of Cognitive Functioning Scale is a widely accepted method of describing the process of cognitive recovery from coma, through emergence from posttraumatic amnesia/delirium, and up to near-normal cognitive functioning (eSlide 43.8).

It is widely adopted to assess patient functioning for the purposes of rehabilitation planning and treatment and to explain patient progress to families.

Inpatient Rehabilitation Assessment and Management

The focus of inpatient rehabilitation following TBI is to assist each patient in improving functional independence. The basic rehabilitation team comprises an interdisciplinary group of specialists, including physiatrists, physical therapists, occupational therapists, speech language pathologists, neuropsychologists, and other hospital staff, such as nurses and case managers. As cognitive and behavioral issues associated with TBI may pose unique challenges to the provision of rehabilitation treatment, all members of the team should ideally be specially trained to work with patients who have sustained a TBI.

MEDICAL REHABILITATION EVALUATION, COMPLICATIONS, AND MANAGEMENT

A physiatrist or rehabilitation specialist should conduct a thorough neurologic examination during the initial evaluation of a new patient admitted to the inpatient rehabilitation unit. The evaluation is often performed in multiple sessions, depending on a patient's medical and cognitive status. Medical complications can still occur while patients are in the rehabilitation unit, despite medical stability having been achieved at the time of transfer to inpatient rehabilitation.

Posttraumatic Seizures. Posttraumatic seizures (PTSs) have been classified as immediate (<24 hours after injury), early (24 hours to 7 days after injury), and late (>7 days after injury). Late PTSs are also defined as posttraumatic epilepsies. Up to 86% of patients with one seizure after TBI will have a second seizure within 2 years of their injury. Risk factors for PTSs include a penetrating brain injury, depressed skull fracture, GCS score <8, and focal mass lesion with a midline shift. Phenytoin is commonly used for early prophylaxis against the development of PTSs, as well as for the treatment of these seizures. It is recommended that asymptomatic patients with a moderate to severe TBI receive prophylactic treatment with phenytoin for 7 days after their injury.

Heterotopic Ossification. Heterotopic ossification (HO), the formation of ectopic bone outside the skeleton, is a common complication occurring after TBI. The pathophysiology of HO after TBI is poorly understood, but evidence suggests that central nervous system processes facilitate HO formation. The incidence of HO after TBI ranges from 11% to 28%. Patients at greater risk are those with more severe TBI, immobility, spasticity, fractures, and dysautonomia. X-rays can identify HO (eSlide 43.9) in more advanced cases, but a triple phase bone scan is sensitive for identifying early and asymptomatic HO. Common prophylactic methods include antiinflammatory medications, irradiation, and calcium binding chelating agents; however, the efficacy of these strategies is not well established. Surgical excision is the most effective treatment for HO after TBI, which is performed after maturation of the ossification is complete.

Deep Venous Thrombosis. The estimated incidence of deep venous thrombosis (DVT) after TBI is 40%. Patients at highest risk for DVT include those with an advanced age, a severe injury, prolonged immobilization, significant fractures, and presence of a clotting disorder. Evidence supports the use of either unfractionated heparin or low molecular weight heparin within 24–72 hours after severe TBI as DVT prophylaxis. Caution should be used when considering prophylaxis or anticoagulation for patients at risk of bleeding or falling (e.g., because of their behavior patterns). In patients with a risk of bleeding, mechanical compression devices can be used instead. The length of DVT prophylaxis in the TBI population is similar to the duration used for general rehabilitation patients: continued prophylaxis until the patients can consistently ambulate greater than 100 feet.

Swallowing and Nutrition. Moderate to severe TBI is associated with specific nutritional needs because of hypermetabolism, increased energy expenditure, and increased protein loss. The focus of nutritional support is progressive institution of oral feeding, caloric and nutriceutical supplementation, and early institution of enteral nutritional support, if needed. A percutaneous feeding tube is placed if a patient is not expected to tolerate oral nutrition for more than 30 days.

Bowel and Bladder Dysfunction. Injury to cortical and subcortical structures can lead to bladder and bowel dysfunction. Patterns of dysfunction include an uninhibited overactive bladder, poor perception of bladder fullness, and poor sphincter control. Treatment options include behavioral interventions, such as timed voiding and anticholinergic medications. For bowel dysfunction, constipation is more common than incontinence. Bowel programs to manage dysfunction include stool softeners, stimulant suppositories, and hydration.

Airway and Pulmonary Management. Pulmonary complications after TBI may be directly related to the trauma (e.g., pneumothorax, hemothorax, flail chest, and rib fractures) or the degree of neurologic injury (e.g., respiratory failure, pulmonary edema, and airway complications). Pneumonia occurs in 60% of patients in acute care and rehabilitation. The presence of respiratory failure and the need for tracheostomy increase hospital length of stay and reduce functional status at 1 year. Early tracheostomy (≤8 days) is an option to reduce morbidity and shorten the time to initiation of acute rehabilitation. A step-wise decannulation approach should be considered when patients with TBI regain sufficient pulmonary and neurologic functions.

Spasticity and Contractures. In population with severe TBI, the incidence of spasticity measured using the modified Ashworth Scale or the Tardieu Scale (eSlide 43.10) has been reported to be as high as 84%. Risk factors for developing spasticity include more severe injury (lower GCS score), motor dysfunction (hemiplegia or tetraplegia), associated anoxic injury, spinal cord injury, and increased age. Management of spasticity is often multimodal and may include the use of splinting devices with passive range of movement exercises, a stretching program, physical modalities, serial casting, or pharmacotherapy. Commonly used medications are dantrolene, baclofen, benzodiazepines, tizanidine, and clonidine. Somnolence and cognitive effects often limit the usefulness of these medications in the TBI population; thus focal chemodenervation using phenol or botulinum toxin may be preferred for focal spasticity.

Normal Pressure Hydrocephalus. Normal pressure hydrocephalus is a treatable neurosurgical complication after severe TBI, with an estimated incidence of 45%. Clinical presentation of acute hydrocephalus includes headache, nausea, vomiting, and lethargy. The symptoms of delayed hydrocephalus or normal pressure hydrocephalus are more subtle and include the clinical triad of dementia, gait ataxia, and urinary incontinence. These symptoms are amenable to shunting of the CSF, but patients with concomitant cerebral atrophy are less likely to be responsive to shunting.

Endocrine Dysfunction Associated With Traumatic Brain Injury. Neuroendocrine disorders affect a significant portion of the TBI population regardless of the injury severity, with anterior pituitary dysfunction being more common than posterior pituitary dysfunction. The pathology is attributed to primary injury, secondary injury, or both to the hypothalamus and pituitary gland. In patients with cognitive decline, slow recovery, and decreased energy levels, anterior pituitary hormone levels, specifically thyroid hormone and growth hormone levels, should be evaluated. The syndrome of inappropriate antidiuretic hormone secretion and neurogenic diabetes insipidus are examples of posterior pituitary dysfunction.

Posttraumatic Headache. Posttraumatic headache is the most common secondary headache disorder and a cardinal feature of the postconcussive syndrome. Headache types after TBI are diverse and include tension and migraine or probable migraine types. Acetaminophen or nonsteroidal antiinflammatory drugs (NSAIDs) have been used for treatment with variable success. Patients with migraine or probable migraine headaches may need to use more traditional migraine abortive agents (e.g., triptans and long-acting NSAIDs) and/or preventive agents (e.g., tricyclics, β-blockers, calcium channel blockers, and anticonvulsants).

Neurodegenerative Disorders and Chronic Traumatic Encephalopathy. There is increased awareness of the long-term neurodegenerative consequences of repetitive TBI; however, definitive research is still under way.

FUNCTIONAL EVALUATION AND TREATMENT CONCEPTS IN REHABILITATION

Vestibular Dysfunction. The incidence of dizziness and imbalance is between 30% and 60% in post-TBI populations, with the highest incidence in patients with a temporal bone fracture. Etiologies for these symptoms include peripheral vestibular injuries, such as benign paroxysmal positional vertigo, labyrinthine concussion, or hearing loss and vertigo, which can be managed with vestibular and balance rehabilitation. Central causes of dizziness, which have worse outcomes, can include direct trauma to the brainstem, cerebellum, or both. Rehabilitation techniques for these conditions aim to induce adaptation in the central nervous system, decrease symptoms, and promote active function and postural stability.

Visual and Perceptual Dysfunction. Injury may occur to the optic nerve, visual cortex, visual processing centers, or oculomotor nerves and lead to various symptoms, such as diplopia, photophobia, difficulties with tracking and fixation, and visuoperceptual complaints. The most common cranial nerve palsy after TBI is a third nerve palsy, followed by fourth and sixth cranial nerve palsies. Assessment of visual problems should include visual acuity testing, visual field examination, functional testing, and a neuro-ophthalmologic evaluation. Adaptive strategies include prisms, computer-based treatments, biofeedback, and stereoscopic devices.

Exercise and Traumatic Brain Injury. Increasing evidence suggests that voluntary exercise may provide neurotrophic support to the injured brain. However, physical exertion too early after an injury may be detrimental to recovery. Measures should be taken to reintroduce exercise programs in a graded fashion to limit the patient's symptoms. There are unique challenges in implementing an exercise program in TBI patients with behavioral dysfunction, such as agitation, impulsivity, and aggression.

COGNITION AFTER TRAUMATIC BRAIN INJURY

Arousal, attention, memory, and executive control are areas of cognitive functioning commonly impaired following TBI. Research has supported the use of methylphenidate to improve attention and amantadine to enhance general cognition and attention in patients with moderate and severe TBI. Initiation of neuropsychological assessment can begin during the early stages of emergence from coma, continue through the period of PTA, and be completed during long-term recovery. Administering full neuropsychological test batteries should be postponed until the patient is medically stable and able to tolerate formal testing. Awareness of a patient's current cognitive status by family members and all staff is critical for providing optimal therapeutic care. Training families of the patients' regarding cognitive and behavioral issues associated with TBI is an important part of the rehabilitation process. Patient interventions are individualized and may include reorientation, step-by-step instructions, and use of consistent therapy staff. Helpful behavioral and cognitive strategies for common issues following TBI are reviewed in eSlide 43.11.

BEHAVIORAL, EMOTIONAL, AND MOOD ISSUES IN REHABILITATION

Agitation. Agitation, an excess of one or more behaviors that occur during an altered state of consciousness (e.g., PTA), is common in the acute phase of recovery from TBI. These behaviors can include aggressive physical or verbal behaviors, restlessness, and disinhibition. The Agitated Behavior Scale (eSlide 43.12) is effectively used to describe the agitation, monitor the patient's progression through recovery, and evaluate the effectiveness of interventions to manage agitation. Medications should be chosen carefully and used in conjunction with other behavior management techniques for maximum effect. Pharmacologic treatment for agitation may be beneficial, but potential adverse effects on neurologic recovery should be considered. Commonly used medications include atypical antipsychotics (e.g., quetiapine), β-blockers (e.g., propranolol), and selective serotonin (5-HT) reuptake inhibitors and 5-HT2 receptor antagonists (e.g., trazodone).

Hypoarousal and Sleep Disturbance. Patients with hypoarousal complain of fatigue, may fall asleep in the midst of a task, or frequently ask to return to their room or bed. The timing of administration and the sedating side effect profiles of existing medications should be reviewed. Treatment of hypoarousal includes using psychostimulants, evaluating the therapy schedule, establishing patient therapy routines, providing rest breaks in the schedule, and scheduling the most challenging tasks during periods of the day when the patient appears to be most alert. Sleep disturbances after TBI include alterations in circadian rhythms, sleep patterns, and sleep quality, which can result from pharmacologic treatments, associated neuropsychiatric conditions, agitation, drug withdrawal, pain, preexisting sleep disorders, and environmental overstimulation. Pharmacologic intervention is often needed to effectively treat TBI-mediated sleep disorders. Trazodone is frequently used in the TBI population, as it promotes natural sleep cycles. Cognitive-behavioral therapies, including stimulus control, sleep restriction, and sleep hygiene education, are beneficial.

Psychiatric Issues. Depression is the most common psychological problem after TBI, with the highest prevalence in the first year after injury, especially in individuals with moderate to severe injury. It is associated with impaired cognitive function and poor outcomes and may mimic the effects of the TBI itself. Posttraumatic stress disorder may develop, especially in military blast-related injuries. Treatments for these issues are the same as for individuals without TBI.

BEHAVIORAL MANAGEMENT

Behavioral management involves interactions designed to promote positive behaviors and/or decrease negative behaviors. Any observed patterns of antecedents, behaviors, and consequences may be used to create an individualized behavior plan to promote desired behaviors.

PEDIATRIC POPULATION

Assaults, child abuse, and falls are commonly associated with pediatric TBI, especially in children under the age of 7 years. Cognitive deficits may become more apparent as the child ages, supporting the need for serial neuropsychological testing and increased educational support. The neuropsychological test findings most correlated with long-term dependency are memory deficits. Social difficulties stem from deficits in executive functioning and behavior, and they are more apparent in children injured during their teens. Social functioning is an important predictor of quality of life.

• OUTCOMES, COMMUNITY INTEGRATION, AND PREVENTION

Demographic factors, severity scores, and other clinical, biochemical, and physiologic markers are used as acute predictors of TBI outcome. Neuroimaging techniques are being explored to assist clinicians with TBI prognosis (eSlides 43.13 and 43.14). There are numerous outcome measures available to track TBI patient progress and recovery during the acute care and rehabilitation phases, and on return to the community. The Functional Independence Measure tracks progress in rehabilitation, the Glasgow Outcome Scale-Extended measures general recovery and outcome, and the Disability Rating Scale rates changes in functioning from coma to community reentry. Quality of life in the TBI population is assessed using the 36-Item Short Form Health Survey and the Sickness Impact Profile-5. Community integration, which includes self-care, mobility, physical function issues, and participation in vocational, social, and community roles, is the ultimate goal for patients with a TBI and can be objectively assessed using measures such as the Community Integration Questionnaire. Vocational rehabilitation is effective in helping patients return to employment after TBI. While transportation is one of the most important links to community integration, driving is a complex cognitive task, which requires skill sets in which TBI patients may have deficits. A formal driving evaluation using driving simulators and on-road tests is recommended for some patients with TBI.

TBI prevention focuses on three aspects: (1) primary prevention (i.e., preventing the event through legislation and policymaking), (2) secondary prevention to decrease bodily harm caused by an injury (e.g., mandatory use of protective helmets), and (3) tertiary prevention, which is the care and rehabilitation of those already injured to further reduce the consequences of their injury. Telerehabilitation is an example of tertiary prevention.

Clinical Pearls

1. The syndrome of inappropriate antidiuretic hormone secretion is a common cause of hyponatremia after traumatic brain injury (TBI), and initial management for the syndrome includes fluid restriction.
2. Key criteria for the diagnosis of mild TBI include a Glasgow Coma Scale score of 13–15 after 30 minutes and at least one of the following: confusion, disorientation, loss of consciousness <30 minutes, posttraumatic amnesia <24 hours, or other transient focal neurologic abnormalities.

BIBLIOGRAPHY
The complete bibliography is available on ExpertConsult.com.

Stroke Syndromes 44

Mooyeon Oh-Park, Mauro Zampolini, and
Jason Bitterman

Stroke is the leading cause of serious disability worldwide. Early and accurate rec-ognition of stroke syndromes will enable clinicians to implement interventions for the optimal functional outcome of this population. Visualization of the brain has improved substantially with the advancement of neuroimaging. However, stroke syndromes are diagnosed primarily based on the history and physical examination, especially for individuals with negative brain images. Therefore clinicians should have a thorough knowledge of the functional neuroanatomy and vascular anatomy of the brain to make an accurate diagnosis of stroke syndromes. This chapter sum-marizes neuroanatomy, vascular anatomy, and specific stroke syndromes.

• CLINICAL IMPORTANCE AND RELEVANCE OF STROKE SYNDROMES

Stroke affects 800,000 individuals in the United States. Some stroke syndromes are subtle at the onset yet result in profound functional deficits later. Therefore it is essential for clinicians to be familiar with the symptoms and signs of specific stroke syndromes for prompt diagnosis and optimal intervention.

• FUNCTIONAL NEUROANATOMY

The brain is conventionally divided into four distinct regions: cerebrum, dienceph-alon, cerebellum, and brainstem.

The cerebrum has the cortex (frontal, parietal, occipital, temporal lobes; eSlide 44.1), basal ganglia, and limbic system. The frontal lobe controls skeletal movement, executive function, and behavioral expression. The parietal lobe receives somatic sensation, spatial cognition (particularly the nondominant side), and houses some optic radiations. The temporal lobe involves hearing and olfactory function and also houses optic radiations. The occipital lobe receives optic radiations, and lesions of the occipital lobe cause vision dysfunction. Because the optic radiation travels through the parietal and temporal lobes, superior or inferior contralateral vision loss may occur from a stroke affecting the parietal or temporal lobe, respectively.

The diencephalon consists of the thalamus, hypothalamus, pituitary, and pineal glands. The thalamus is connected to all of the major areas of the brain. It receives sensory information from the face and body before it is relayed to the cerebrum, acting as a "switch board." The thalamus also plays an important role in sleep and wakefulness. The hypothalamus controls the functions related to basic survival, including hunger, thirst, and autonomic and endocrine functions. The cerebellum is involved in the fine tuning of movement and balance.

The brainstem consists of the midbrain, pons, and medulla. The brainstem is responsible for vital functions, including respiration, circulation, wakefulness, and swallowing. This explains the high rate of early mortality in patients with

TABLE 44.1 Summary of Structures of the Brainstem

	Neural Structures	Associated Neurologic Deficit
4 Medial structures beginning with **M**	Motor pathway (corticospinal tract) crossing midline at the level of foramen magnum	Contralateral weakness of the arm and leg
	Medial lemniscus (continuation of posterior columns crossing midline at the level of foramen magnum)	Contralateral loss of vibration and proprioception in the arm and leg
	Medial longitudinal fasciculus	Ipsilateral internuclear ophthalmoplegia (failure of adduction of ipsilateral eye and lateral nystagmus in the opposite eye)
	Motor nucleus and nerve	Ipsilateral loss of cranial nerve (III, IV, VI, XII)
4 Lateral structures beginning with **S**	Spinocerebellar pathways	Ipsilateral ataxia of arm and leg
	Spinothalamic pathway	Contralateral deficit of pain and temperature of arm and leg
	Sensory nucleus of the 5th cranial nerve	Ipsilateral deficit of pain and temperature of face
	Sympathetic pathway	Ipsilateral Horner syndrome (partial ptosis, miosis)
Cranial nerves in the medulla (motor nuclei)	IX Glossopharyngeal	Ipsilateral loss of pharyngeal sensation
	X Vagus	Ipsilateral palatal weakness
	XI Spinal accessory	Ipsilateral weakness of trapezius and sternocleidomastoid muscles
	XII Hypoglossal (midline)	Ipsilateral weakness of the tongue
4 Cranial nerves in the pons	V Trigeminal	Ipsilateral deficit of pain, temperature, and light touch on face sparing angle of the jaw
	VI Abducent (midline)	Ipsilateral weakness of abduction of the eye
	VII Facial	Ipsilateral facial weakness
	VIII Cochlear	Ipsilateral deafness
4 Cranial nerves in the midbrain	Oculomotor (III)	Impaired adduction, supraduction, infraduction of ipsilateral eye Dilated pupil may be present
	Trochlear (IV)	Inability for ipsilateral eye to look down when the eye is adducted

Reference: Gates P: The rule of 4 of the brainstem: a simplified method for understanding brainstem anatomy and brainstem vascular syndromes for the non-neurologist, *Intern Med J* 35(4):263–266, 2005.

brainstem strokes. Gates described the rule of four regarding the brainstem structures and corresponding functions (eSlide 44.2). There are four longitudinal structures in the midline beginning with "M" and four longitudinal structures in the lateral beginning with "S" (Table 44.1). The cranial nerve nuclei are horizontal structures spread out in the midbrain (III, IV), the pons (V, VI, VII, VIII), and the medulla (IX, X, XI, XII). The midbrain involves coordination of eye movement. The medulla houses motor pathways (corticospinal track), which decussate at this

TABLE 44.2 Stroke Syndromes of Posterior Circulation

Vascular Territory	Neuroanatomic Location	Clinical Presentations
Posterior cerebral artery (PCA)	Occipital lobe	Contralateral homonymous hemianopsia
	Concomitant involvement of splenium of corpus callosum	Alexia (inability to read)
	Ventral occipital cortex	Achromatopsia (inability to differentiate color)
Bilateral PCA	As above	Cortical blindness
		Anton syndrome (denial of blindness combined with confabulation)
Posterior inferior cerebellar artery (PICA)	Inferior cerebellar hemisphere and vermis, lateral medulla (cranial nerve V nuclei, restiform body,	Wallenberg syndrome
		Ipsilateral deficit of facial temperature, pain, and light touch
		Ataxia
	cerebellar peduncle	Ipsilateral cerebellar signs
	vestibular nucleus,	Vertigo, nystagmus, nausea/vomiting
	nucleus of ambiguous	Hoarseness, dysphagia
	spinothalamic tract, sympathetic tract)	Contralateral hemisensory loss of arm and leg
		Hiccups, Horner syndrome
Basilar artery	Pons	
	Corticospinal pathway	Limb weakness (often bilateral), upper motor neuron signs (hyperreflexia, extensor response of Babinski)
	Corticobulbar pathway	Facial weakness, dysarthria, dysphagia, increase gag reflex
	Oculomotor	Diplopia, gaze palsies, nystagmus
	Medial Longitudinal Fasciculus	Internuclear ophthalmoplegia
	Reticular activating system	Reduced consciousness

Adapted from Nouh A, Remke J, Ruland S: Ischemic posterior circulation stroke: a review of anatomy, clinical presentations, diagnosis, and current management, *Front Neurol* 5:30, 2014.

location and are responsible for movement of the opposite side of the body. Combined examination of longitudinal and horizontal structures aids the diagnosis of brainstem stroke syndromes (eSlide 44.2).

• VASCULAR SUPPLY OF BRAIN

The internal carotid artery divides into the middle and anterior cerebral arteries (MCA and ACA). The MCA supplies the parietal, occipital, and temporal lobes, as well as a small portion of the frontal lobe (eSlide 44.3). The lenticulostriate arteries from the MCA supply the internal capsule and basal ganglia. The ACA supplies the frontal pole and medial frontal lobe (Fig. 44.1). The vertebral arteries supply the posterior circulation of the brain. They form the basilar artery at the junction between the medulla and the pons, supplying the brainstem and cerebellum. The basilar artery eventually divides into bilateral posterior cerebral arteries (PCAs) and posterior communicating arteries, which connect with anterior circulation completing the circle of Willis (eSlide 44.4). The paramedian branches from the basilar artery and three long circumferential branches: the anterior inferior cerebellar artery (AICA), the superior cerebellar artery (SCA), and the posterior inferior cerebellar artery (PICA). The AICA and SCA stem from the basilar artery at the pons and the PICA from the vertebral artery at the medulla.

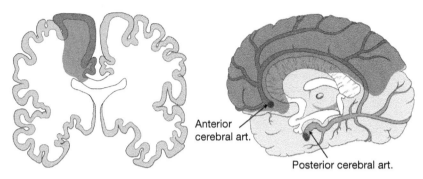

FIG. 44.1 Brain territory supplied by the anterior cerebral artery (art.) supply.

• EMBOLIC, THROMBOTIC, LACUNAR, AND WATERSHED STROKES

The embolus sources include cardiac thrombus, carotid artery plaque, fat, and air. Embolic stroke tends to occur while a person is awake and causes marked deficit at onset. The thrombotic stroke occurs from formation of clot typically at the locations of the cerebral vessels where they bifurcate or converge. Common locations of thrombus formation include the bifurcation of the common carotid artery into internal and external carotid, the origin of the MCA, the converging point of the vertebral arteries forming the basilar artery, the division of the basilar artery into the PCA, and the posterior communicating arteries (eSlide 44.4). Thrombotic strokes tend to cause a gradual increase in neurologic deficit over a period of hours to days, and this often occurs during sleep.

The lacunar infarct refers to a stroke caused by occlusion of the small, deep, penetrating arteries. Lacunar strokes of the posterior limb of internal capsule may present with pure motor hemiparesis. In contrast, lacunar strokes in the thalamus or parietal white matter may cause a pure sensory deficit in the contralateral face, arm, and leg. Lacunar stroke of the pons may result in *dysarthria-clumsy hand*.

The infarct of the watershed area of the brain may occur following hypoxia or hypotension. Anterior border watershed infarct may cause aphasia and weakness of the leg and proximal arm. The posterior border watershed infarct may cause visual deficit.

• STROKE CHAMELEONS AND STROKE MIMICS

Stroke chameleons are disorders that resemble other disorders but are actually stroke syndromes. Stroke mimics are disorders that look like strokes but are not stroke syndromes. The rates of stroke chameleons and stroke mimics are approximately 26% and 31%, respectively. Common stroke chameleons and mimics are summarized in eSlides 44.5 and 44.6.

• SPECIFIC STROKE SYNDROMES

Middle Cerebral Artery Occlusion

Occlusion of the MCA results in paralysis and sensory loss of the contralateral face, upper limb, and, to a lesser degree, lower limb; homonymous hemianopsia; global aphasia if the dominant side is involved; and spatial neglect if the nondominant side is involved (eSlide 44.7). Occlusion of the superior or inferior branch of the MCA affects Broca area causing nonfluent aphasia (frontal lobe) or Wernike area causing fluent aphasia (temporal lobe), respectively.

Anterior Cerebral Artery Occlusion

ACA occlusion results in sensory loss and paralysis of the contralateral lower limb, sparing the face and the upper limb. The patient may also have frontal lobe deficits including indifference about his or her condition, disinhibition, primitive frontal lobe reflexes, and incontinence (Fig. 44.1; eSlide 44.8).

Posterior Cerebral Artery Occlusion

Patients with PCA infarct present with contralateral homonymous hemianopia, visual agnosia, and ipsilateral sensory loss (Fig. 44.3). If the infarct is bilateral,

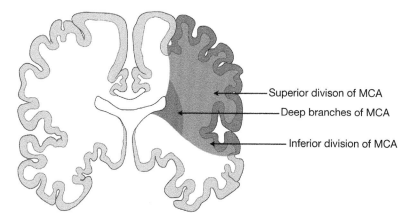

FIG. 44.2 Brain territory supplied by middle cerebral artery (MCA).

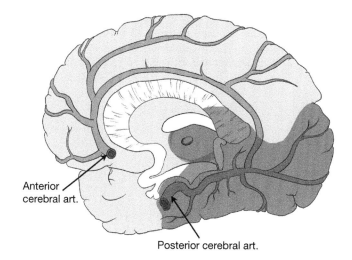

FIG. 44.3 Brain territory supplied by posterior cerebral artery (art.).

patients may have blindness and inability to form new memories. If the dominant side is involved, alexia (inability to read words or sentences) with or without agraphia (inability to write) may be present. There is no paralysis or aphasia although there may be some sensory loss.

Brainstem Stroke Syndromes

The face arm speech test (FAST), a widely used prehospital stroke recognition instrument, may not be sensitive for brainstem strokes. The cardinal features of brainstem stroke include vertigo, nausea, cranial nerve symptoms and signs, presence of crossed signs (e.g., ipsilateral facial weakness with contralateral limb weakness), oculomotor involvement, bilateral deficit of sensory or motor function (e.g., one-side weakness first followed by contralateral side weakness), and ataxia. Presence of upper motor neuron signs in patients with suspected brainstem strokes indicates involvement of motor pathway (corticospinal tract) in the midline (medial brainstem strokes; Table 44.1; eSlide 44.9). In terms of longitudinal localization of medial brainstem strokes, involvement of midline cranial nerve nuclei can be helpful: oculomotor (midbrain), trochlear (midbrain), abducens (pons), and hypoglossal (medulla; eSlide 44.10).

LATERAL MEDULLARY SYNDROME (WALLENBERG SYNDROME)

This is the most common brainstem stroke, and it results from occlusion of the PICA. Symptoms include pain and temperature sensation deficits of ipsilateral face and contralateral body, vertigo/nystagmus, ipsilateral hemiataxia, dysarthria, ipsilateral Horner syndrome (ptosis, miosis, anhidrosis), and dysphagia from involvement of lateral cranial nuclei (glossopharyngeal, vagus). The patient may have ipsilateral occipital or neck pain due to swelling and mass effect. There is no weakness of face or limbs (eSlides 44.11 and 44.12).

BASILAR ARTERY OCCLUSION

Atherostenosis and basilar artery occlusion often cause bilateral symptoms and signs or crossed findings involving one side of the face and the contralateral limbs (Table 44.1). Patients with acute basilar artery occlusion have a high mortality rate (more than 40%) and severe disability upon survival. More than half of the patients with basilar artery occlusion initially present with transient ischemic attack but eventually progress to full brainstem strokes. Locked-in syndrome is a result of complete pontine infarction presenting with quadriplegia, anarthria, and preserved consciousness.

Clinical Pearls

1. Knowledge of neuro and vascular anatomy is essential for diagnosis of stroke syndromes.
2. Posterior circulation stroke diagnosis is more challenging than anterior circulation stroke diagnosis. Clinicians should be aware of cardinal symptoms and signs of posterior circulation strokes (e.g., vertigo, crossed neurologic signs).
3. Clinicians should be aware of stroke chameleons and stroke mimics in order to implement appropriate interventions for stroke patients.

BIBLIOGRAPHY

The complete bibliography is available on ExpertConsult.com.

Degenerative Movement Disorders of the Central Nervous System

45

Andrew Malcolm Dermot Cole

• DEGENERATIVE MOVEMENT DISORDERS OF THE CENTRAL NERVOUS SYSTEM (eSlide 45.1)

Neurodegenerative disorders are characterized by abnormal protein aggregates accumulating in the nervous system. They commonly present clinically as excess movement (hyperkinetic) or paucity of voluntary and automatic movement (hypokinetic) disorders. Normal extrapyramidal system modulation of motor function is disturbed. Hyperkinetic disorders include restless leg syndrome (RLS), tremor, dystonia, myoclonus, chorea, and tic. Hypokinetic disorders include Parkinson disease (PD) and "Parkinson plus" syndromes, including progressive supranuclear palsy (PSP), multiple system atrophy (MSA), and corticobasal ganglionic degeneration (CBGD). Repeated clinical examinations and video recordings can be helpful in clarifying the clinical diagnosis.

RLS (eSlide 45.2) is a disorder characterized by deep, ill-defined, leg discomfort or dysesthesia, accompanied by the urge to move the legs. This urge is worse when the person is sitting or lying down and most often occurs immediately before or during asleep. The urge to move is relieved by movement (e.g., walking or stretching), for as long as the movement lasts. RLS may be primary, or it may be secondary to diabetes mellitus, uremia, carcinoma, pregnancy, malabsorption, or chronic obstructive airway disease. The estimated prevalence of RLS is 2%–15%, with the disorder being slightly more common in women than men and in individuals of Northern European descent. In one-third of patients, symptom onset occurs before 20 years of age. First-line treatment of RLS involves long-acting dopaminergic compounds and iron supplements, particularly in patients with a low serum ferritin. Other treatment includes anticonvulsants (gabapentin, pregabalin, or carbamazepine), benzodiazepines, and sometimes opioids.

Tremor (eSlide 45.3) is a rhythmic, oscillatory movement produced by contractions of antagonist muscle pairs. It may be fast or slow and may occur at rest, while a posture is being maintained, or with active movement. Factors that can exacerbate tremors include anxiety, fatigue, hypoglycemia, thyrotoxicosis, alcohol withdrawal, lithium use, sympathomimetic drugs, caffeine, and sodium valproate.

Essential tremor (ET) is the most common movement disorder. It begins at any age and is inherited in more than 50% of individuals. ET often occurs in the hands (with flexion-extension hand movements), and it may be combined with head, trunk, voice, tongue, and lip tremors as well; it may be asymmetric. Small quantities of alcohol improve most ETs; this is often used as clinical challenge to aid diagnosis, but its usage as treatment is not recommended. Mild abnormalities of muscle tone, posture, and balance may be seen on examination.

Dystonia (eSlide 45.4) refers to sustained abnormal muscle contractions, producing twisting or repetitive movements and abnormal postures. Often autosomal dominant in inheritance, dystonia may involve a single part of the body (focal dystonia), noncontiguous parts of the body (multifocal dystonia), half of the body, or it may be generalized. Dystonia may occur at rest or with movement, such as writer's or musician's cramp, and it is often relieved by sleep. Dystonia may be primary (idiopathic), with preservation of verbal cognition, or it may be secondary (in 30% of patients) to other conditions, such as Parkinsonism. A unique phenomenon is that some people are able to modify their dystonia; for example, blepharospasm may be relieved by touching the skin around the eye.

Myoclonus (eSlide 45.5) presents as sudden, shocklike, jerky movements of variable intensity. Positive myoclonus involves active muscle contractions and may occur when falling asleep (hypnagogic jerks). It can occur in local spinal segments or in the palate and laryngeal muscles. Either occurring spontaneously or triggered by touch, light, or noise, positive myoclonus can begin at any age. There may be a family history of myoclonus. Positive myoclonus may be primary (idiopathic) or secondary to other disorders, such as seizures. Negative myoclonus (asterixis) involves brief lapses of tone in antigravity muscles. It may be seen in metabolic encephalopathies, during general anesthetic reactions, and with anticonvulsants.

Chorea (eSlide 45.6) presents with irregular, unpredictable, brief, jerky, fidgeting low-amplitude movements, resulting from basal ganglia pathology. Chorea may include various types of movements, from facial grimacing or unstable dance-like postures to a continuous flow of disabling violent movements. The movements fluctuate according to stress, as well as physical and mental activities. Chorea may arise from genetic disorders (e.g., Huntington disease), or it may be secondary to infectious, autoimmune, iatrogenic, or metabolic causes (e.g., Wilson disease).

Tics (eSlide 45.7) are abnormal movements (motor tics) or sounds (phonic tics) that are brief, involuntary, rapid, and nonrhythmic. An irresistible urge builds tension that produces the tic, with relief occurring with execution of the tic. If motor and phonic features are present, then the term *Tourette syndrome* is used. Tics vary in frequency, amplitude, and duration. They are made worse by stress, anxiety, and fatigue and may be relieved by concentrating on a task or undertaking absorbing activities. Tics are best treated with comprehensive behavioral intervention programs.

Simple motor tics are abrupt and brief, such as a blink, facial grimace, shoulder shrug, or head jerk. Simple vocal tics may include throat clearing, grunts, coughs, snorting, or animal sounds. Complex motor tics include stereotypic facial expressions or coordinated movements, such as grooming, scratching, kicking, or obscene gesturing, and they may be difficult to distinguish from associated obsessive-compulsive behavior or attention deficit hyperactivity disorder. Complex vocal tics include phonic features, such as words, phrases, obscene utterances (coprolalia), or religious profanities.

PD (eSlide 45.8) is the most common movement disorder, affecting 10–20 in every 100,000 people worldwide and >1% of people over 60 years of age in the United States. PD prevalence increases with age. About 90% of cases are sporadic, with some genetic and environmental causes identified. Midbrain neurons progressively lose dopamine; other areas are affected later. The diagnosis of PD is made by clinical evaluation of motor, nonmotor, and autonomic nervous system (ANS) symptoms. The "TRAP" motor features of PD (tremor, rigidity, akinesia or bradykinesia, and postural instability) and similar warning signs may be perceived by patients and family as a normal part of aging because of their insidious onset and variable progression (eSlide 45.9).

Nonmotor symptoms (eSlide 45.10) include depression (20%-40%), anxiety (30%-50%), and visual hallucinations. Cognitive defects in problem-solving, visuospatial function, and memory retrieval interact, adding significant disability to motor difficulties as PD progresses. The relative risk of dementia in people with PD is about five times that of matched controls. Lewy body dementia starts early, with hallucinations and delusions, whereas PD-type dementia usually starts at least 1 year after the onset of motor symptoms. Disturbed sleep is common, with insomnia, nightmares, and daytime sleepiness. ANS symptoms include urinary frequency or urgency, sweating, genital dysfunction, and constipation. Orthostatic hypotension will develop in one-third of PD patients.

The unified Parkinson's disease rating scale (UPDRS) is a helpful, widely used clinical instrument for consistent recording of disease severity. Levodopa is the most effective initial monotherapy for motor symptoms; however, with its short half-life, many people experience "on–off" phenomenon, in which symptoms worsen prior to a dose and are relieved thereafter. Catechol-O-methyl transferase (COMT) inhibitors, monoamine oxidase B (MAO-B) inhibitors, and dopamine agonists prolong levodopa's half-life and may help control the on–off phenomenon. These may be used first in younger patients, to avoid levodopa-induced dyskinesias (Video 45.1), which eventually affect more than 40% of patients receiving levodopa treatment for more than 6 years. Amantadine has established antidyskinetic efficacy, but it may induce cognitive dysfunction. Pharmacologic motor treatment options for PD are listed by class in eSlide 45.11, and nonmotor treatment options are listed in eSlide 45.12.

Definitive evidence for speech or occupational therapy and acupuncture efficacy is still lacking, but physical therapy is well accepted as a symptomatic adjunct therapy for gait and balance problems. Deep brain stimulation by an electrode implanted in the subthalamic nucleus or globus pallidus provides continuous, high-frequency electrical stimulation to treat resistant dyskinesias and severe tremor in PD. Caregivers have an important supportive role, often being the effective leader of the care team, helping with activities of daily living, safety, medication compliance, and social involvement. As first-hand observers of treatment effects, they can clarify communication. Providing support for caregivers is vital to successful overall patient care at home. Team members must be alert for any signs of caregiver stress and intervene to provide assistance when necessary for the welfare of the caregiver and patient alike.

PSP (eSlide 45.13) usually commences with postural instability and falls, and later produces axial rigidity, bradykinesia, cognitive deficits, and supranuclear vertical gaze palsy. PSP is often poorly responsive to levodopa therapy. Other findings are marked micrographia, stuttering, palilalia (abnormal repetition of syllables, words, or phrases), and early dysphagia. The facies in PSP may resemble the appearance of perpetual astonishment because of sustained frontalis contraction and a low blink rate. The disease generally occurs sporadically. The prevalence is 5.3 per 100,000 people, and the incidence increases sharply from about 45 years of age onward.

MSA (eSlide 45.14) is a progressive, adult-onset (age >30 years) neurodegenerative disorder, which affects both sexes equally. The estimated prevalence is 3 per 100,000 people. It is usually sporadic and associated with degeneration of the thalamus, pons, and cerebellum. Motor phenomena may initially resemble akinetic parkinsonism (MSA-P, the more common variant) or show cerebellar variant damage with ataxia, dysarthria, or nystagmus (MSA-C). Signs of severe autonomic failure occur within 2 years in more than half of patients with MSA. Only one-third of patients with MSA show a response to levodopa, which is almost always atypical. Pursuing treatment with dopamine agonists or amantadine may produce a better response in some people, but there is no consistently effective treatment for cerebellar manifestations. Autonomic problems are more amenable to measures such as increasing salt and fluid intake and adopting specific body postures.

CBGD (eSlide 45.15) is the least well understood of the Parkinson plus syndromes, and it is less common than either PSP or MSA. Nearly always sporadic, CBGD develops insidiously and gradually. CBGD findings occur in three groups (motor, cerebellar, and other manifestations) and are often strikingly asymmetric. Motor manifestations include fixed dystonias with painful deformities, postural instability, athetosis, and orofacial dyskinesias. Other signs of dysfunction include apraxia, cortical sensory loss, the alien limb phenomenon, dementia, and the presence of frontal lobe reflexes. Brain imaging will demonstrate asymmetric atrophy. There is no specific treatment for CBGD; therapy is purely symptomatic at present.

• CONCLUSION (Table 45.1)

Movement disorders present a significant challenge to the diagnostic and management skills of physiatrists and are common enough to likely be encountered by most physiatrists in all types of clinical settings. There is still a lack of evidence-based and patient-specific rehabilitative interventions for individuals diagnosed with movement disorders. Although anecdotal studies focusing on different

TABLE 45.1 Symptom Manifestations of Various Movement Disorders

	PD	ET	MSA	PSP	Hunt	RLS
Resting tremor	++	+/−	−	+/−	+/−	−
Action tremor	+/−	++	+	−	+/−	−
Rigidity	+	−	+	+/−	−	−
Postural instability	+	−	++	+++	++	−
Cognitive decline	+	−	++	++	++	−
Sleep disorder	+	−	+/−	+	+	+
Visual hallucinations	+/−	−	+/−	+/−	+/−	−
Response to PD medications	+++	+	−	−	−	+/−
Mood disorders	++	+/−	−	−	+/−	−
Motor fluctuations	+	−	−	−	−	−

ET, essential tremor; *Hunt*, Huntington disease; *MSA*, multiple system atrophy; *PD*, Parkinson disease; *PSP*, progressive supranuclear palsy; *RLS*, restless leg syndrome.

rehabilitative exercise programs have suggested that the quality of life for patients with a movement disorder may be significantly improved by participation in such programs, further research is needed to confirm this contention.

Clinical Pearls

Essential tremor is a common movement disorder, is inherited in more than 50% of patients, and may be temporarily improved by small quantities of alcohol. Parkinson disease (PD) prevalence increases with age, and the presence of TRAP (tremor, rigidity, akinesia, postural instability) features in an older person and should not be discounted as a normal part of aging.

Rehabilitation is important in the care of PD and related disorders. Physiotherapy is well accepted as symptomatic adjunct therapy for gait and balance problems, whereas psychologists and social workers provide vital support for caregivers at home. Depending on symptoms and patient needs, occupational and speech therapy also have important roles to play.

BIBLIOGRAPHY
The complete bibliography is available on ExpertConsult.com.

46 Multiple Sclerosis

Mohd Izmi Bin Ahmad

Multiple sclerosis (MS) is a chronic, inflammatory, neurodegenerative disorder of the central nervous system (CNS) with heterogeneous presentations. The pathogenesis and characteristics of MS, as well as pharmacologic and rehabilitative options for people with MS (PwMS), are summarized in this chapter and the accompanying eSlides.

• EPIDEMIOLOGY

MS is the most common cause of nontraumatic disability affecting young Caucasians in temperate areas (peak age: 20–40 years). Females are affected two to three times more frequently than males. Males with MS exhibit a much worse prognosis in terms of disease course and disability.

• PATHOGENESIS

MS is triggered by an autoimmune process in susceptible individuals. The etiology is multifactorial, involving both genetic and environmental factors.

Immunology

Autoreactive T and B cells are activated in the periphery and subsequently cross the blood-brain barrier, triggering an autoimmune cascade that leads to damage of the myelin sheath surrounding axons within the CNS. The activating mechanism or antigen(s) have not been fully established.

Subtypes

Relapsing-remitting multiple sclerosis (RRMS) is the most common subtype, which affects 85% of PwMS. Secondary progressive multiple sclerosis (SPMS) develops when a patient with RRMS no longer has exacerbations and has persistent accumulation of disability over time. Primary progressive multiple sclerosis (PPMS) is characterized by disease progression without noticeable exacerbations. It affects males and females equally and makes up 10%–15% of PwMS. The least common (affecting 5% of PwMS) and most aggressive type is progressive relapsing (PRMS) (eSlide 46.1).

Diagnosis

Clinical presentations in MS are summarized in eSlide 46.2. The currently accepted criteria for MS diagnosis are the Revised McDonald 2010 Magnetic Resonance Imaging (MRI) criteria (eSlides 46.3 and 46.4). Two clinical attacks at two separate points in time fulfill the criteria for clinically definite MS.

Clinical Decision-Making

MRI is the mainstay of investigations for MS. T1 images with and without contrast, T2 images, and fluid-attenuated inversion recovery (FLAIR) sequencing are used for diagnostic workup. The short T1 inversion recovery sequence is a new technique used to better visualize the spinal cord. New T2 or FLAIR lesions help determine the efficacy of disease-modifying therapy (DMT) and correlate with long-term disability accumulation. In the setting of a patient with no abnormal or nonspecific MRI findings, cerebrospinal fluid (CSF) analysis (looking for oligoclonal bands) and evoked potential studies may be needed for additional diagnostic support. Oligoclonal bands are present in 83%–94% of patients with MS when the test is performed with isoelectric focusing. When accompanied by the onset of optic neuritis, the presence of oligoclonal bands is predictive of the diagnosis of MS. Testing of evoked potentials measures electrical activity in the brain. Slowing of conduction is due to demyelination. Currently, only visual evoked potentials are included in the MS diagnostic guidelines.

Differential Diagnosis

Other conditions that mimic the presentation of MS are summarized in eSlide 46.5. The relevant characteristics of neuromyelitis optica, acute transverse myelitis, acute disseminated encephalomyelitis, and clinically isolated syndrome are presented in eSlide 46.6. The steps in MS diagnosis are depicted in eSlide 46.7.

Measuring Progression

The Expanded Disability Status Scale (EDSS) is the gold standard for grading disability in MS; it focuses primarily on mobility. EDSS is based on a detailed neurologic examination and includes functional systems. The levels range from 0 (no impairment) to 10 (death from MS), with half-point levels along the way. The time to reach a selected level of EDSS is the best way to measure disease progression (eSlides 46.8 and 46.9).

• PHARMACOLOGIC MANAGEMENT

First-Generation Disease-Modifying Therapies

Interferon β (IFN-β) treatments include Rebif and Betaseron, which are administered via subcutaneous injection three times per week, and Avonex injection, which is given once per week. These drugs are thought to modulate T cell, B cell, and cytokine functions (producing antiinflammatory effects). The most common side effects are flulike symptoms, fatigue, and injection site reactions. All IFNs are associated with possible blood and bone marrow abnormalities, liver dysfunction, hypothyroidism, and mood dysfunction.

Glatiramer acetate's mechanism is unclear, but it is probably attributable to the stimulation of Treg cells. The most common adverse events are flushing, palpitations, and shortness of breath.

Both IFNs and glatiramer acetate have similar efficacy, exhibit favorable long-term safety profiles, and remain the first-line treatment for MS. Patients with progressive disability may require escalation therapy.

Oral Therapies

Fingolimod has been associated with a 50% reduction in relapse rate (in RRMS) compared with placebo. It is a sphingosine 1-phosphate receptor modulator that prevents the migration of potentially autoreactive lymphocytes from lymph nodes into the CNS. Potential adverse effects include bradycardia, other arrhythmias, lymphopenia, macular edema, elevated liver enzymes, and certain opportunistic infections, particularly varicella zoster.

Teriflunomide exerts immunologic effects by selectively inhibiting dihydroorotate dehydrogenase, leading to reduction in the proliferation of activated T and B lymphocytes. Common side effects include lymphopenia, elevated transaminases, acute renal failure, and alopecia. Teriflunomide is teratogenic and contraindicated in pregnancy.

Dimethyl fumarate is a fumaric acid metabolite that is approved for twice-daily oral DMT for relapsing MS. It is thought to have antioxidant and antiinflammatory properties mediated through activation of the nuclear-related factor-2 transcriptional pathway. It is generally safe but may cause flushing, gastrointestinal upset, lymphopenia, and elevated liver enzymes.

Intravenous Therapies

Natalizumab is a highly specific α4-integrin antagonist that acts as the blood-brain barrier to inhibit leukocyte migration across the barrier. It has been shown to reduce relapse rates and improve functional outcomes. With regard to the reported risk of progressive multifocal leukoencephalopathy, factors such as prior immunosuppressant treatment, duration of natalizumab therapy, and evidence of previous John Cunningham virus exposure should be taken into consideration when deciding whether natalizumab should be used in a patient with RRMS. Additional potential adverse effects are a mildly increased risk of infections (especially urinary and upper respiratory tract infections) and hepatotoxicity.

Mitoxantrone is a chemotherapeutic agent that has been approved to treat aggressive RRMS and SPMS. It is a cytotoxic agent that inhibits B cell, T cell, and macrophage proliferation. It is administered as an intravenous infusion four times per year. Its safety is acceptable, provided that the cumulative dose, cardiac function, hematologic profile, and liver enzymes are monitored closely. If patients have not completed their family planning, they should be informed of the possibility that the drug may cause sterility.

Alemtuzumab is a monoclonal antibody against CD52 antigen, which is found on the surface of lymphocytes and monocytes. Appropriate frequent monitoring is required to detect potential adverse effects, such as thyroid disease and idiopathic thrombocytopenia (eSlide 46.10).

• REHABILITATION, EXERCISE, AND SYMPTOM MANAGEMENT

Physical Activity

Recent studies have demonstrated the safety and benefits of exercise in PwMS. The intensity, duration, and frequency must be coupled with a patient's symptoms, heat intolerance, strength, and endurance.

Gait Impairment

Approximately 75% of PwMS have mobility challenges. The timed 25-foot walk test is a validated measure of walking speed in MS. A 20% change in walking speed is considered significant. Dalfampridine is an oral potassium channel agonist with the ability to enhance nerve conduction in areas of demyelination, which has been approved for the use in PwMS with walking impairment. Dalfampridine lowers the seizure threshold and has other potential adverse events, including an increased frequency of urinary tract infections, vertigo, insomnia, headache, and falls.

Fatigue

Fatigue is very common in PwMS. Primary fatigue is attributable to the disease process, and secondary fatigue is the result of other causes, including metabolic, endocrine, and hematologic abnormalities; depression; and medication side effects. The fatigue severity scale, fatigue impact scale, and modified fatigue impact scale are the most commonly used methods for assessing fatigue. In addition to energy conservation and avoidance of triggers (heat, stress, or overexertion), pharmacologic treatment is advised to help maintain energy and focus (eSlide 46.11).

Sleep Disorders

Approximately 50% of PwMS report difficulty with sleep initiation, sleep maintenance, or early morning awakening. MS symptoms that may interfere with sleep include spasticity, pain or paresthesias, and nocturia. Side effects of DMT, particularly IFNs, may lead to sleep disruption. Mood disorders should also be screened for. Guided imagery, biofeedback, and cognitive-behavioral therapy have demonstrated beneficial effects in treating sleep disorders associated with MS. Pharmacologic agents include zolpidem, trazodone, benzodiazepine, sedating antidepressants, and antihistamines.

Mood Disorders

The most common mood disorder in MS is depression, which occurs in at least 50% of patients. The Beck Depression Inventory and Beck Depression Inventory—Fast Screen are validated scales to screen for depression in PwMS. Treatment should be individualized, using pharmacologic therapy, psychological counseling, or both.

Spasticity

Spasticity affects up to 85% of PwMS. The MS spasticity scale has been validated for use in PwMS. Treatment follows standard approaches. Commonly prescribed drugs for MS are summarized in eSlide 46.12. Oral cannabis has also been demonstrated to significantly improve pain, spasm, and spasticity. Botulinum toxin (BoNT) injections had been shown to improve focal spasticity in MS. Intrathecal baclofen therapy via an implanted drug delivery device is indicated when oral or injectable treatments become ineffective. Phenol injections or surgical intervention may be used in patients with severe mobility or contractures who have failed conservative therapies.

Pain

Neuropathic pain has a prevalence of 50% in PwMS and is believed to be due to the presence of plaques in the CNS. Anticonvulsants efficacious for pain are gabapentin and pregabalin. Tricyclic antidepressants are also helpful choice of drugs. Intrathecal morphine and ziconotide have demonstrated significant neuropathic pain reduction compared with placebo and can be the considered for patients who do not respond well to oral medications. Trigeminal neuralgia (TN) affects 2%–6% of patients with MS. Treatment options include anticonvulsants, antispasmodics, and in rare instances, narcotics. Misoprostol, a prostaglandin E analogue, has been shown to relieve pain in patients with TN and can be considered as a treatment approach. BoNT injections, rhizotomy, or gamma knife procedure are reserved for those who fail other treatments. Painful optic neuritis can be treated with steroids. L'hermitte's sign and the "MS hug" are other types of neuropathic pain symptoms in PwMS, for which anticonvulsants can be beneficial.

• NEUROGENIC BLADDER

Approximately 75% of PwMS have bladder dysfunction. Screening guidelines for bladder dysfunction include performing an appropriate history and evaluating the postvoid residual volume. Nonpharmacologic treatments, such as fluid management, timed voiding, pelvic floor exercises, and catheterization, may be offered for initial management. Pharmacologic treatment consists of antimuscarinic agents for treating disorders of storage. α-Antagonists are recommended for the treatment of voiding disorders. Desmopressin may be indicated for symptoms of nocturia. Intravesical injections of BoNT-A are approved by the US Food and Drug Administration (FDA) for the treatment of neurogenic detrusor overactivity in PwMS. Neuromodulation strategies, such as posterior tibial nerve stimulation and sacral nerve stimulation, are indicated in patients who have failed or are unable to tolerate conservative treatment for overactive bladder.

• NEUROGENIC BOWEL

Neurogenic bowel in PwMS presents as constipation or fecal incontinence. Constipation is caused by immobility, reduced parasympathetic input, drug side effects, fluid restriction due to bladder frequency, and a low-residue diet. Fecal incontinence may be attributable to loss of control of the external anal sphincter, abnormal rectosigmoid compliance, or rectoanal reflexes. The use of probiotics can help both constipation and incontinence. Recommendations for an effective bowel program are listed in eSlide 46.13.

• SEXUAL DYSFUNCTION

Sexual dysfunction (SD) is present in 42%–90% of PwMS. Women commonly report decreased libido and loss of lubrication. Men report erectile and ejaculatory dysfunction. Both sexes report challenges with achieving orgasm. Side effects of DMT and symptomatic treatments (e.g., antidepressants, antispasmodics, α-antagonists), as well as underlying psychological issues, may contribute to SD. The MS Intimacy and Sexuality Questionnaire can be used to assess the perceived influence of MS symptoms on sexual activity. Treatment includes education, psychological counseling, and reducing the dependence on medications that impair libido or energy. Sildenafil citrate is effective for male patients with erectile dysfunction.

• COGNITIVE IMPAIRMENT

Cognitive impairment (CI) affects 40%–70% of PwMS. eSlide 46.14 illustrates impairments affecting the cognitive domain in PwMS. Certain MRI findings, such as increased cortical atrophy, widening of the third ventricle, and overall loss of brain volume, have been correlated with CI in PwMS. Subcutaneous IFN-β has been shown to stabilize or delay the progression of CI. One year of natalizumab treatment was also demonstrated to significantly improve CI. Psychostimulants, such as methylphenidate and L-amphetamine, have been shown to improve attention, learning, and focusing ability. There is no specific evidence to suggest that memantine and donepezil are beneficial for the treatment of memory disorders associated with MS. Cognitive-behavioral therapy may be beneficial for CI in PwMS, but its long-term benefit is unknown.

Swallowing

Dysphagia in MS is likely due to involvement of corticobulbar, cerebellar, or brainstem regions and occurs in 33%–43% of PwMS. The Dysphagia in Multiple Sclerosis Questionnaire has been validated to assess the risk of dysphagia in MS. A videofluorographic swallow study is the tool of choice for evaluating the presence of silent aspiration. Compensatory strategies, such as changing the posture, modifying the volume of food boluses, and changing food consistency, are effective strategies for dysphagia. Injection of BoNT into the cricopharyngeal muscle has been reported to be effective for the treatment of upper esophageal hyperactivity. Pharyngeal electrical stimulation to treat oropharyngeal dysphagia significantly reduces the amount of glottis penetration and aspiration.

• MULTIPLE SCLEROSIS IN PREGNANCY

MS has no direct effect on pregnancy and fetal well-being, as pregnancy is considered an immune-tolerant state. DMTs should not be used in PwMS who are pregnant or trying to become pregnant. When needed, glatiramer acetate has the most favorable safety rating (class B). Acute relapses can be treated with a short course of high-dose glucocorticoids, as determined by the practitioner. Symptomatic medications should be minimized during pregnancy. During the 3 months postpartum, the relapse rate rebounds to 70% above the prepregnancy level, then returns to the prepregnancy rate. There are conflicting data regarding the potential benefits of breastfeeding in reducing MS activity. Although it is not FDA approved for this purpose, intravenous immunoglobulin G has been shown in some studies to reduce the risk of postpartum relapse.

• CONCLUSION

The varying nature of MS symptoms presents unique challenges for PwMS, their families, and clinicians. The disease is progressive, and PwMS are faced with variable disabilities. Because MS is a lifetime disease, lifelong management and rehabilitation have a significant role in improving the quality of life of PwMS.

1. The most common symptom of multiple sclerosis (MS) is fatigue, which is most pronounced in the afternoon.
2. The major enhancer of neuroplasticity in patients with MS is slow-wave deep sleep, as cortical neurons undergo slow oscillations in membrane potential during much of deep sleep.
3. Energy conservation through rationing activities according to the patient's optimum hours of function and total capacity for daily exertion improves self-efficacy, quality of life, and social participation.
4. There is strong evidence that aerobic training improves maximum exercise capacity for ambulatory individuals with MS, whereas there is less evidence regarding the effects of exercise in semiambulatory and nonambulatory individuals with MS.
5. Tremor is reported in nearly 30% of patients with MS and can be one of the most difficult symptoms to manage.
6. When compared with healthy people, patients with MS display slower walking rates, increased steps per minute (cadence), less rotation at the hips, and increased trunk flexion.
7. Meticulous attention must be paid to treating depression, fatigue, and heat intolerance because all these can contribute to cognitive impairment.
8. Dysarthria is reported in 14%–19% of patients with MS and is most often found in more neurologically impaired individuals.
9. Factors that contribute to the challenge of rehabilitation in patients with MS include progression of the disease, the varying nature of MS symptoms and disability, uncertainty regarding the future, and a variety of vocational and social issues.

BIBLIOGRAPHY
The complete bibliography is available on ExpertConsult.com.

Cerebral Palsy 47

Desiree L. Roge

Cerebral palsy (CP) is a group of permanent disorders that includes abnormal development of movements and postures that cause activity limitations. It is attributed to nonprogressive disturbances that occur in the developing fetal or infant brain. Comorbidities include disturbances of sensation, cognition, communication, behavior, epilepsy, and secondary musculoskeletal problems.

• EPIDEMIOLOGY, ETIOLOGY, AND RISK FACTORS

CP is the most common cause of disability in developed countries. There are five major categories of risk factors associated with the diagnosis of CP, which are shown in eSlide 47.1.

• CLASSIFICATION

CP can be classified in various ways. One classification system uses the topography or distribution of the affected limbs (eSlides 47.2 and 47.3). CP can also be classified by motor signs (eSlide 47.4) or functions (eSlide 47.5).

• DIAGNOSIS

The term CP is a description of clinical findings. The detailed history must include the medical history, birth history, developmental and functional history, family history of blood clots or stroke, and presence of risk factors for CP. The medical examination must include detailed neurologic, musculoskeletal, and functional components. Primitive reflexes, areas of weakness, alterations of tone, and movement abnormalities should be identified. Milestones may be delayed in premature children until the age of 2 years; hence, in the young child or infant, repeat examinations should be conducted. Regression of milestones suggests a neurodegenerative process and the need for a metabolic or genetic disease workup (Fig. 47.1 and eSlide 47.6).

• FUNCTIONAL PROGNOSIS

A positive predictor of ambulation is being able to sit independently by the age of 2 years or having less than three primitive reflexes by 18–24 months; not sitting independently by 4 years is a negative predictor. Ambulation will occur in 80%–90% of children with diplegia, 50% of those with quadriplegia, and 75% of children with dyskinesia.

• MEDICAL MANAGEMENT

Feeding, Growth, and Nutrition

Dysphagia increases the risk of feeding inefficiency, malnutrition, and aspiration. Gastrostomy tubes may be necessary to avoid malnutrition. Malnutrition

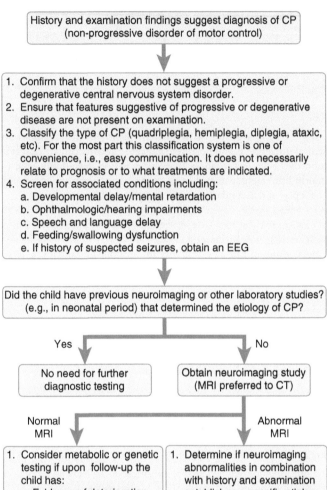

FIG. 47.1 Diagnostic algorithm for a child with suspected cerebral palsy. *CP,* cerebral palsy; *CT,* computed tomography; *EEG,* electroencephalogram; *MRI,* magnetic resonance imaging. (Redrawn from Ashwal S, Russman BS, Blasco PA, et al: Practice parameter: diagnostic assessment of the child with cerebral palsy: report of the Quality Standards Subcommittee of the American Academy of Neurology and the Practice Committee of the Child Neurology Society, *Neurology* 62:851–863, 2004.)

increases the risk of growth disturbances, infections, skin breakdown, osteopenia, and reduces life expectancy.

Pulmonary

Repeated aspiration events, infections, decreased mucociliary clearance, scoliosis, and airway obstruction result in cumulative injury to lung tissue. Preventative measures include immunizations. Prevention of pulmonary aspiration may require modified feeding consistencies, gastrostomy tubes, and treatment of reflux and sialorrhea. Upper airway obstruction may require continuous positive airway pressure, surgery, or both. Lower airway obstruction may respond to bronchodilators and continuous positive airway pressure. Sleep-disordered breathing, characterized by snoring or irregular breathing patterns and apneic episodes, is common. Hypoventilation secondary to neuromuscular weakness may require noninvasive ventilator support and external aids for mobilization of secretions and generation of a cough. Scoliosis surgery may improve restrictive lung disease but must be carefully considered given its risks.

Neurologic Issues

The CP population has an increased risk of epilepsy, intellectual disability, and cognitive impairment. Attention deficit and communication difficulties are common, and screening for their presence is recommended. Vision deficits include retinal damage, strabismus, myopia, and cortical visual impairment. Hearing deficits may be conductive, sensorineural, or both in etiology.

Genitourinary

Voiding dysfunction may result from impaired processing of sensory feedback and detrusor sphincter dyssynergia. Urinary retention may lead to urinary tract infections. Chronic high intravesical pressure resulting in hydronephrosis requires clean intermittent catheterizations.

Gastrointestinal

Gastroesophageal reflux disease (GERD) and constipation are very common. Severe cases of GERD may result in dysmotility, with delayed gastric empting and esophagitis.

Musculoskeletal Pain and Osteopenia

Impaired mobility results in an increased risk of contractures, bony deformities, musculoskeletal pain, osteopenia, and fragility fractures. Common sites of musculoskeletal pain include the hips, spine, knees, ankles, and feet. Risk factors for osteopenia include decreased weight bearing, use of anticonvulsants, and malnutrition. Supplementation with calcium and vitamin D is common, but their effectiveness is unclear. Bisphosphonates improve bone mineral density but are not without risk. They are reserved for children who have experienced a fragility fracture.

THERAPEUTIC MANAGEMENT

The treatment of a person with CP requires a multidisciplinary team.

Childhood Disabilities and Education

Table 47. 1 shows the important legislation and laws for children with disabilities.

TABLE 47.1 Important Legislation and Laws for Children With Disabilities[24]

Law or Legislation	Summary
The Handicapped Children's Early Education Assistance Act of 1968, or Public Law (PL) 95-538	Provides for educational programs for young children with disabilities. Funds research institutes to study the behavioral, cognitive, and emotional functioning of children.
The Vocational Rehabilitation Act of 1973, or PL 93-112	Provides for services for individuals with physical or mental handicaps that promote independence and employability. Section 504 provides protection against discrimination of children who might not meet "special education" definitions but require classroom accommodations, such as extra time for test taking or frequent breaks.
The Education of All Handicapped Children Act of 1975, or PL 94-142	Requires that no child, regardless of disability type or severity, can be excluded from a school education. Mandates that every child with a disability have an individualized educational plan that ensures appropriate accommodations, but also includes detailed plans and goals of education.
The Individuals with Disabilities Education Act (IDEA) of 1990, or PL101-476	Provides funding for infant and toddler early intervention programs. Replaces the word "handicapped" with "disabled." Ensures infants and toddlers with disabilities from birth to 2 years of age with developmental delay receive early intervention services. Requires that children aged 3–21 years receive special education and services.
The No Child Left Behind Act of 2002	Changes the distribution of federal funds from volume-based metrics to student performance-based metrics.
The Individuals with Disabilities Education Act (IDEA) revisions of 2004	Updates PL101-476 to include a requirement that children with disabilities be prepared for further education, employment, and independent living.

Therapy Interventions

There are many forms of therapy interventions (eSlides 47.7 and 47.8).

Stretching: The goal of stretching is to reduce the risk of contracture development as a result of muscle imbalances and hypertonicity. Sustained stretching can be achieved through the use of positioning devices, orthoses, and serial casting.

Strengthening: Strengthening does not increase spasticity or reduce range of movement.

Aerobic Exercise: Aerobic exercise improves physiologic measures of aerobic fitness, without producing adverse effects such as increased spasticity, fatigue, or musculoskeletal trauma.

Constraint-Induced Movement Therapy: Constraint-induced movement therapy is a treatment for hemiparesis designed to improve motor function in the affected upper limb. The unaffected limb is restrained with a removable cast, and the child undergoes intensive, structured therapy.

Functional Electrical Stimulation: Neuromuscular electrical stimulation is the application of an electrical current of sufficient intensity to elicit muscle contraction. When applied during a functional activity, it is referred to as functional electrical stimulation.

Robotic and Partial Body Weight Support Treadmill Training: These forms of therapy involve an overhead harness system to support the child's body weight on a treadmill while a therapist or robot facilitates the kinematic, kinetic, and temporal features of walking.

Durable Medical Equipment

The goals when prescribing durable medical equipment for individuals with CP should focus on maximizing function, improving safety, and enabling independence. Examples include standing frames and specialized seating devices for toileting, feeding, and bathing. A wheelchair becomes necessary when a child either outgrows commercially available strollers or requires additional support to facilitate interaction with the environment and minimize deforming forces secondary to postural abnormalities. For children with adequate head and trunk support, a gait trainer, walker, or crutches might facilitate gait training. For the dependent individual, families might benefit from lift systems to facilitate transfers. Meaningful communication and expression of needs may be facilitated with the use of augmentative adaptive equipment. Splinting and orthoses are used in individuals with CP to manage spastic yet flexible dynamic deformities of the limbs. A variety of passive and dynamic splints are available.

Management of Hypertonia

Tone management should translate into mobility improvement, self-care, skin breakdown prevention, ease of care, and comfort.

ORAL MEDICATIONS

Generalized hypertonia is often treated with oral medications, such as baclofen, diazepam, dantrolene, tizanidine, and clonazepam. All of these, except dantrolene, can cause sedation.

Pediatric dosing is variable, and the side effects of these medications limit their use. Generalized secondary dystonia responds poorly to oral medications. Commonly used drugs include trihexyphenidyl, oral baclofen, and levodopa/carbidopa.

CHEMODENERVATION

Botulinum toxin intramuscular injections and phenol neurolysis are used in the treatment of focal hypertonicity (spasticity and dystonia). Botulinum toxin and phenol can be used at the same time to maximize the dose and number of muscles treated (eSlide 47.9).

Chemoneurolysis should start at a young age when gait patterns and motor function are still flexible to allow for gross motor function learning.

INTRATHECAL BACLOFEN THERAPY

Intrathecal baclofen (ITB) is a United States Food and Drug Administration–approved method of treating moderate to severe generalized spasticity of cerebral or spinal origin. ITB can also treat generalized moderate to severe dystonia. ITB is delivered through a programmable pump placed subfascially in the abdominal wall and connected to a catheter that is tunneled into the intrathecal space. This method allows the delivery of small doses of baclofen intrathecally, which reduces the side effects seen with larger doses of oral baclofen. The pump requires replacement every 6–7 years owing to its battery life. Potential complications of

ITB include infections, cerebrospinal fluid leaks, and catheter problems. Abrupt withdrawal of ITB is a medical emergency and may present with increased tone, spasms, diaphoresis, agitation, and pruritus. If untreated, it can progress to rhabdomyolysis and multisystem failure. Treatment includes high doses of oral baclofen, benzodiazepines, and cyproheptadine.

SELECTIVE DORSAL RHIZOTOMY

Selective dorsal rhizotomy is a surgical procedure used for spasticity. The surgical technique involves single-level or multilevel laminectomies to expose the L2-S2 nerve roots, followed by selective cutting of a percentage of the dorsal rootlets that exhibit an abnormal response during electrophysiologic monitoring. The ideal candidate is a child between 3 and 8 years with diplegic CP and predominantly spastic tone (Gross Motor Function Classification System [GMFCS] levels I-III), little upper limb involvement, sufficient underlying strength, and good selective motor control. Weakness can be unmasked postoperatively by reducing the spasticity, making intensive physical therapy a necessity. Positive outcomes include reduced spasticity, increased range of movement, improved gait pattern, and decreased oxygen cost, making gait more efficient. Complications, such as sensory dysfunction, bladder or bowel dysfunction, or back pain, are infrequent.

• ORTHOPEDIC MANAGEMENT

The abnormalities in muscle tone present in children with CP restrict the range of movement of the affected joints, and when coupled with musculoskeletal growth, result in muscle contractures and bony deformities. Surgeries designed to improve ambulation are preferred in patients at GMFCS levels I-III, whereas surgeries aimed toward improving care and comfort are performed in those with GMFCS levels IV and V. Typically, orthopedic surgical intervention is delayed until the age of 7-9 years because of the high risk of recurrence, unless there is evidence of hip subluxation. Before this age, the focus should be on therapies and tone management.

Hips

It has been estimated that one in three children with CP will have hip displacement. The highest risk is in the nonambulatory population. Annual or semiannual surveillance films are recommended. Monitoring the acetabular index and migration percentage are the most effective parameters. Children with a migration percentage greater than 33% or an acetabular index over 30 degrees are likely to need further treatment (eSlide 47.10).

For the ambulatory child with CP, the goal of preserved ambulation requires a contained and stable hip. In the nonambulatory child with CP, the goals include prevention of hip dislocation, maintenance of sitting balance, and facilitation of hygiene. For those with painful hip subluxation or dislocation, temporary relief with intraarticular steroid injections has been reported. Salvage surgical procedures are available.

Lower Limbs

In CP, biarticular muscles (e.g., psoas, rectus femoris, hamstrings, and gastrocnemius) are more commonly contracted than monoarticular muscles (eSlide 47.11).

Orthopedic surgeries for contractures include lengthenings and transfers. These procedures are more effective if integrated into a single-event multilevel surgery. The ultimate goal is to achieve satisfactory joint position during gait, without restriction (eSlides 47.12, 47.13, and 47.14).

In the nonambulatory cohort, the goals include facilitating sitting (hamstrings) and perineal care (adductors), as well as containment of the hips (psoas and adductors), without performing bony surgery.

Abnormal long-bone torsions (lever arm dysfunction [LAD]) are the result of abnormal muscle forces and delays in walking. With time and growth, untreated LAD will produce further malalignment of bone and unwanted gait compensations. Soft tissue and bony procedures are available for foot and ankle deformities, with the goal of obtaining a plantigrade, braceable foot and stable base of support for standing and gait.

Upper Limb

Upper limb surgical procedures are recommended to improve function, ease of care in patients with severe contractures, and sometimes cosmesis. Common functional impairments include deficiencies in sensation, pinch, grasp and release, and reach. The ideal candidate for surgical intervention would be a motivated child with volitional use of the hand, spasticity without fixed contractures, and reasonable sensory function. Patients with significant athetosis and dystonia do not benefit from upper limb surgery, given the unpredictability of the outcomes.

Spine

The reported incidence of scoliosis in CP has been estimated as 21%–76%. Scoliosis is more prevalent in the nonambulatory cohort. Onset occurs between 3 and 10 years of age, and rapid progression occurs during the adolescent growth spurt. A physical examination should be performed every 6–12 months, and a radiograph obtained if a curve is detected. Observation is warranted for flexible curves less than 40 degrees that do not compromise sitting balance. Bracing traditionally has a very limited role in decreasing curve progression. Spinal instrumentation and fusion are considered when there is significant curve progression and loss of sitting balance. Surgical complications are high.

Clinical Pearls

- Cerebral palsy (CP) is a nonprogressive condition; the brain injury does not worsen over time.
- Children with progressive neurologic disorders have regression and loss of developmental skills; children with CP do not have regression of developmental skills.
- Secondary musculoskeletal comorbidities in children with CP may worsen with growth, resulting in decline in function.

BIBLIOGRAPHY
The complete bibliography is available on ExpertConsult.com.

48 Myelomeningocele and Other Spinal Dysraphisms

Rashidah Ismail Ohnmar Htwe

Neural tube defects (NTDs) affect 0.5–2 per 1000 established pregnancies worldwide and are the second most common group of severely disabling birth defects after congenital heart defects. Myelomeningocele (MMC) is the most complex congenital anomaly compatible with life and the second most common disabling condition in childhood after cerebral palsy. In this chapter, we summarize the etiology, advances in prevention, approaches to maximizing health-related outcomes, transitioning to adult-based health care systems, and improving activity and participation at the societal level and comprehensive management at different ages.

• EPIDEMIOLOGY

MMC accounts for more than 98% of "open" spinal dysraphic states and exists in the spectrum of NTDs. Studies have reported a 17%–30% incidence of spina bifida occulta, depending on the population studied (eSlide 48.1). Spinal dysraphisms are classified into open and closed spinal dysraphisms (eSlide 48.2).

A subcutaneous mass, such as a lipomyelomeningocele, is often associated with closed spinal dysraphisms. Hydrocephalus and Chiari II malformations are generally associated with open spinal dysraphisms. The incidence of spinal dysraphisms worldwide is approximately 1–10 per 1000 births, depending on the region; in the United States, the incidence is less than 0.7 per 1000. The decreasing prevalence of MMC can be attributed to the advent of prenatal screening and elective termination of pregnancy. The most influential factor has been the increased consumption of folic acid among women of childbearing age. Supplementation with folic acid (4 mg/day) has been shown to prevent 72% of NTDs in women with a previously affected pregnancy.

• RISK FACTORS AND ETIOLOGY (Table 48.1)

Possible risk factors for NTDs are vitamin B_6 and vitamin B_{12} deficiency, geographic location, low socioeconomic status, increased maternal age, maternal hyperthermia, maternal obesity, maternal diabetes mellitus, and certain drug exposures (e.g., carbamazepine, valproic acid).

• GENETIC FACTORS (eSlide 48.3)

NTDs recur within families, with first-degree relatives of a patient with a NTD possessing a 3%–5% risk of having offspring with an NTD, and second-degree

TABLE 48.1 Established and Suspected Risk Factors for Neural Tube Defects

Risk Factors	Relative Risk
Established Factors	
History of previous affected pregnancy with same partner	30
Inadequate maternal intake of folic acid	2 to 8
Pregestational maternal diabetes	2-10
Valproic acid and carbamazepine exposure	10–20
Suspected Factors	
Maternal vitamin B_{12} status	3
Maternal obesity	1.5–3.5
Maternal hyperthermia	2
Maternal diarrhea	3–4
Maternal age	>35 years: OR = 5.21, 95% CI = 2.42–11
	<25 years: OR = 3.36, 95% CI = 1.89–5.36
Paternal and maternal occupation and exposure to agrochemicals and pesticides	Appears increased but not firmly established
Gestational diabetes	Appears increased but not firmly established
Fumonisin (fungal protein) exposure	Appears increased but not firmly established
Acetaminophen exposure	Seems to have a protective effect

Data from references 15, 29, 40, 42, 44, 47, 60, 60a, 65, 72, 94, 98, 114, 115, 116, 117, 121, 127, 131, 139a, 148, 150, 160, 187.
CI, confidence interval; *OR,* odds ratio.

relatives having a 1%–2% risk. Women with two or more affected pregnancies have a higher risk (approximately 10%) of recurrence during subsequent pregnancies.

Embryology (eSlide 48.4) NTDs are known to occur as a result of failure of neurulation. Neurulation is the folding process in vertebrate embryos that occurs between the seventeenth and thirtieth days of gestation.

• PRENATAL DIAGNOSIS AND MANAGEMENT

Ultrasound (US) is the current "gold standard" for the prenatal diagnosis of MMC, with three-dimensional US and fetal magnetic resonance imaging (MRI) further enhancing characterization of these lesions.

• NEONATAL AND EARLY MANAGEMENT

Back Defect

Closure within 72 hours of delivery reduces the risk of infection in the central nervous system.

Hydrocephalus

Most infants with MMC require ventriculoperitoneal (VP) shunting for hydrocephalus after their back defect is closed, and approximately 15% who are born with severe hydrocephalus require immediate shunting. Infants without shunts should be monitored for the presence of signs of increased intracranial pressure. Thoracic lesions are associated with a higher incidence of hydrocephalus than lumbar or sacral lesions.

Early Bladder Management

Greater than 90% of infants with MMC will have a neurogenic bladder. Closure of the spinal lesion within 24 hours of birth seems to provide the best chance for favorable lower urinary tract function. The importance of aggressive urinary management should be stressed to the family before the child leaves the hospital. Baseline investigations should include renal-bladder sonography and a voiding cystourethrogram. Infants who are unable to void should begin intermittent catheterization programs. If an infant is able to void, he or she should be evaluated for complete bladder emptying by checking the postvoid residual volume, either by catheterization or bladder scan.

Assessment of the Neurologic Level

The best motor examination can be obtained by observation, palpation, and postural changes.

Therapy

The goal of any interdisciplinary MMC team should be to develop and implement a comprehensive plan that enables the affected child to attain a maximal level of function in all areas. Physical and occupational therapists, orthotists, and speech-language pathologists play a key role. Throughout the patient's life span, the MMC therapy team will educate and coordinate with community therapists to optimize the development and implementation of a comprehensive plan of care.

• CHILDHOOD MANAGEMENT

Shunts (eSlide 48.5)

Almost all children with MMC require placement of a VP shunt for management of hydrocephalus. The two most common shunt complications are infection and obstruction. Recurrent and frequent shunt infections adversely affect cognitive function.

Arnold-Chiari II Malformations (eSlides 48.6A and 48.7)

An Arnold-Chiari II malformation is characterized by variable displacement of cerebellar tissue into the spinal canal, accompanied by caudal dislocation of the lower brainstem and fourth ventricle. It is easily identified on MRI studies.

Hydromyelia (eSlide 48.6B)

Hydromyelia refers to dilatation of the central canal of the spinal cord. It is a relatively common occurrence in children with MMC.

Tethered Cord Syndrome (eSlide 48.8)

In children with MMC, the spinal cord can be fixed or "tethered" at one point, causing traction on the cord as the child grows. This leads to progressive urologic, orthopedic, or neurologic decline.

Neurogenic Bladder (eSlides 48.9, 48.10, and 48.11)

In MMC, more than 90% of patients have partial or complete denervation of the bladder, with poor compliance and contractibility that result in unacceptably high residual urine volumes. The urethral sphincter is incompetent in 86% of patients, and approximately one-third of patients have detrusor sphincter dyssynergia. The external sphincter is usually partially functional and can improve in the first year after birth.

Neurogenic Bowel

Patterns of neurogenic bowel involvement in children with MMC vary from normal bowel control (in approximately 20% of children) to incontinence caused by impaired rectal sensation, impaired sphincter function, and altered colonic motility (in the remaining children). The goal of a bowel management program is to achieve efficient, regular, and predictable emptying before the rectum becomes full enough to stimulate reflex relaxation of the internal anal sphincter in children with intact innervation. This will enhance a smooth transition into preschool and kindergarten. Peristeen transanal colonic irrigation should be considered as the first line of treatment for children with bowel incontinence when simple pharmacologic interventions are ineffective; it should be attempted before proceeding with surgical interventions. Surgical options, such as the antegrade continence enema procedure and colostomy, are available when conservative treatment has failed.

Latex Allergy

The prevalence of latex allergy (immunoglobulin E–mediated response) among children with MMC ranges from 20%–65%.

Endocrine Disorders

Complex central nervous system abnormalities and hydrocephalus place patients with MMC at risk for hypothalamic-pituitary dysfunction, including central precocious puberty (in 12%–16% of children) and growth hormone deficiency, further contributing to their short stature. Precocious puberty occurs more commonly in girls with MMC than in boys.

Musculoskeletal Considerations

MOTOR INNERVATION

The level of motor function in MMC does not necessarily correspond to the anatomic vertebral level on radiographic studies. The majority of children with MMC have lumbosacral-level vertebral lesions, with a quarter having midlumbar-level lesions, and one-fifth having sacral-level involvement.

HIPS

Hip flexion contractures create anterior pelvic tilt, which increases lumbar lordosis and can interfere with ambulation. Hip dislocations in children with MMC are present at birth or may occur later as a result of unopposed action of the hip flexor and adductor muscles.

KNEES

Children with MMC can develop knee flexion or extension contractures, especially if they have a thoracic-level lesion. Valgus knee stress is a major contributor to anterior-medial knee laxity and pain.

FEET

The most common foot deformities in children with MMC are equinus contracture, clubfeet, vertical talus, and calcaneal deformities; clubfeet occur in almost 50% of infants. Calcaneal deformities result from unopposed contraction of foot dorsiflexors and can be present at birth or develop later. The goal in treating these children is to achieve a plantigrade foot. Valgus deformities of the foot and ankle are common problems encountered in the ambulatory child with MMC.

SPINE

Spinal deformities are more likely to occur in individuals with thoracic lesions (>90%). Potential indications for surgical intervention include scoliosis greater than 50 degrees, inability to be managed with a brace, and individuals older than 10–12 years of age who wish to maximize their adult spinal height. Kyphotic deformities can cause severe seating and skin problems. Lordosis is usually related to hip flexion contractures.

FRACTURES

Children with MMC are susceptible to pathologic fractures in the lower limbs. Fracture rates range from 11% to 30% in children with spina bifida.

MOBILITY (eSlides 48.12 and 48.13)

"Will my child walk?" is a common question posed by most parents of children with MMC in infancy and early childhood. Most patients with lumbar lesions will achieve some level of ambulation (household or community), but those with high lumbar lesions tend to lose this ability during adolescence.

ORTHOSES

There are four typical goals or objectives when prescribing an orthotic device for a child with MMC: (1) to prevent deformity, (2) to support normal joint alignment and mechanics, (3) to control range of movement during gait, and (4) to improve function. An ankle-foot orthosis is the most commonly prescribed orthotic device for children with MMC.

Skin Breakdown

Skin breakdown is a very common occurrence in children and adults with MMC. The prevalence steadily increases between infancy and 10 years of age.

Obesity

Obesity rates are higher among adults with spina bifida (38%), particularly in women. A lower metabolic rate and lower energy expenditure predisposes patients with spina bifida to obesity.

Psychological and Social Issues

COGNITIVE FUNCTION

Children with MMC have specific behavioral and cognitive issues that need to be addressed, or at least recognized, by parents, health care providers, and school personnel. Children with MMC have lower intelligence quotient (IQ) scores compared with their able-bodied peers and usually demonstrate a higher verbal IQ than performance IQ. IQ scores are adversely affected by central nervous system infections but not necessarily by recurrent shunt revisions.

BEHAVIOR (eSlide 48.14)

Many individuals with MMC have much better verbal skills than written skills. It is often described as verbose, but irrelevant, conversation ("cocktail party chatter"). They often speak off-topic and use many routine social phrases.

• MYELOMENINGOCELE IN ADULTS

Transition to Adult Health Care

As a result of advances in medical care, 75%–85% of individuals with MMC now survive into early adulthood.

General Issues, Health, and Participation (eSlide 48.15)

The standard International Classification of Functioning, Disability and Health is used.

Late Neurologic Changes

Late changes may be due to VP shunt infections and malfunctions, syringomyelia, a symptomatic tethered cord, or a symptomatic type II Chiari malformation.

Late Musculoskeletal Considerations

Shoulder pain is very common in wheelchair users. Rotator cuff disorders and bicipital tendonitis are the most common injuries in chronic wheelchair users. Charcot joints can develop in the lower limbs as a result of lack of sensation and demineralization. Charcot osteoarthropathy is most commonly seen in the foot and ankle, followed by the hip and knee.

Renal and Urologic Damage

With the high prevalence of bladder dysfunction in individuals with spina bifida, renal damage remains one of the most common causes of morbidity and mortality among individuals with MMC.

Fertility, Sexuality, and Reproductive Issues

Menstruation and fertility among women with MMC are thought to be normal, and affected individuals are capable of becoming pregnant. Many men with MMC are infertile and demonstrate poor semen quality.

Educational Issues, Vocational Issues, and Independent Living

Most adolescents with MMC complete high school, and approximately 50% move on to further education. One long-term follow-up survey reported that 85% of children who survived to adulthood either attended or graduated from high school and/or college, with 36% requiring special education services. Forty-five percent of survey participants were employed, and 15% lived independently.

Palliative Care and Neural Tube Defects

Perinatal palliative care begins soon after diagnosis, follows through the decision-making process, involves a family birth plan, and extends into the bereavement period.

• CONCLUSION

The majority of fetuses with meningomyelocele are live born, and survival to adulthood is now common with proper treatment. MMC presents lifelong challenges to affected patients, their families, and clinicians. Vigilant surveillance and education are required to prevent life-threatening events and to decrease morbidity related to VP shunt malfunction, Chiari II malformation, renal failure, latex allergy, and infection. Monitoring for decline in motor function, preventing deformity, providing training in self-care and independent mobility, teaching independence with a bowel and bladder program, giving emotional and social support, and providing educational and vocational guidance are essential to maximize the functional independence of individuals with MMC.

Clinical Pearls

1. Preventive measures, especially folic acid supplementation, have a protective effect against neural tube defects (NTDs).
2. Maternal diabetes mellitus, maternal obesity, and maternal hyperthermia have all been associated with NTDs.
3. Less than 10% of children with myelomeningocele (MMC) have normal urinary control.
4. Cord tethering can result in weakness, scoliosis, pain, urologic dysfunction, and orthopedic deformities.
5. Intelligence quotient scores are adversely affected by central nervous system infections but not necessarily by recurrent shunt revisions.
6. There is an increased incidence of precocious puberty in individuals with MMC.
7. A multidisciplinary team approach is mandatory for managing children with spina bifida.
8. The International Classification of Functioning, Disability and Health model of functioning should be kept in mind when caring for individuals across their life span, addressing not only their medical needs but also other contextual factors so that function and participation are maximized.

BIBLIOGRAPHY
The complete bibliography is available on ExpertConsult.com.

Spinal Cord Injury 49

Chen-Yu Hung

In this chapter, I summarize the basic anatomy, classification system, and rehabilitation approaches for spinal cord injury (SCI) and the management of secondary conditions.

• EPIDEMIOLOGY

Age at Time of Injury and Gender

The incidence of traumatic SCI is bimodal, being highest among young adults and older individuals (>65 years). The majority of traumatic SCIs occur in males (70%–80%). The ratio of male to female SCIs is equal until the age of 5 years, after which the ratio begins to favor males, exceeding 80% between 16 and 20 years of age. However, with age, the ratio begins to fall again, especially in people older than 65 years.

Causes of Spinal Cord Injury

The most common causes of SCI worldwide, in descending order of incidence, are transport crashes, falls, violence, and sports. Although transport crashes remain a significant cause of SCI in all age groups, falls are the most common cause of SCI in people older than 60 years. High falls (from >1 m) are more common in young people, whereas low falls (from <1 m) are more common in people older than 45 years. SCI in older individuals is often related to cervical spinal stenosis and caused by a relatively minor trauma, such as a fall at home. The causes for children parallel those for younger adults, with a greater percentage of injuries (over 30%) related to sports being the exception; diving is the most common sports-related cause. Compared with older children and adults, children younger than 8 years have a significantly higher incidence of SCI without radiologic abnormalities, delayed onset of neurologic deficits (ranging from 0.5 hour to 4 days), and more neurologically complete lesions.

Life Expectancy and Causes of Death (eSlides 49.1 and 49.2)

Life expectancy for people with SCI remains below that of people without SCI. People with an SCI are two to five times more likely to die prematurely. Diseases of the respiratory system, especially pneumonia, are the leading cause of death during both the first postinjury year and subsequent years. Heart diseases (hypertensive and ischemic heart diseases, plus "other" heart diseases) are the second most common cause of death. Other heart diseases are thought to reflect deaths that are apparently caused by heart attacks in younger people without obvious underlying heart or vascular disease and cardiac dysrhythmias.

• ANATOMY, MECHANICS, AND SYNDROMES OF TRAUMATIC INJURY

Because the bony vertebral column elongates more than the spinal cord during embryologic development, the spinal cord terminates at the level of the L1-L2 intervertebral disk. As a result, the individual spinal cord segments do not line up with the corresponding bony levels of the same number (eSlide 49.3). The anatomy of the spinal cord, neurologic tracts, and vascular supply and the association between spinal cord and spine are depicted in eSlides 49.4–49.10.

Spinal Mechanics and Stability

The three-column spinal stability model is depicted in eSlide 49.11.

• CLASSIFICATION OF SPINAL CORD INJURY

Determining the most inferior intact sensory and motor level can reliably and accurately determine the neurologic level of injury (NLI). A complete injury is defined by the International Standards for Neurologic Classification of Spinal Cord Injury (ISNCSCI) as an injury in which there is a lack of any sensory or motor function in the lowest sacral segment; this includes pressure sensation within the anus, sensation at the anal mucocutaneous junction, or voluntary contraction of the external anal sphincter. An incomplete injury is defined as an injury in which there is at least partial sensory or motor function in the lowest sacral segment.

The sensory portion of the neurologic examination includes testing of a key point in each of the 28 dermatomes on each side of the body for both light touch and pinprick. Sensation is rated as absent, impaired, or normal. The motor portion of the neurologic examination includes the testing of a key muscle function for strength on a 6-point scale in each of 10 myotomes on each side of the body, as well as testing for contraction of the external anal sphincter. The NLI is defined as the most caudal segment of the spinal cord, with normal sensation and motor function bilaterally. The American Spinal Injury Association Impairment Scale (AIS), which classifies an SCI into five categories of severity, labeled A through E, is based on the degree of motor and sensory loss. A complete SCI, without any motor and sensory function at S4-S5, would be designated as AIS A. An SCI in which sensation is preserved in sacral segments S4-S5, but there is no motor function caudal to three segments below the NLI, is an AIS B injury. An SCI in which sensation is preserved in sacral segments S4-S5, but more than half of the key muscles below the NLI have a muscle grade less than 3/5, has an AIS grade of C. An SCI in which sensation is preserved in the sacral segments S4-S5, and at least half of the key muscles below the NLI have a muscle grade greater than or equal to 3/5, is classified as an AIS grade of D. When both sensory and motor function are normal, the AIS grade is E.

• NEUROLOGIC RECOVERY AND AMBULATION

A combination of age (<65 years versus ≥65 years), motor score of the stronger quadriceps femoris muscle, motor score of the stronger gastrocsoleus muscle, and light touch sensation at the L3 and S1 dermatomes shows excellent discrimination in distinguishing people who will be able to walk and those who will not be able to walk at 1 year after SCI (eSlides 49.12 and 49.13).

• ACUTE PHASE OF INJURY

The first step in the treatment of a person with a suspected spinal injury is ensuring an adequate airway, breathing, and circulation. Patients with cervical cord injuries are at high risk for respiratory failure and must be monitored closely for the need for ventilatory support. All people with suspected acute SCI should have their spines immobilized in a neutral supine position, regardless of the position the individual was found in after the accident. Neurogenic shock, which is associated with cervical and high thoracic injuries, is the result of sympathetic denervation. It is characterized by hypotension and bradycardia in the setting of flaccid paralysis. Once the patient is stabilized medically, a thorough evaluation of neurologic status and spinal stability is performed. Serial ISNCSCI examinations should be performed to detect neurologic status deterioration or improvement, particularly in the first 3 days after injury and after manipulations, such as transport, closed reduction, or surgical treatment. Operative treatment of acute spinal injury is generally performed to either stabilize an unstable spine or decompress compressed neural elements.

REHABILITATION AND CHRONIC PHASE

Vocational Training

Only approximately 25% of all individuals with SCI are employed after their injury. Predictors of employment after an SCI include being employed before the SCI, having a less physically demanding occupation before the SCI, being younger at the time of the SCI, having a less severe SCI, having lived more years with the SCI, having more education before the SCI, being motivated to work, and being white.

Reconstructive Surgery of the Upper Limbs

Functional upper limb surgical reconstruction has historically been delayed for 1 year after injury to allow neurologic recovery in the targeted muscles. Tendon transfer, as an example, refers to detaching the tendon of an expendable innervated muscle from one of its attachment sites, and reattaching that innervated muscle and tendon to another tendon that lacks an innervated muscle, but whose regained function is sought. Muscles are chosen for transfer if they have a strength grade of 4 or 5, because one grade of muscle strength is usually lost with the transfer. Transferred muscles with a strength grade of less than 3 generally do not improve function. Muscles should not be chosen for transfer if their loss would result in functional decline. Common tendon transfers and tenodesis procedures are stratified according to the ISNCSCI motor level and the more specific international classification for surgery of the hand in tetraplegia motor group (eSlide 49.14).

QUALITY OF LIFE

There is no relationship between the neurologic level, completeness of SCI, and subjective quality of life. Some factors are thought to positively affect quality of life, such as mobility and independence in activities of daily living, emotional support, good overall health, self-esteem, absence of depression, physical and social activities, and integration. Other factors are being married and employed, having completed more years of education, and living at home.

SECONDARY CONDITIONS

Pulmonary System

SCI can lead to alterations in lung, chest wall, and airway mechanics, and the degree of dysfunction is strongly correlated with the NLI and degree of motor impairment. The pulmonary function profile of people with chronic tetraplegia and high paraplegia reveals decreased lung volumes and decreased thoracic wall compliance as a result of the restriction caused by respiratory muscle weakness, as well as airway hyperreactivity. Spirometric and lung volume studies in people with tetraplegia and high levels of paraplegia demonstrate significant reduction of vital capacity (VC), total lung capacity, expiratory reserve volume, and inspiratory capacity, along with a significant increase in residual volume (RV) and little or no change in functional residual capacity. The diaphragm, innervated by the anterior horn cells located in the C3-C5 segments, is the major primary muscle of inspiration. The sternocleidomastoid and trapezius muscles, innervated by the spinal accessory nerve and the C2-C4 and C1-C4 roots, respectively, are accessory muscles of inspiration and can be necessary to allow adequate ventilation in people with a higher-level SCI (eSlide 49.15). People with a neurologic level of C2 or above with a complete SCI usually have no diaphragmatic function and require mechanical ventilation or diaphragmatic or phrenic nerve pacing. People with a complete C3 SCI have severe diaphragmatic weakness and commonly require mechanical ventilation, at least temporarily. People with a complete C4 SCI also often have severe diaphragmatic weakness and can also require mechanical ventilation, at least temporarily. People with a complete C5-C8 SCI are usually able to maintain independent breathing, but because of loss of innervation to the intercostal and abdominal muscles, they remain at high risk for pulmonary complications.

The VC of people with tetraplegia or high paraplegia is posturally dependent, being up to 15% lower in the upright position than in the supine position. In the sitting position in people with paralyzed abdominal muscles, the effect of gravity on the abdominal contents leads to an increased RV. Use of an abdominal binder in the sitting position helps reverse this effect by pressing the abdominal contents into the diaphragm, allowing a more efficient diaphragmatic resting position. Treatment of atelectasis includes lung expansion and secretion mobilization and clearance. Intermittent positive-pressure breathing, bilevel positive airway pressure, or continuous positive airway pressure devices can all be used, with or without tracheostomy tubes to help lung expansion and to prevent or treat atelectasis. Secretion mobilization techniques include postural drainage and chest percussion or vibration. Secretion clearance techniques include suctioning, manually assistive cough, use of a mechanical insufflator-exsufflator, and bronchoscopy. The insufflator-exsufflator supplies a positive pressure to the airway, followed immediately by a negative pressure, delivered either through the mouth or via a tracheostomy tube. This rapid pressure change induces a high expiratory flow rate similar to a cough. Medications are useful adjuncts in treating and preventing atelectasis. Bronchodilators reduce airway hyperreactivity and inflammation that contribute to atelectasis formation and sputum production, and they stimulate the secretion of surfactant. Use of beta-2-adenergic medications has been shown to improve expiratory pressures, which can lead to a more effective cough. Mucolytics can be given orally (e.g., guaifenesin) or via a nebulizer (e.g., acetylcysteine). Adequate hydration thins pulmonary secretions.

Deep Vein Thrombosis

Deep vein thrombosis (DVT), one type of venous thromboembolism (VTE) along with its potential sequela pulmonary embolism (PE), develops in approximately 50%–75% of people with SCI who do not receive VTE prophylaxis. The risk of

DVT is greatest between days 7 and 10 after the injury. Identified risk factors for DVT include complete motor injuries and injuries at the thoracic level and below. Because of the high incidence of DVT and the potentially fatal outcome of a PE, VTE prophylaxis is the standard of care. Several large trials comparing subcutaneously administered low-molecular-weight heparin (LMWH) and fixed-dose unfractionated heparin have shown LMWH to be more effective in preventing both DVT and PE after SCI. Guidelines recommend that pharmacologic prophylaxis continue for 8–12 weeks after injury, with the addition of distal lower extremity pneumatic compression garments during the first 2 weeks after injury. The treatment regimen for DVT or PE typically involves therapeutic anticoagulation, unless contradicted. Treatment is generally continued for 6 months after a DVT is diagnosed to prevent progression and recurrence of thrombosis. Inferior vena cava (IVC) filters are indicated for people who have failed anticoagulant prophylaxis by developing a DVT or PE despite adequate anticoagulation or for people with a thromboembolus within the IVC or iliac veins.

Autonomic Dysreflexia

Autonomic dysreflexia (AD) is a syndrome and clinical emergency that affects people with an SCI at the characteristic defining of level T6 or above. It is attributed to preservation of the splanchnic outflow innervation below T6 level. AD is triggered by a noxious stimulus below the injury level, which elicits a sudden reflex sympathetic activity that is uninhibited by supraspinal centers and results in profound vasoconstriction and other autonomic responses. The symptoms of AD are somewhat variable but include a pounding headache; systolic and diastolic hypertension; profuse sweating and cutaneous vasodilatation, with flushing of the face, neck, and shoulders; nasal congestion; pupillary dilatation; and bradycardia. The hypertension can be profound and result in intracerebral hemorrhage, status epilepticus, myocardial ischemia, and even death. The noxious stimulus responsible for AD frequently stems from the sacral dermatomes, most often from a distended bladder. Other causes include fecal impaction, pathology of the bladder or rectum, ingrown toenails, labor and delivery, surgical procedures, orgasm, and a variety of other conditions. AD occurs more commonly in people with complete injuries (>90%) than in those with incomplete injuries (approximately 25%) and is more likely to occur in the chronic phase of injury.

Treatment of acute AD must be prompt and efficient to prevent potential morbidity and mortality. The individual should be placed in a sitting position, constrictive clothing and garments should be loosened, the blood pressure should be monitored every 2–5 minutes, and evacuation of the bladder should be performed promptly to ensure continuous drainage of urine. If symptoms are not relieved by these measures, fecal impaction should be suspected and, if present, resolved. If hypertension is present, fast-acting antihypertensive agents should be administered, preferably with something that can be removed if it causes hypotension, such as a topical nitrate. Alpha-adrenoceptor antagonists, alpha- and beta-adrenoceptor antagonists, or the centrally acting alpha-2-adrenoceptor agonist clonidine are occasionally required for patients with chronic recurrent symptoms of AD.

Calcium Metabolism and Osteoporosis

An imbalance between bone formation and resorption occurs after SCI. The potential adverse clinical effects of this imbalance are osteoporosis-related fractures, hypercalcemia, and renal calculi resulting from hypercalciuria. During this time of prominent bone resorption, the release of calcium and phosphorus from bone tissue into the blood causes a significant decrease in parathyroid hormone (PTH) secretion. Decreased PTH levels are thought to act in the kidney to decrease calcium resorption and inhibit the synthesis of $1,25(OH)_2D$ (the active form of vitamin D), which indirectly decreases intestinal calcium absorption; both mechanisms act to minimize the possibility that the skeletal calcium loss will lead to hypercalcemia. However, in adolescent boys, who seem to have especially high bone turnover, hypercalcemia is not uncommon within the first 3–4 months after SCI. Symptoms of hypercalcemia include abdominal pain, nausea, vomiting, malaise, polyuria, polydipsia, and dehydration. Management of hypercalcemia includes hydration with saline infusions, administration of diuretics, and bisphosphonates. Reducing calcium intake is not typically effective for lowering elevated serum or urinary calcium concentrations, and restrictions of dietary calcium and vitamin D intake are not recommended.

People with chronic SCI are often vitamin D deficient because of inadequate nutritional intake or reduced sunlight exposure. Supplementation with calcium and vitamin D (which can improve calcium resorption), particularly in the chronic phase when hypercalcemia is not present, can be effective for minimizing bone loss. Individuals with SCI who perform passive weight-bearing standing with the aid of a standing device might have better-preserved bone mineral density (BMD) in their lower limbs than those who do not stand. Functional electrical stimulation cycle ergometry has been shown to slow the rate of bone loss. Several bisphosphonate antiresorptive therapies have been shown to be effective in either maintaining lower extremity BMD after acute SCI or improving low BMD.

Bowel Management

Parasympathetic innervation to the portion of bowel extending from the esophagus to the splenic flexure of the colon, which modulates peristalsis, is provided by the vagus nerve. Parasympathetic innervation to the descending colon and rectum is provided by the pelvic nerve, which exits from the spinal cord at segments S2-S4. The somatic pudendal nerve, also originating from segments S2-S4, innervates the external anal sphincter and pelvic floor musculature. An SCI that damages segments above the sacral segments produces a reflexic or upper motor neuron (UMN) bowel, in which defecation cannot be initiated by voluntary relaxation of the external anal sphincter, although there can be reflex-mediated colonic peristalsis. In contrast, an SCI that includes destruction of the S2-S4 anterior horn cells or cauda equina produces an areflexic or lower motor neuron (LMN) bowel, in which there is no reflex-mediated colonic peristalsis. There is only slow stool propulsion coordinated by the intrinsically innervated myenteric plexus. The anal sphincter of an LMN bowel is typically atonic and prone to leakage of stool.

A bowel program is a treatment plan for managing neurogenic bowel with the goal of allowing effective and efficient colonic evacuation while preventing incontinence and constipation. A bowel program should be scheduled at the same time every day, usually in the morning. Two mechanical methods are used to evacuate the rectum: digital stimulation and digital evacuation. If an effective bowel routine cannot be achieved with the above techniques, pulsed water irrigation has been shown to be effective for some people in decreasing the time it takes to complete a bowel routine and reducing the incidence of bowel accidents and constipation.

Neurogenic bladder

Parasympathetic innervation to the bladder, which modulates contraction of the urinary bladder with opening of the bladder neck to allow voiding, is provided by the pelvic splanchnic nerves. These nerves exit the spinal cord at segments S2-S4. Sympathetic innervation to the bladder and bladder neck or internal urethral sphincter, which modulates relaxation of the body of the bladder and narrowing of the bladder neck to inhibit voiding, is provided by the hypogastric nerves. These nerves exit the spinal cord at segments T11-L2. The somatic pudendal nerve, also originating from segments S2-S4, innervates the external urinary sphincter. An SCI that damages segments above the sacral segments produces a reflexic or UMN bladder, in which urination cannot be initiated by voluntary relaxation of the external urinary sphincter, although reflex voiding can occur. In contrast, an SCI that includes destruction of the S2-S4 anterior horn cells or cauda equina produces an areflexic or LMN bladder, in which there is no reflex voiding. The external urinary sphincter of an LMN bladder is typically atonic and prone to leakage of urine. Because central coordination of normal voiding is thought to occur at the level of the pons, in a person with a UMN bladder resulting from an SCI, coordination of contraction (or relaxation) of the bladder with relaxation (or contraction) of the external urinary sphincter is lost. This leads to a pattern of simultaneous reflex contractile activity called detrusor-sphincter dyssynergia, which often results in elevated bladder pressures.

The goal of management of a neurogenic bladder is to achieve a socially acceptable method of bladder emptying while avoiding complications such as infections, hydronephrosis with renal failure, urinary tract stones, and AD. During the immediate postinjury period, an indwelling catheter is placed within the bladder because virtually all people with SCI have urinary retention. Intermittent bladder catheterization (IC) is generally accepted as the best option, other than regaining normal voiding, for the long-term bladder management of people who can perform IC themselves. This is because of the physiologic advantage of allowing for regular bladder filling and emptying, the social acceptability of not needing a drainage appliance, and fewer complications than with other methods. Reflex voiding is another viable option for men with a UMN bladder in whom bladder pressures generated are greater than that of the outlet pressures of the sphincters, thereby allowing spontaneous voiding. A condom catheter is applied to the penis and connected via tubing to a leg bag or bedside bag. Reflex voiding can sometimes be triggered by suprapubic tapping. The completeness of voiding can be determined by measurement of a postvoid residual urine volume. High RVs predispose to urinary tract infection (UTI) and bladder stone formation. Furthermore, reflex voiding is often associated with elevated voiding pressures, which can predispose to vesicoureteral reflux, hydronephrosis, and eventual renal failure. It is critically important for reflex voiders to undergo regular imaging with a renal ultrasound to identify the presence of reflux or hydronephrosis. When accompanying urination, the symptoms and signs of AD typically indicate that high-pressure (within the detrusor) voiding is occurring. Alpha-adrenergic receptor antagonist medications, such as prazosin and terazosin, are often effective in decreasing bladder outlet resistance, bladder pressures, and postvoid RVs. Long-term bladder drainage with an indwelling catheter is a reasonable option for people with tetraplegia who are unable to perform IC or for men who are unable to effectively maintain an external catheter on their penis. Use of an indwelling catheter inserted through the urethra is associated with an increased risk of UTIs, bladder stone formation, epididymitis, prostatitis, hypospadias, and bladder cancer. Placement of a suprapubic cystostomy tube in people requiring long-term indwelling catheters can avoid some of these complications.

Sexuality and Fertility

The ability to have psychogenic erections in men and psychogenic vaginal vaso-congestion and lubrication in women is mediated by the sympathetic and para-sympathetic nervous systems and directly related to the degree of light touch and pinprick sensory preservation within the T11-L2 dermatomes. The ability to have reflex erections in men and reflex vaginal vasocongestion and lubrication in women is mediated by the parasympathetic nervous system and related to sacral reflex pres-ervation. If a hyperactive bulbocavernosus (BC) reflex is present, reflex erections and lubrication are usually possible, although the quality of arousal might differ from that experienced before the injury. If there is a hypoactive BC reflex with some preservation of sensation within the S4-S5 dermatomes, reflex erections and lubrication are usually possible. However, if the BC reflex is absent and there is no sensation within the S4-S5 dermatomes, the ability to have reflex erections and lubrication is lost, and the ability to generate erections and lubrication psychogeni-cally is related to T11-L2 sensory preservation. The neurologic control of orgasm is generally believed to be a spinal-level reflex response that can be inhibited or excited by the brain. If on physical examination the BC and anocutaneous reflexes are absent and there is no sensation at S4-S5, attainment of orgasm is unlikely. Approximately 40% of men and women with SCI report orgasm.

Effective treatments for male erectile dysfunction, not ejaculatory dysfunction, resulting from SCI include oral medications (type 5 phosphodiesterase inhibitors, such as sildenafil, vardenafil, and tadalafil), vacuum tumescence devices, intracav-ernous (penile) injections, and penile implants. Treatment of infertility in men with SCI is initially focused on producing an ejaculate, because only 10%–20% of men are able to ejaculate naturally after SCI. Interventions, including manual or partner masturbation, penile vibratory stimulation, and electroejaculation, can lead to success in ejaculation in 95% of individuals. Significant deterioration of semen quality, including reduced numbers of spermatozoa, decreased sperm motility, and the presence of inhibitory factors within the seminal fluid, occurs within the first 2 weeks after SCI. Women with SCI are not thought to have decreased fertility. Most women experience temporary amenorrhea after injury that lasts for an aver-age of 4 months. Labor might not be perceived by women with injury levels above T10. Uterine contractions during labor have been associated with AD in women with injury levels above T6, and this needs to be differentiated from the blood pres-sure elevations seen with preeclampsia.

Pressure Ulcers

During acute rehabilitation, pressure ulcers occur in the following areas: sacrum, 39%; calcaneus, 13%; ischium, 8%; occiput, 6%; and scapula, 5%. Muscle is the tissue most susceptible to pressure damage over a bony promi-nence. The higher distribution of ulcers in the sacrum and calcaneus in the acute SCI population is probably because of the increased time spent supine in bed soon after the injury, as opposed to more time sitting in a wheelchair at a later stage. Risk factors for pressure ulcers following SCI include urinary or bowel incontinence, severe spasticity, diabetes mellitus, smoking, respiratory disease, hypotension, depression, and improper support surfaces. Assessment of a pressure ulcer should include notation of the location, stage of the wound, its size, characteristics of the ulcer cavity, and characteristics of the surrounding skin. Different categories or stages of wounds require different components to heal. Category/Stage II ulcers might need only epithelialization, whereas a category/stage III or IV ulcer can require matrix synthesis and deposition, angiogenesis, fibroplasia, and contraction.

Removal of necrotic tissue of pressure ulcers can be performed by a number of different methods of débridement, including autolysis and chemical, sharp, and mechanical débridement. Dressings are topical products used to protect a pressure ulcer from contamination and trauma, apply medication, débride necrotic tissue, and provide an environment in which tissue hydration levels and viability of the wound tissue are maintained by something other than the skin. The major dressing categories include transparent films, hydrocolloids, hydrogels, foams, alginates, and gauze dressings. Adequate nutrition is essential for healing of a pressure ulcer. Caloric requirements are increased for a person with SCI who has a pressure ulcer. An estimate of the difference in basal energy expenditure between people with SCI who have severe pressure ulcers and those who do not have pressure ulcers is approximately 5 kcal/kg of body weight/day. Protein requirements are increased for a person with an SCI and pressure ulcers; recommendations for increased protein intake range from 1.25–2 g protein/kg of body weight/day.

Spasticity

Spasticity is a syndrome with different components, including velocity-dependent increased resistance to passive motion, involuntary muscle contractions or spasms, and hyperreflexia. Although spasticity can cause difficulties with mobility, positioning, and comfort, and might even predispose to skin breakdown, it can also be helpful for ambulating and performing activities of daily living. Prolonged static stretching and proper positioning of spastic muscles are the mainstays of treatment for spasticity for virtually all people with SCI. In addition, many pharmacologic options are available for the treatment of spasticity. Many practitioners consider oral baclofen to be the first-line pharmacologic treatment for spinal spasticity. Baclofen is a structural analog of gamma-aminobutyric acid (GABA), the main inhibitory transmitter of the spinal cord; baclofen binds to $GABA_B$ receptors. Starting doses are typically 5–10 mg given 2–4 times per day, with gradual increases as clinically indicated. The maximum recommended dose is 80 mg/day. Adverse effects of baclofen include fatigue and dizziness, and seizures can occur with abrupt withdrawal. Diazepam and other benzodiazepines bind to $GABA_A$ receptors. Benzodiazepines can cause physical dependence, as well as lethargy and diminished concentration. Tizanidine hydrochloride is a central alpha-2-adrenergic agonist that has been shown to be effective in treating spasticity after SCI. Adverse effects of tizanidine include sedation and liver function abnormalities. When only a few specific muscles are affected by problematic spasticity, targeted injections of these muscles with a neurotoxin (e.g., botulinum toxin) can be performed. Botulinum toxin injected into a muscle binds to receptor sites on the presynaptic nerve terminal of the neuromuscular junction, inhibiting the release of acetylcholine and preventing neuromuscular transmission. Needle electrical stimulation to localize motor points or electromyography to identify motor endplates can improve the effectiveness of these injections. Clinical effects of a botulinum toxin injection can be noted within 2 to 3 days and persist for 3 to 6 months.

- The majority of spinal cord injuries (SCIs) occur in males (70%–80%), and the most common causes, in descending order of incidence, are transport crashes, falls, violence, and sports.
- Respiratory and heart diseases are the two most common primary causes of death in people with an SCI.
- A complete injury is defined as an injury in which there is a lack of pressure sensation within the anus, sensation at the anal mucocutaneous junction, and voluntary contraction of the external anal sphincter.
- Neurogenic shock, which is associated with cervical and high thoracic injuries, results from sympathetic denervation and is characterized by bradycardia, hypotension, hypothermia, and flaccid paralysis.
- Vital capacity of patients with tetraplegia or high paraplegia is greater in the supine position than in the sitting position because of a more optimal diaphragm position when supine.
- Pharmacologic prophylaxis for venous thromboembolism is the standard of care following acute SCI.
- Autonomic dysreflexia is a syndrome that affects people with an SCI at T6 level or above.
- The goal of management of a neurogenic bladder is to achieve a socially acceptable method of bladder emptying while avoiding associated complications.

BIBLIOGRAPHY
The complete bibliography is available on ExpertConsult.com.

Auditory, Vestibular, and Visual Impairments

50

Ding-Hao Liu

Auditory, vestibular, and visual impairments are among the most common sensory issues that can adversely affect a person's rehabilitation process. This chapter will briefly describe the diagnosis and rehabilitation of auditory, vestibular, and visual sensory impairments.

• AUDITORY IMPAIRMENTS

Approximately 30 million Americans (13%), age 12 years or older, have bilateral hearing loss. In general, increased age is associated with the development of hearing loss, and men are more likely to experience hearing loss than women. Disabling hearing loss has been reported by 2% of the population in the 45- to 54-year-old range, increasing to 8.5% in the 55- to 64-year-old range, 25% in the 65- to 74-year-old range, and 50% in those 75 years and older.

• ANATOMY AND PHYSIOLOGY OF THE AUDITORY SYSTEM

Sound travels to the middle ear, which houses two major ear structures: the tympanic membrane (eardrum) and the ossicular chain that consists of the malleus, incus, and stapes. Sound vibrates the tympanic membrane and then sets the ossicular chain into motion. This amplifies the sound by making the ossicular chain act as an impedance-matching transformer, which is an important step to prevent energy loss when sound travels from air (in the middle ear) to a fluid medium (in the inner ear). The inner ear is a fluid-filled space within the temporal bone and is connected to the stapes of the ossicular chain via the oval window and to the eighth cranial nerve (vestibulocochlear nerve) through hair cells (eSlide 50.1).

• EXAMINATION OF THE AUDITORY SYSTEM

Various audiologic tests are performed to evaluate the hearing status and help establish the diagnosis for detected abnormalities. eSlides 50.2 and 50.3 summarize typical audiologic tests and sites evaluated by each test.

Degree of Hearing Loss

The degree of hearing loss describes the severity of hearing impairment. eSlide 50.4 shows classification of degree of hearing loss. There is no uniform classification system for the degree of hearing loss, but 25 dB hearing loss or less is usually considered normal hearing in adults.

Types of Hearing Loss

There are three types of hearing loss: conductive, sensorineural, and mixed. Hearing loss caused by damage to the outer ear, middle ear, or both is called conductive hearing loss. It is characterized by normal bone-conduction thresholds and elevated air-conduction thresholds, with an air-bone gap (difference between air-conduction and bone-conduction thresholds) of 15 dB or greater. This type of hearing loss can be caused by obstruction of the ear canal by a foreign body or cerumen, outer or middle ear disorders, deformation of the outer or middle ear, mechanical injury to the outer or middle ear, and other middle ear disorders, such as otosclerosis and cholesteatoma. The clarity of sounds is mostly preserved, but the conductive hearing loss decreases the intensity of sounds. Sensorineural hearing loss (SNHL) is characterized by elevated air-conduction thresholds, with an air-bone gap of 10 dB or less. This type of hearing loss is the result of damage to the cochlea, retrocochlear pathway, or both. Clarity and intensity of sound are both degraded. SNHL is permanent in most cases and can be caused by various auditory disorders, such as tumors involving the eighth cranial nerve, Meniere disease, and deformation of the cochlea or eighth cranial nerve. Other factors that contribute to the development of SNHL are aging, acoustic trauma from loud noise, ototoxic drugs or chemicals, hypoxia, traumatic brain injury, infections, immune system disorders, and genetics. Systemic diseases, such as neurofibromatosis type II and multiple sclerosis, can also cause this type of hearing loss. Mixed hearing loss is characterized by elevated air-conduction and bone-conduction thresholds, with an air-bone gap of 15 dB or greater. It is a mixture of conductive hearing loss and SNHL.

Immittance Audiometry

Tympanometry measures the mobility of the tympanic membrane and the middle ear pressure, but it does not measure perceptual hearing. The results from tympanometry are plotted as a graph called a tympanogram (eSlide 50.5). There are three main types of tympanograms: A, B, and C. A Type A tympanogram indicates normal middle ear status. Reduced mobility of the tympanic membrane caused by a stiffened middle ear system can cause a shallow peak on the tympanogram, called a Type A_s tympanogram. If the middle ear system is overly compliant because of ossicular chain discontinuity or a flaccid tympanic membrane, the peak will be very high or off the chart, which is shown as a Type A_d tympanogram. A Type B tympanogram shows no clear peak pressure and is relatively flat. If the ear canal volume is normal, the Type B tympanogram may be reflective of an advanced stage of otosclerosis or a middle ear filled with an effusion (possibly caused by an ear infection). If the ear canal volume is abnormally small and a Type B tympanogram is observed, this is suggestive of blockage of the ear canal because of cerumen impaction. If the ear canal volume is abnormally large and the tympanogram is peakless, this is a sign of a perforation in the tympanic membrane. Finally, a Type C tympanogram indicates a significantly negative peak pressure, which is possibly caused by Eustachian tube dysfunction or a developing or resolving middle ear infection.

Otoacoustic Emissions

Otoacoustic emissions (OAEs) are retrograde transmissions of energy from the cochlea to the ear canal. Clinically, OAEs are used for differential diagnosis, infant and pediatric hearing screening, and ototoxicity monitoring. There are two major types of OAEs that have been used clinically: transient evoked OAEs and distortion product OAEs.

Auditory Brainstem Response

The auditory brainstem response (ABR) measures neural activities along the auditory pathway from the eighth cranial nerve up to possibly the inferior colliculus in response to auditory stimuli delivered via insert earphones. ABR waveforms are produced as a result of synchronous neural discharges and are used for analysis. In adults with normal hearing, the ABR has seven distinct peaks, labeled sequentially from I to VII. Typically, only waves I, III, and V are used clinically (eSlide 50.6). ABR testing is used for differential diagnosis (e.g., detection of the effects of an acoustic tumor), intraoperative monitoring during tumor removal surgery, auditory threshold estimation, and infant hearing screening.

• CAUSES OF HEARING IMPAIRMENTS

Causes of hearing impairments include acquired hearing loss, ototoxic drugs, chemically induced hearing loss, noise-induced hearing loss, age-related hearing loss, auditory processing disorders, and tinnitus.

• RED FLAGS: WARNING OF EAR DISEASE

The 10 red flags of ear disease are listed in eSlides 50.7 and 50.8. Patients who show any evidence of red flags should be referred to a physician or specialist (i.e., otolaryngologist or otologist) for further evaluation and treatment of ear diseases.

• AUDITORY REHABILITATION

Hearing Aid Consultation and Selection

Ear diseases should be treated medically and surgically if treatments are available. Acknowledgment of hearing loss and the degree of motivation to do something about hearing loss are strongly correlated with how frequently patients wear their hearing aids. eSlide 50.9 shows different styles of hearing aids.

Hearing Assistance Technology

Hearing assistance technology (HAT) refers to personal devices that help an individual with or without hearing loss communicate more effectively (eSlides 50.10 and 50.11). A personal frequency modulation (FM) system is a very popular HAT that transmits a speaker's voice directly to an individual's ear; it can be used in academic and group settings, including classrooms, churches, and restaurants. The speaker must wear a microphone and FM transmitter, and the listener has to wear an FM receiver that can be coupled directly to the listener's ear via earphones, ear buds, an induction loop, hearing aids, or a cochlear implant.

• VESTIBULAR IMPAIRMENTS

Approximately 4% of American adults (almost 8 million) report chronic problems with balance, and an additional 1.1% (2.4 million) report chronic problems with dizziness alone.

• ANATOMY AND PHYSIOLOGY OF THE VESTIBULAR SYSTEM

The vestibular neurons of the eighth cranial nerve project centrally to both the cerebellum and the vestibular nuclei, where they synapse and transmit afferent vestibular inputs and contribute to vestibular reflex pathways. There are three main vestibular reflexes: the vestibulospinal reflex (for body stabilization), vestibulocollic reflex (for head stabilization), and the vestibuloocular reflex (VOR; for visual gaze stabilization). The presence of nystagmus (involuntary eye movements) can be related to vestibular dysfunction. Jerk nystagmus consists of eye drift in one direction (slow phase) and a quick corrective eye movement (fast phase). These involuntary eye movements can occur in a side-to-side (horizontal nystagmus), up-and-down (vertical nystagmus), or circular (torsional or rotary nystagmus) pattern.

Physical Examination

Gaze testing involves monitoring for the presence of nystagmus or other abnormal eye movements while the patient fixates on stationary visual targets. Gaze nystagmus is considered abnormal if it is present with appropriately positioned visual targets. It can be interpreted with the Alexander law, which states that gazing in the direction of the fast phase enhances the nystagmus. For the Romberg test, the patient stands with his or her feet together and arms to the side and is instructed to maintain this position with the eyes open and then closed. The maximum time taken by the patient in maintaining the position with eyes open and eyes closed is compared with normative data from healthy control subjects. The Fukuda stepping test assesses labyrinthine function through the vestibulospinal reflexes. The patient steps in place on a marked grid with the eyes closed and arms outstretched forward. Measurements of rotation and displacement are obtained after 50–100 steps and compared with data from healthy control subjects. The Dix-Hallpike maneuver can be used to assess for the effects of displaced otoconia in the posterior semicircular canal (SSC). Abnormal migration of otoconia into the SSC system results in benign paroxysmal positional vertigo (BPPV). In the Dix-Hallpike maneuver, the patient is seated on the examination bed with the head rotated 45 degrees to the lesion side. The patient is then quickly lowered backward to the supine position, with the head hanging over the edge of the bed by 30 degrees. This places the patient in a position that aligns the posterior SSC in a vertical orientation. Any debris in the posterior SSC is influenced by gravity, thus producing abnormal fluid movement within the affected canal. Nystagmus with a predominant torsional component is present in classic BPPV. If nystagmus appears, the position is maintained until the nystagmus terminates before quickly returning the patient to an upright position. The signs and symptoms of BPPV are fatigable; therefore if nystagmus and vertigo are present, the maneuver should be repeated immediately to assess whether fatigue occurs (eSlide 50.12).

• COMPUTERIZED VESTIBULAR TESTING

A variety of sophisticated computerized vestibular tests are available for those cases of dizziness in which the history and physical examination alone are inadequate or when there is a need for further corroborative data to confirm a diagnosis. These tests can provide information related to the site of dysfunction and can also be applied after treatment to provide information regarding the potential functional benefits of vestibular rehabilitation.

Electronystagmography and Videonystagmography

Electronystagmography and videonystagmography use computer-based systems that assess the vestibular system by recording horizontal and vertical eye movements.

Random Saccade Testing

Saccades are rapid movements of the eyes. During saccadic testing, the patient's eye movements are compared with the fast, random movement of the target stimuli.

Smooth Pursuit Testing

During smooth pursuit testing, the patient tracts a visual target moving in a sinusoidal pattern that varies in frequency over time.

Positional Testing

Positional testing is used to identify the presence of nystagmus during maintenance of a provocative head or body position. Measures must be taken to prevent visual fixation and central suppression.

Caloric Testing

The caloric test is performed by applying cool and warm irrigations of water or air in the external auditory canal. The patient is positioned such that the horizontal or lateral SSC is perpendicular to the ground. The temperature gradient induces endolymph flow in the horizontal or lateral SSC, which then activates the VOR. The ensuing nystagmus should follow the "COWS" (Cold Opposite, Warm Same) mnemonic.

• ROTATIONAL CHAIR TESTING

Rotational chair testing involves stimulation of the horizontal SSCs or superior vestibular nerves by spinning the patient along a vertical axis in a quantifiable sinusoidal, pseudorandom, or constant-velocity manner (eSlide 50.13).

• COMPUTERIZED DYNAMIC POSTUROGRAPHY

Computerized dynamic posturography (CDP) uses a movable platform and visual surround. The patient's motor reactions and postural stability are recorded as the support surface and the visual surround move. The Sensory Organization Test (SOT) and the Motor Control Test are the components of CDP. eSlide 50.13 illustrates the six SOT sensory conditions.

• CERVICAL AND OCULAR VESTIBULAR EVOKED MYOGENIC POTENTIAL

Intense sound stimuli, such as clicks or tone pips, can stimulate sensory tissue within the otolithic organs. The cervical vestibular evoked myogenic potential (cVEMP) can be recorded with electrodes placed over the sternocleidomastoid muscle. The cVEMP is based on the vestibulocollic reflex and is thought to originate in the saccule. The ocular vestibular evoked myogenic potential (oVEMP) is believed to originate in the utricle; it involves the superior division of the vestibular nerve. oVEMP can be recorded using electrodes placed over the inferior oblique muscle in the contralateral infraorbital region. eSlide 50.14 outlines the cVEMP abnormalities encountered in various otologic and neurologic disorders.

• VIDEO HEAD IMPULSE TEST

The video head impulse test can be used to assess the dynamic function of the individual SSCs.

• SUBJECTIVE ASSESSMENTS

The Dizziness Handicap Inventory and the Activities-Specific Balance Confidence Scale are subjective assessments of postural instability.

• RISK FACTORS, COMORBIDITIES, AND EPIDEMIOLOGY OF VESTIBULAR DISORDERS

The most common vestibular disorders include BPPV, vestibular neuritis, vestibular migraine, and Meniere disease. Vestibular neuritis was the second most common cause of dizziness after BPPV identified in general practice clinics. Meniere disease is characterized by recurring episodes of long-lasting vertigo, fluctuating sensorineural hearing loss, tinnitus, and aural fullness.

• VESTIBULAR REHABILITATION

Habituation

Habituation is the process by which symptoms are decreased through repeated exposure to provocative stimuli. A peripheral vestibular lesion can create a sensory discrepancy caused by unequal vestibular inputs from the vestibular labyrinths. Repetitive movement may reduce this asymmetry of vestibular input.

Vestibuloocular Reflex Adaptation

The VOR is an important three-neuron vestibular reflex affected by stimulation of the SSCs, which creates conjugate eye movement equal to and in the opposite direction of movement of the head. The VOR allows for stabilization of the image on the retina, leading to clear vision when the head is moved. The gain of the VOR is the ratio of eye velocity to head velocity. The ideal gain in a normal patient is 1:1. A vestibular disorder can cause a decreased gain of the VOR, which in turn would result in a blurred image when the head is moved rapidly.

Sensory Substitution

Sensory substitution refers to the use of an alternative intact sense for an impaired sense. Visual and somatosensory cues are critical components of this facet of vestibular rehabilitation therapy. Enhancing the use of visual and somatosensory cues for balance and postural control may not adequately compensate for the vestibular impairment, but it may assist in functional recovery.

Canalith Repositioning Treatment for Benign Paroxysmal Positional Vertigo

Canalith repositioning treatment for BPPV (eSlide 50.12B) is the most effective vestibular rehabilitation technique.

• VISUAL IMPAIRMENTS

Vision rehabilitation focuses on restoration of function in individuals who are blind or visually impaired. Most people with vision loss are aged 50 years and older and have age-related eye disease (e.g., age-related macular degeneration, diabetic retinopathy, glaucoma). However, vision loss can occur at any age because of congenital conditions, other diseases, or injury to the eye, orbit, or brain. The approach taken in vision rehabilitation is functional restoration of the capacity to perform activities of daily living.

Definitions of Blindness and Visual Impairment

"Legal blindness" is defined as best corrected visual acuity of 20/200 or worse in the better eye or the presence of a visual field limitation, such that the widest diameter of the visual field in the better eye subtends an angle of no greater than 20 degrees.

• ANATOMY AND PHYSIOLOGY OF VISION

Vision is most commonly associated with the eye; however, the human visual system is a complex set of structures, extending from the eye back to the visual cortex and then forward to sensory association areas, as well as the motor, memory, cognitive, emotional, and other areas of the brain. eSlide 50.15A illustrates the structures of the eyeball, and eSlide 50.15B illustrates the optic pathways from the retina to the visual cortex.

• RISK FACTORS FOR VISION IMPAIRMENT

Risk factors for developing vision impairment include age-related macular degeneration, diabetic retinopathy, glaucoma, and brain injury–related vision loss.

• EXAMINATION

Vision rehabilitation assessments usually consist of two components. The first is the low-vision examination provided by a low-vision clinician, optometrist, or ophthalmologist. This examination will include a patient history and assessments of visual acuity, visual field, contrast sensitivity, color vision, and other visual functions, as well as eye health. Based on the results of this examination, the clinician will make recommendations (e.g., magnification, training in eccentric viewing or overcoming field loss) for the second component, which is the functional assessment performed by vision rehabilitation specialists.

• VISION REHABILITATION

The most frequently used vision rehabilitation devices are low-vision optical devices (e.g., magnifiers, telescopes), nonoptical devices (e.g., bold-lined paper, typoscopes), computer assistive devices, orientation and mobility aids, and activities of daily living aids. Recently, smartphones and tablets have become accessible to both blind and low-vision individuals.

Near Vision Activities

In low-vision settings, reading rehabilitation is one of the most common patient requests, and it has been shown to improve reading ability. Optical magnifiers have historically been important because they are low cost and portable. More recently, electronic devices, including both portable and desktop closed-circuit television systems, have become widely used. Patients with central visual field loss may benefit from eccentric viewing training. This uses a protocol to identify the parafoveal or peripheral area of the retina (preferred retinal locus [PRL]) that will provide the best reading performance and also training in the use of the PRL for reading. Smartphone and tablet technologies are surprisingly accessible for the visually impaired individual, with features and applications that enlarge text, provide global positioning information, convert text to speech, and exhibit many other useful features.

Distance Vision Activities

Orientation and mobility is the term used in the rehabilitation of visually impaired individuals to restore independent travel in their environment; the white cane has become synonymous with such travel. The cane, first systematically developed in the late 1940s, serves as a tactile preview of the environment in the traveler's immediate path.

• CONCLUSION

The diagnosis and rehabilitation of the most common sensory impairments involving the auditory, vestibular, and visual domains have been described. Dual sensory impairments, affecting both the auditory and visual domains, can have devastating effects on the person's ability to compensate and participate in the rehabilitation process. Multiple sensory impairments may also compromise the recovery process; they should be addressed early by the rehabilitation team.

Clinical Pearls

- Realizing the anatomy and physiology of auditory, vestibular, and visual systems
- Specific examination and testing of auditory, vestibular, and visual systems
- Auditory rehabilitation: hearing aid and hearing assistance technology
- Vestibular rehabilitation: habituation; vestibular reflex adaptation; sensory substation; auditory, vestibular, and visual system
- Visual rehabilitation: near vision activity, distance vision activity

BIBLIOGRAPHY
The complete bibliography is available on ExpertConsult.com.

Index

Page numbers followed by *f* indicate figures; *t*, tables; *b*, boxes.

365

Rheumatoid arthritis, 69, 209–210
rehabilitation intervention for, 212
Rheumatologic disease, sexual dysfunction and, 151
Rheumatologic rehabilitation, 208–213.e3
Right hemisphere stroke, 19
Riluzole, 283
Risk adjustment, performance measures/metrics and, 42
RLS. see Restless leg syndrome
ROM. see Range of movement
Romberg test, 11
for visual impairments, 360
Rotational chair testing, for vestibular impairments, 361
Rotator cuff tendonitis and impingement, 245
RPP. see Rate pressure product
RRMS. see Relapsing-remitting multiple sclerosis
RSIs. see Repetitive strain injuries
"Rule of nines," 178
Running, biomechanics of, 272

S
Sacral orthoses, 89–90
Sacral plexopathies, 200
Sacroiliac orthoses, 89–90
Salix alba (white willow bark), 231–232
Sarcopenia, 187, 204
Satiety, early, management of, 146
SBS. see Shaken baby syndrome
Scapholunate instability, 247
SCC. see Spinal cord compression
Scheuermann disease, 236
SCI. see Spinal cord injury
Sciatic mononeuropathy, 297

Scintigraphy, in low back pain, 230
Scoliosis, orthoses for, 90
thoracolumbosacral low-profile, 90
Scooters, 100
Scott-Craig orthosis, 81
Seating principles, 97–98
Seating systems, 92–101.e4
Secondary hyposexual disorder, 154
Secondary injuries, assistive technology (AT) devices for, 130–131
Secondary progressive multiple sclerosis (SPMS), 326
Security, performance measures/metrics and, 42
Segmental dysfunction, lumbar, 229
Segmental pressure, in arterial evaluation, 173–174
Seizures, posttraumatic, TBI and, 310
Selective dorsal rhizotomy, for hypertonia, 338
Selective nerve root blocks (SNRBs), for cervical radiculopathy, 221
Selective nerve root injections (SNRIs), for cervical radiculopathy, 221
Selective serotonin reuptake inhibitors (SSRIs)
for chronic pain, 262
premature ejaculation and, 155
Sensorineural hearing loss, 358
Sensory examination, 10
Sensory nerve action potential (SNAP), 44, 288
Sensory substitution, vestibular, 362
Seronegative spondyloarthropathies (SSAs), 210
Serotonin-norepinephrine reuptake inhibitors, for chronic pain, 262
Serotonin syndrome, 262
Sesamoiditis, 255
Sexual behavior, 150
and aging, 150

Sexual dysfunction, 150–156.e11
in chronic disease, 151–152
diagnostic evaluation of, 153
in disability, 151–152
evaluation of, 152–153
in multiple sclerosis, 330
related to medication use, in individuals with disability, 152, 152t–153t
treatment of, 154–156
types of, 150
Sexual history taking, for sexual dysfunction evaluation, 152
Sexual response, 150
Sexuality, 150
spinal cord injury and, 354
Shaken baby syndrome (SBS), 306
Sheltered workshops, 36
Shiatsu, 117
Shoes
for lower limb orthoses, 75
pediatric, 77
Shortwave, 122
contraindications and precautions for, 122
indications and evidence basis for, 122
physics of, 122
Shoulder disarticulation, 52
Shoulder dysfunction, 244–246
Shoulder harnesses, wheelchair essentials, 98t–100t
Shoulder injuries, in disabled athletes, 277
Shoulder pain, 244–246
in myelomeningocele, 345
Shunts, for children with myelomeningocele, 342
Sialorrhea, in amyotrophic lateral sclerosis (ALS), 284
Sickness Impact Profile-5, 314
Silesian belt suspensions, 59–60
Simple motor tics, 322
Single-photon emission computed tomography (SPECT), in low back pain, 230

Skin breakdown
in children with
myelomeningocele,
344
in disabled athletes, 277
Skin disorders, in disabled
athletes, 278
Sleep, chronic pain and, 260
Sleep disorders, in multiple
sclerosis, 329
Sleep disturbance, TBI and,
313
Sliding filament mechanism,
104
Slow transit constipation,
267
SMA. *see* Spinal muscle
atrophy
Smooth pursuit testing, 361
SNAP. *see* Sensory nerve
action potential
SNRBs. *see* Selective nerve
root blocks
SNRIs. *see* Selective nerve
root injections
Social history, 5
of pediatric patients, 15
Social Security Disability
Insurance (SSDI), 29
Socket, upper limb, 54
Socket designs, for lower
limb amputation, 59
prescription criteria of,
63
Soft tissue techniques, 113
Solid ankle cushion heel
(SACH) foot, 60
Solid organ transplant
recipients,
rehabilitation in,
193–194
Somatic dysfunction, 112
Somatosensory cortex, 144
Sonophoresis, 121–122
Spasticity, 157–163.e13, 11
in ALS patients,
treatment of, 283
biomechanical assessment
of, 160
clinical assessment in, 159
in disabled athletes, 278
epidemiology of, 157
goal-setting in, 159
maladaptive plasticity
and, 158
management of, 160–163
in multiple sclerosis, 329
pathophysiology of,
157–158
problem identification in,
158–159

Spasticity *(Continued)*
spinal cord injury and,
355–356
surgical intervention for,
163
TBI and, 311
SPECT. *see* Single-photon
emission computed
tomography
SPEED program. *see*
Spinal proprioceptive
extension exercise
dynamic (SPEED)
program
Sphincter
electromyography, for
neurogenic bladder
dysfunction, 139
Sphincter muscle,
characteristics of, 137
Spinal accessory nerve
palsy, 202
Spinal afferents, 144
Spinal anatomy, 85–86
Spinal cord compression
(SCC)
epidural, 199–200
malignant, 199
Spinal cord injury (SCI),
347–356.e7
acute phase of, 348–349
anatomy, mechanics,
and syndromes of,
347–448
causes of, 347
chronic phase of, 349
classification of, 348
epidemiology of, 347
neurogenic bowel
dysfunction and, 143
neurologic recovery and
ambulation in, 348
orthoses for, 71
and pulmonary
dysfunction, 193
quality of life in, 349
rehabilitation for, 349
secondary conditions of,
349–356
sexual dysfunction and,
151
Spinal deformities,
in children with
myelomeningocele, 344
Spinal dysraphisms,
340–346.e11
Spinal extension exercise,
for osteoporosis, 242
Spinal fractures, 232–234
Spinal muscle atrophy
(SMA), 279–281

Spinal proprioceptive
extension exercise
dynamic (SPEED)
program, 242
Spinal traction, 120–121
Spiral groove, radial
neuropathy at, 295–296
Spirituality, 5
Splint, 66
examples of, 67–72
SPMS. *see* Secondary
progressive multiple
sclerosis
Spondyloarthropathies, 234
Spondylolisthesis, 233
Spondylolysis, 232
in young athletes, 236
Sporadic inclusion body
myositis, 300
Sport knee orthoses, 82
Sports
biomechanics of, 271–273
as causes of spinal cord
injury, 347
pharmacology in, 273
Sports concussion, 274
Sports medicine, 270–278
emergency assessment
and care in, 274
injury prevention and
rehabilitation in, 271
specific diagnoses in,
274–275
specific populations in, 275
team physician in, 270
Sportsman's hernia, 249
Sprains
acromioclavicular joint,
244
ankle, 254–255
cervical, 217–218
medial collateral
ligament, 253
splints for, 68
ulnar collateral ligament,
246
SSAs. *see* Seronegative
spondyloarthropathies
SSI. *see* Supplemental
Security Income
SSRIs. *see* Selective
serotonin reuptake
inhibitors
Stair mobility, assessment
of, 4
Stance control orthosis, 81
Stand-up wheelchairs, 100
Standing frame, 82
State worker's
compensation systems,
29–30

Printed and bound by CPI Group (UK) Ltd, Croydon, CR0 4YY

08/06/2025

01896876-0001